RICHARD N. TODD, M. D.
3500 HADLEY PLACE - USA
ARCATA, CALIFORNIA 95521

GAMUTS IN RADIOLOGY

Comprehensive Lists of Roentgen Differential Diagnosis

by

MAURICE M. REEDER, M.D.

Colonel, Medical Corps, United States Army,
Chief, Department of Radiology, Walter Reed Army Medical Center, and
Radiology Consultant to The Surgeon General, United States Army,
Washington, D.C.; formerly Associate Radiologist, Registry of
Radiologic Pathology, Armed Forces Institute of Pathology,
Washington, D.C.

and

BENJAMIN FELSON, M.D.

Professor, Department of Radiology,
University of Cincinnati College of Medicine and Medical Center;
Consultant to Cincinnati and Dayton Veterans Administration Hospitals;
National Consultant to the Medical Corps of the United States
Air Force, Army, Navy, and Veterans Administration,
United States Public Health Service,
Armed Forces Institute of Pathology,
and Walter Reed General Hospital

With Contributions by

Elias G. Theros, M.D.

Chairman, Department of Radiologic Pathology,
and Registrar of the American Registry of Radiologic Pathology,
Washington, D.C.

Herbert E. Parks, M.D.

Department of Radiology,
Community Hospital, Indianapolis, Indiana

and

George B. Greenfield, M.D.

Professor and Chairman, Department of Radiology,
Chicago Medical School, Mount Sinai Hospital Medical Center,
Chicago, Illinois

Published by
Audiovisual Radiology of Cincinnati, Inc.
P.O. Box 8942
Cincinnati, Ohio 45208

Library of Congress Catalog Card Number: 74-27229

2 3 4 5 6 7 8 9 10 /79 78 77

Printed in the United States of America

DEDICATION

*This book is dedicated to Colonel William LeRoy Thompson,
Medical Corps, U.S. Army (retired)*

Colonel Thompson, legendary teacher of morphology in radiology and originator of the Gamut concept, received his M.D. degree from the University of Pennsylvania in 1917, and began a long and illustrious career in the U.S. Army Medical Corps that same year. He had various assignments in general medicine and administration and later became one of the early Army radiologists.

It was during his last year before retirement from the Army (1951), however, that he began his most important work, his major contribution to medicine: the organization of the Registry of Radiologic Pathology at the Armed Forces Institute of Pathology. After retirement, he offered his services, without remuneration, to continue as full-time Registrar and Chief of Radiologic Pathology.

In the ensuing 16 years, Colonel Thompson worked laboriously in accessioning new material and collating the material already in the files of the Institute. He was sustained in this labor by hours of daily contact with his "students." It was here, in seminar form at the viewbox, that Colonel Thompson drew upon a lifetime of accumulated knowledge and experience to educate residents, fellows, and practicing physicians from all over the world who came to study under his guidance. In this role, Colonel Thompson was the catalyst, igniting in his students a love of learning and an understanding of the vital role that pathology plays in the discipline of radiology. He was primarily a morphologist, and accepted as such by his colleagues and peers at the AFIP.

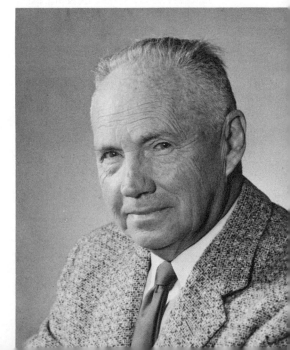

Colonel Thompson's down-to-earth nature, his éclat in interpersonal relationships, his obvious deep regard for his students as well as for medicine, and his abundant and abiding warmth as a human being have made him truly beloved by all who have come to know him.

PREFACE

The word *gamut* is defined as the whole range of anything. As used in this book, it indicates a complete list of causes of a particular roentgen finding or pattern. Colonel William L. Thompson, to whom this book is dedicated, was probably the first to employ it in this sense. For many years, he distributed a small collection of Gamuts to his "students" in the Radiology Registry of the Armed Forces Institute of Pathology.

Although many others have also created and collected such lists, no extensive compilation has ever been published. The two authors of this book, disciples of Colonel Thompson, had been collecting radiology Gamuts for years, independently and without each other's knowledge. Good friends that we were, we eventually discovered the mutuality of our endeavor and decided to combine forces. This book is the product of our collaboration.

The Gamuts were accumulated from a variety of sources: from books and articles, from our own experience, and from the creative efforts of other individuals and groups. Dr. Herbert E. Parks, during his radiology fellowship, began recording Gamuts during the roentgen conferences at the University of Cincinnati, and eventually added a number of his own. Similarly, Dr. Elias G. Theros, who succeeded Colonel Thompson as Chief of the Registry of Radiologic Pathology at the AFIP, added new Gamuts and enlarged on several of the original ones. Both graciously donated their collections to us. For several years, each daily roentgen conference at the University of Cincinnati began with a five minute "Gamut Session." A resident would display on the blackboard a Gamut of his own creation or one he had culled from the literature. The entire group would then add and delete items, and at the end of the session the edited Gamut was copied down for later distribution to the residents and staff. Similar group projects took place at Tripler Army Hospital in Honolulu and Walter Reed Army Hospital in Washington, D.C. Most of the Gamuts produced thereby have been incorporated in our book.

Many of you have a tendency to use the "Gamut approach" without calling it that. You see a solitary calcification in the skull and immediately start groping in your memory bank for causes. You recall perhaps six causes, then eliminate two because of rarity or incompatible roentgen pattern. Then, with the clinical information at your elbow in the form of an x-ray requisition or a clinician, you weed out two more that don't fit the clinical setting, leaving you with two likely diagnoses, both of which may prove to be incorrect. How frustratingly incomplete these cerebral gamuts really are!

The purpose of the Gamut Book is to provide you with more complete and more accurate lists. It is intended as an unobstrusive consultant, quickly available whenever you interpret films or prepare a presentation. In each patient, the possibilities are narrowed down to those that fit the roentgen signs and the clinical and laboratory findings. Of course, all the pertinent data on the film must be analysed to find the appropriate roentgen sign or pattern. Study well — to identify a pattern incorrectly will land you in the wrong Gamut, which could be a disaster!

Despite our painstaking efforts, the Gamut Book has its imperfections. This is not surprising, considering that we have arrogantly undertaken a task requiring a breadth of knowledge we don't possess, memory and judgment beyond our capacity, and the luxury of time none but the idle can afford. However, we firmly believe the book as it now stands is usable and useful, practical and practicable, and pledge a continuing effort to create an even more accurate, complete, and versatile second edition.

Toward this end, we hope to involve many of you in the project. Please help us expand, cull, and revise the material in this first edition. Specifically, we request that you edit the present Gamuts, create new ones, and add to the bibliography. We will be delighted to receive and acknowledge your contributions and to act as a clearing house for this information.

HOW TO USE THE GAMUT BOOK

1. SECTIONS

The Gamuts are grouped into eight *Sections*, conforming to the eight body systems utilized in the American College of Radiology *Index for Roentgen Diagnoses*. Each Section is denoted by an alphabetical letter. Thus, under *D* you will find all the Gamuts that deal with the skeletal system.

2. TABLE OF CONTENTS

This book has no Index. Instead, each Section has its own *Table of Contents*, the pages of which have been black-edged for quick recognition. You can identify the appropriate Table of Contents by referring to page xv or counting down the black hashmarks along the free edge of the closed book.

It will pay you to take a few minutes to look over the Subheadings in the Table of Contents of each Section. We have grouped the Gamuts in what we consider a logical manner. Since our logic may not be your logic, if you don't find a Gamut where you think it belongs, scan the entire Table of Contents of that Section before assuming that it is absent.

3. SUBGAMUTS

A *Subgamut* amplifies some part of the Gamut to which it belongs. Be sure to refer to it after you have finished with the parent Gamut.

4. INCIDENCE

In most of the Gamuts, the entities are subdivided into two groups, *Common* and *Uncommon*. These terms refer to the relative, rather than the absolute incidence of the disease. Although a bone blister (Gamut D-37) is an uncommon roentgen finding, if you do see one the diagnosis will generally prove to be giant cell tumor or nonossifying fibroma (the two conditions listed under *Common*). Conversely, an acute disseminated alveolar pattern (Gamut F-6) is encountered daily in a busy hospital as a result of the prevalence of pulmonary edema and of pneumonia; yet pulmonary hemorrhage, listed under *Uncommon*, is certainly not a rare condition but is simply a less common cause of that pattern.

The prevalence of many disorders varies both geographically and from one type of institution to another. Amebiasis is one of the commonest entities in the world, but it is hardly ever seen in Cincinnati. Histiocytosis X is much more common at Walter Reed Army Hospital than it is in a county hospital. To avoid such discrepancies, we have based our incidence estimates on our experience at Theoretical General Hospital, Midland, U.S.A.

Admittedly, some of the Gamuts deal with seldom seen roentgen signs, but it is in just this type of situation that a Gamut is most welcome. It substitutes someone else's experience for your own lack of it.

5. ALPHABETICAL LISTING

The entries in each Gamut have been alphabetized for your convenience. Since the entry may not be listed in the form that first comes to your mind, be sure to read the entire Gamut before assuming that a condition is not included.

6. SUPPLEMENTARY GAMUTS

Most of the Gamuts refer to a roentgen sign, pattern, or complex. However, interspersed throughout the book are classifications, anatomic and physiologic Gamuts, and other information we considered useful to the radiologist. Typical examples are Gamuts D-46 (Age Incidence of Bone Tumors) and D-29 (Sites of Predilection and Eponyms for Aseptic Necrosis).

7. TERMINOLOGY

We have usually selected the most widely used term for each disease, often furnishing a synonym or eponym as well.

The term *generalized* indicates more or less diffuse involvement (eg, thalassemia of the skeleton); *widespread* means extensive but spotty involvement (eg, Paget's disease of the skeleton); *multiple* means more than one lesion but less than widespread (eg, large metastatic nodules in the lung).

In order to shorten the Gamut lists, we have combined similar or related conditions. They are often separated by a comma or semicolon (eg, scleroderma; dermatomyositis). Inclusive group designations, such as *primary anemia*, *lymphoma*, and *mesenchymal tumor* are often utilized. In these instances, we have commonly added parenthetical examples of individual conditions included under the group designation. To illustrate: Anemia, primary (eg, sickle cell, thalassemia, iron deficiency).

The term *lymphoma* is intended to include Hodgkin's disease, reticulum cell sarcoma, lymphosarcoma, leukemia, and Burkitt's tumor. *Mesenchymal tumor* encompasses fibroma, lipoma, myoma, angioma, combinations thereof, as well as their malignant counterparts. If one member of any of these groups is a more likely cause of a particular roentgen finding, it is specifically listed.

viii

8. BRACKETS

These are used to indicate a condition that does not actually cause the gamuted roentgen finding, but can produce roentgen changes that simulate it. In Gamut E-38 (Dilatation of the Main Pulmonary Artery Segment), *mediastinal or left hilar mass*, not a cause but a mimic, is bracketed.

9. SYNDROMES

S. stands for Syndrome. We must apologize for the great number of congenital syndromes we have included. Since the information was available, we could hardly ignore it. Lump them together? The pediatric roentgenologists had just split them apart. We had a huge tiger by the tail, an animal with variegated stripes and swollen gamuts. Shawl scrotum, Cockayne, and Prader-Willi syndromes, indeed! They should have their own Gamut Book. We can only advise those of you who seldom see and don't care much about dwarfs and other little people to ignore these entries. For those who do care, it will be useful to consult Taybi's syndrome book* for definitions of these congenital disorders.

10. REFERENCES

We have referenced only articles, books, and other contributions that have provided us with a number of the disease entities listed in a Gamut. To document each entity is a collosal task and would have caused an inordinate delay in publication while adding little to the usefulness of the Gamuts.

11. ALTERATIONS

We are fully aware that there are omissions on the Gamut lists; that there are some inconsistencies in terminology, coverage, and unity; and that there are factual inaccuracies. We hope to correct these flaws in the future.

But we need your assistance. Please correct errors as you encounter them; delete entities that you feel do not belong on a Gamut; insert additional disorders and add new Gamuts as you discover them in the literature or in your practice; and create some Gamuts yourself. You can make these alterations in longhand or use typewriter "strips" in your own Gamut Book. New Gamuts can be stored in a looseleaf notebook. Then send us your changes, with documentation, so that we can incorporate them in the next edition.

---

*Taybi H: Radiology of Syndromes. Chicago, Year Book Medical Publishers, 1975.

ACKNOWLEDGEMENTS

We have borrowed freely from many sources. Where records or recollections were clear, we have acknowledged them on this page or in the references. Of those whose contributions we have slighted, we beg forgiveness. Lost notes and jaded memories, not ingratitude, are to blame.

The following radiographic textbooks and articles provided invaluable source material in the preparation of this book. Their excellent tables and lists formed a nucleus for many of our own Gamuts.

DuBoulay GH: Principles of X-ray Diagnosis of the Skull. Washington, Butterworths, 1965.

Eaton SB, Ferrucci JT Jr: Radiology of the Pancreas and Duodenum. Philadelphia, WB Saunders Co, 1973.

Edeiken J, Hodes PJ: Roentgen Diagnosis of Diseases of Bone, ed 2. Baltimore, Williams & Wilkins Co, 1973.

Edwards JE, Carey LS, Neufeld HN, Lester RG: Congenital Heart Disease. Philadelphia, WB Saunders Co, 1965.

Emmett JL, Witten DM: Clinical Urography, ed 3. Philadelphia, WB Saunders Co, 1971.

Eversole LR, Rovin S: Differential radiographic diagnosis of lesions of the jawbones. Radiology 105:277-284, 1972.

Felson B: Chest Roentgenology. Philadelphia, WB Saunders Co, 1973.

Felson B, Editor: Dwarfs and Other Little People. Semin Roentgenol, April, 1973.

Fraser RG, Paré JAP: Diagnosis of Diseases of the Chest. Philadelphia, WB Saunders Co, 1970.

Greenfield GB: Radiology of Bone Diseases. Philadelphia, JB Lippincott Co, 1969.

Kreel L: Outline of Radiology. New York, Appleton-Century-Crofts, 1971.

Meszaros WT: Cardiac Roentgenology. Springfield, Charles C Thomas, 1969.

Murray RO, Jacobson HG: The Radiology of Skeletal Disorders. Baltimore, Williams & Wilkins Co, 1971.

Newton TH, Potts DG: Radiology of the Skull and Brain. St. Louis, Mosby, 1971, vol 1, books 1 and 2.

Poznanski AK: The Hand in Radiologic Diagnosis. Philadelphia, WB Saunders Co, 1974.

Smith DW: Recognizable Patterns of Human Malformation. Philadelphia, WB Saunders Co, 1970.

Teplick JG, Haskin ME: Roentgenologic Diagnosis, ed 2. Philadelphia, WB Saunders Co, 1971, vol 2.

We are immeasurably indebted to the following outstanding individuals for their review of, and valuable additions to many of the Gamuts found in this book.

Dr. John P. Dorst, Professor of Radiology, Johns Hopkins Hospital, Baltimore, Md.

Dr. Marvin E. Haskin, Professor and Chairman, Department of Diagnostic Radiology, Hahnemann Medical College and Hospital, Philadelphia, Pa.

Dr. Harold G. Jacobson, Professor and Co-chairman, Department of Radiology, Albert Einstein College of Medicine, Montefiore Hospital and Medical Center, New York, N.Y.

Colonel Sigurds O. Krolls, USAF, DC, Chief Division of Soft Tissue Oral Pathology, Armed Forces Institute of Pathology, Washington, D.C.

Dr. Joseph M. LoPresti, Radiologist, D.C. General Hospital; former Chief, Department of Radiology, Childrens' Hospital, Washington, D.C.

Dr. David W. Smith, Professor of Pediatrics, University of Washington School of Medicine, Seattle, Wash.

Dr. J. George Teplick, Clinical Professor, Department of Diagnostic Radiology, Hahnemann Medical College and Hospital, Philadelphia, Pa.

Dr. Elias G. Theros, Chief, Radiologic Branch, Armed Forces Institute of Pathology, Washington, D.C.

The authors are also grateful for the help provided in specific areas by Dr. Arthur Clemett of New York, Drs. Sang Oh and Richard Heller of Baltimore, Drs. Robert Whaley, Albert Post, Robert Brannon, and Harvey Neiman of Washington, D.C., and Drs. Jerome Wiot, Harold Spitz, Kenneth Kattan, Corning Benton, Alan Chambers, Robert Luken, and Frederic Silverman, and Mr. Thomas J. Bresnahan, all of Cincinnati. Lastly, this text would not be possible in its present format without the dedicated and meticulous secretarial and typing support provided especially by Mrs. Ruby Kernan of Washington, and also by Mrs. Yuki Takenouchi of Honolulu, and Miss Claire Bittner and Mrs. Margy Himelhoch Potasky, of Cincinnati.

AN APPRECIATION:

TO THE STAFFS AND RESIDENTS OF
The Registry of Radiologic Pathology, Armed Forces Institute of Pathology and Department of Radiology, Walter Reed Army Medical Center, Washington, D.C.

and of

The Department of Radiology, University of Cincinnati College of Medicine and Medical Center, Cincinnati, Ohio.

and to

Our wives, Elaine and Virginia, and families, in whom this endeavor raised a gamut of emotions.

TABLES OF CONTENTS

TABLE OF CONTENTS

A. SKULL AND BRAIN

I. SKULL

ABNORMAL SIZE OR SHAPE

ABNORMAL DENSITY OR THICKNESS

DESTRUCTION

(Continued)

(Continued)

A

A

PREMATURE CRANIOSYNOSTOSIS (CRANIOSTENOSIS)

COMMON

1. Idiopathic (see Subgamut A-1A)

UNCOMMON

1. Acrocephalopolysyndactyly (Carpenter's S.)
2. Acrocephalosyndactyly (Apert's S.)
3. Aminopterin-induced S.
4. Anemia (eg, sickle cell, thalassemia, iron deficiency)
5. Craniofacial dysostosis (Crouzon's disease)
6. Craniotelencephalic dysplasia
7. Down's S. (mongolism)
8. Hyperostosis diseases (eg, Pyle's, Engelmann's, Van Buchem's, osteopetrosis)
9. Hyperthyroidism
10. Hypervitaminosis D
11. Hypophosphatasia (late)
12. Idiopathic hypercalcemia (eg, William's S.)
13. Laurence-Moon-Biedl S.
14. Mandibulofacial dysostosis (Treacher Collins S.)
15. Metaphyseal dysplasia (Jansen type)
16. Microcephaly
17. Mucopolysaccharidosis (eg, Hurler, Hunter, Maroteaux-Lamy); mucolipidosis II, III, generalized gangliosidosis
18. Rickets (hypophosphatemic), treated
19. Rubinstein-Taybi S.
20. Shunting procedure for hydrocephalus

(Continued)

A

PREMATURE CRANIOSYNOSTOSIS
(CRANIOSTENOSIS)
(Continued)

References:

1. Duggan CA, Keener EB, Gay BB Jr: Secondary craniosynostosis. *Am J Roentgenol* 109:277–293, 1970.

2. Newton TH, Potts DG: *Radiology of the Skull and Brain*. St. Louis, Mosby, 1971, vol 1 book 1, pp 222–228.

3. Smith DW: *Recognizable Patterns of Human Malformation*. Philadelphia, WB Saunders Co, 1970.

A

SUBGAMUT A-1A
CLASSIFICATION OF PRIMARY (IDIOPATHIC) PREMATURE CRANIOSYNOSTOSIS

1. Brachycephaly (short head) — premature bilateral closure of coronal and/or lambdoid sutures

2. Oxycephaly, acrocephaly, turricephaly (pointed head) — premature closure of all sutures

3. Plagiocephaly (oblique head) — unilateral premature closure of coronal and/or lambdoid sutures

4. Scaphocephaly (boat head), dolichocephaly (long head) — premature closure of sagittal suture

5. Trigonocephaly (triangular head) — premature closure of metopic suture

Reference:

Newton TH, Potts DG: *Radiology of the Skull and Brain*. St. Louis, Mosby, 1971, vol 1 book 1, p 222.

MICROCEPHALY (MICROCRANIA)

COMMON

1. [Craniostenosis, total]
2. Idiopathic small brain (micrencephaly)
3. Prenatal irradiation or infection (eg, toxoplasmosis, rubella, cytomegalic inclusion disease, herpes, syphilis)

UNCOMMON

1. Bird-headed dwarfism (Seckel's S.)
2. Cat-cry S.
3. Cerebral atrophy
4. Cockayne's S.
5. Cornelia de Lange S.
6. Down's S. (mongolism)
7. Dubowitz S.
8. Fahr's S. (ferrocalcinosis)
9. Familial
10. Fanconi S. (aminoaciduria)
11. G deletion S.
12. Goltz S.
13. Holoprosencephaly (arhinencephaly)
14. Homocystinuria
15. Incontinentia pigmenti
16. Long arm 18 deletion S.
17. Myotonic dystrophy
18. [Normal variant]
19. Phenylketonuria

(Continued)

20. Riley-Day S.
21. Smith-Lemli-Opitz S.
22. Trisomy 13 S.
23. Trisomy 18 S.
24. Tuberous sclerosis
25. XXXXY S.

References:

1. Felson B, Editor: Dwarfs and Other Little People. *Semin Roentgenol* 8:257–258, 1973.

2. Newton TH, Potts DG: *Radiology of the Skull and Brain.* St. Louis, Mosby, 1971, vol 1 book 1, pp 151–152.

3. Smith DW: *Recognizable Patterns of Human Malformation.* Philadelphia, WB Saunders Co, 1970, p 278.

MACROCEPHALY

COMMON

1. [Calvarial thickening (eg, congenital anemias)]
2. Congenital syndromes (see Subgamut A-3A)
*3. Craniostenosis
4. Hydrocephalus (see Gamut A-42 and Subgamut A-42A)
*5. Subdural hematoma

UNCOMMON

1. Aqueduct stenosis
*2. Expansion of middle fossa (see Gamut A-23)
3. Hydranencephaly
*4. Tumor or subarachnoid cyst adjacent to calvarium

*May be asymmetrical

Reference:

Newton TH, Potts DG: *Radiology of the Skull and Brain.* St. Louis, Mosby, 1971, vol 1 book 1, pp 144–151.

SUBGAMUT A-3A
CONGENITAL SYNDROMES
WITH MACROCEPHALY*

COMMON

1. Achondroplasia

2. Cerebral gigantism (Sotos' S.)

3. Hyperostosis diseases (eg, osteopetrosis, Pyle's disease, Engelmann's disease, pyknodysostosis, hyperphosphatasia)

4. Mucopolysaccharidosis (eg, Hurler); mucolipidosis (eg, generalized gangliosidosis)

5. Neurofibromatosis

6. Pituitary dwarfism

UNCOMMON

1. Achondrogenesis

2. Dandy-Walker S. (esp. posterior fossa)

3. Familial macrencephaly

4. Kniest's disease

5. Russell-Silver S.

6. Spondyloepiphyseal dysplasia congenita

7. Thanatophoric dwarfism

8. Wiedemann-Beckwith S.

*Any dwarf may have relative macrocephaly

Reference:

Smith DW: *Recognizable Patterns of Human Malformation.* Philadelphia, WB Saunders Co, 1970, p 278.

ABNORMAL CONTOUR OF THE CALVARIUM

COMMON

1. Achondroplasia
2. Fibrous dysplasia, leontiasis ossea
3. Hemiatrophy or hemihypertrophy of a cerebral hemisphere (eg, Sturge-Weber S.; Davidoff-Dyke-Masson S.)
4. Hydrocephalus
5. Paget's disease (eg, tam-o'-shanter skull)
6. Postoperative
7. Post-traumatic, including obstetrical trauma
8. Postural flattening, usually occipital (eg, cerebral palsy)
9. Premature craniosynostosis (see Gamut A-1 and Subgamut A-1A)
   a. Bathrocephaly
   b. Brachycephaly
   c. Dolichocephaly, scaphocephaly
   d. Oxycephaly, acrocephaly, turricephaly
   e. Plagiocephaly
   f. Trigonocephaly

UNCOMMON

1. Chronic subdural hematoma
2. Craniolacunia
3. Dandy-Walker S.
4. Encephalocele
5. Extradural arachnoid cyst
6. Hyperphosphatasia

(Continued)

7. Microcephaly
8. Neoplasm
9. Neurofibromatosis
10. Porencephalic cyst

ABNORMAL CONTOUR OF THE OCCIPUT (FLAT OR PROMINENT) IN AN INFANT

COMMON

*1. Bathrocephaly (idiopathic)

*2. Dandy-Walker S.; posterior fossa arachnoid cyst

3. Down's S. (mongolism)

4. Postural flattening

UNCOMMON

1. Acrocephalopolysyndactyly (Carpenter's S.)

2. Acrocephalosyndactyly (Apert's S.)

*3. Hajdu-Cheney S. (idiopathic osteolysis)

4. Mucopolysaccharidosis III (Sanfilippo S.)

*5. Occipital cephalohematoma

*6. Occipital meningocele

*7. Otopalatodigital S.

*8. Trisomy 18 S.

9. XXXXY S.

*Prominent occiput; all others are flat

Reference:

   Smith DW: *Recognizable Patterns of Human Malformation*. Philadelphia, WB Saunders Co, 1970, p 278.

FRONTAL BOSSING
(PROMINENT CENTRAL FOREHEAD)

COMMON

1. Achondroplasia
2. Anemia
3. Healed rickets

UNCOMMON

1. Basal cell nevus S. (Gorlin)
2. Mucopolysaccharidosis (eg, Hurler, Hunter); mucolipidosis (eg, Leroy's I-cell disease, generalized gangliosidosis)
3. Oculomandibulofacial S. (Hallerman-Streiff)
4. Orodigitofacial S.
5. Osteopetrosis, severe
6. Otopalatodigital S.
7. Rubinstein-Taybi S.
8. Thanatophoric dwarfism

References:

1. Dorst J: Personal communication.
2. Smith DW: *Recognizable Patterns of Human Malformation.* Philadelphia, WB Saunders Co, 1970, p 279.

BASILAR IMPRESSION

COMMON

1. Congenital (isolated or associated with atlanto-occipital fusion, Klippel-Feil deformity, or stenosis of foramen magnum)
2. Osteogenesis imperfecta
3. Osteomalacia, rickets
4. Paget's disease

UNCOMMON

1. Achondroplasia
2. Aqueduct stenosis
3. Arnold-Chiari malformation
4. Cleidocranial dysplasia
5. Hajdu-Cheney syndrome (idiopathic acro-osteolysis)
6. Histiocytosis X
7. Hydrocephalus, chronic
8. Hyperparathyroidism, primary or secondary
9. Hypoplastic or separate odontoid with atlanto-axial sub-luxation
10. Mucopolysaccharidosis (eg, Hurler, Morquio)
11. Occipital craniotomy in a child
12. Osteopetrosis
13. Osteoporosis
14. Psoriatic arthritis
15. Pyknodysostosis
16. Rheumatoid arthritis; ankylosing spondylitis
17. Syphilis

(Continued)

18. Trauma

19. Tuberculosis

References:

1. DuBoulay GH: *Principles of X-ray Diagnosis of the Skull.* Washington, Butterworths, 1965, p 223–234.

2. Epstein BS, Epstein JA: The association of cerebellar tonsillar herniation with basilar impression incident to Paget's disease. *Am J Roentgenol* 107:535–542, 1969.

HYPOPLASIA OF BASE OF SKULL

COMMON

1. Achondroplasia
2. Cretinism
3. Down's S. (mongolism)

UNCOMMON

1. Achondrogenesis
2. Cranial dysplasia; cleidocranial dysplasia
3. Craniofacial dysostosis (Crouzon's disease)
4. Orodigitofacial S.
5. Short-rib polydactyly S.
6. Thanatophoric dwarfism

References:

1. Dorst J: Personal communication.
2. DuBoulay GH: *Principles of X-ray Diagnosis of the Skull.* Washington, Butterworths, 1965, pp 235–236.

LOCALIZED INCREASED DENSITY OR HYPEROSTOSIS OF THE CALVARIUM

COMMON

1. Anatomic variation (eg, sutural sclerosis)
2. Cephalhematoma
3. [Depressed skull fracture]
4. Fibrous dysplasia
5. Hyperostosis (frontalis) interna
6. Meningioma
7. Metastasis, osteoblastic (eg, prostate, breast)
8. Paget's disease

UNCOMMON

1. Cerebral hemiatrophy
2. Chronic osteomyelitis; tuberculosis
3. [Dural calcification]
4. Hemangioma
5. Ischemic bone flap
6. Neurofibromatosis, with or without meningioma
7. Osteoma, osteochondroma
8. Osteosarcoma
9. Radiation necrosis
10. Tuberous sclerosis

Reference:

DuBoulay GH: *Principles of X-ray Diagnosis of the Skull.* Washington, Butterworths, 1965, pp 106–122.

DIFFUSE OR WIDESPREAD INCREASED DENSITY, HYPEROSTOSIS, OR THICKNESS OF THE CALVARIUM

COMMON

1. Anemia (sickle cell, iron deficiency, thalassemia, hereditary spherocytosis)
2. Fibrous dysplasia, leontiasis ossea
3. Hyperostosis interna generalisata
4. Idiopathic
5. Metastases, osteoblastic (eg, prostate, breast)
6. Paget's disease

UNCOMMON

1. Acromegaly
2. Cerebral atrophy in childhood
3. Chronic increased intracranial pressure in adults (eg, from intermittent congenital obstruction)
4. Congenital cyanotic heart disease, long standing
5. Cranial hemihypertrophy
6. Craniometaphyseal dysplasia; metaphyseal dysplasia (Pyle's disease)
7. Craniostenosis
8. Dilantin medication
9. Dystrophia myotonica
10. Engelmann's disease
11. Fluorosis
12. Hydrocephalus, treated
13. Hyperparathyroidism, primary or secondary (treated)
14. Hyperphosphatasia

(Continued)

15. Hypervitaminosis D

16. Hypoparathyroidism; pseudohypoparathyroidism

17. Idiopathic hypercalcemia (eg, William's S.)

18. Melorheostosis

19. Meningioma

20. Microcephaly

21. Mucopolysaccharidosis (eg, Hurler, Sanfilippo)

22. Mycetoma

23. Myelosclerosis

24. Osteogenesis imperfecta

25. Osteopetrosis

26. Otopalatodigital S.

27. Rickets, treated ("bossing")

28. Secondary polycythemia

29. Syphilitic osteitis

30. Tuberous sclerosis

31. Tubular stenosis (Kenny-Caffey S.)

32. Van Buchem's S.

References:

1. DuBoulay GH: *Principles of X-ray Diagnosis of the Skull.* Washington, Butterworths, 1965, pp 95–106.

2. Teplick JG, Haskin ME: *Roentgenologic Diagnosis,* ed 2. Philadelphia, WB Saunders Co, 1971, vol 2, p xxxvi.

LOCALIZED INCREASED DENSITY
OF BASE OF SKULL
(See also Gamut A-12)

COMMON

1. Fibrous dysplasia
2. Meningioma

UNCOMMON

1. Chordoma (with calcification)
2. Chronic petrositis
3. Lymphoma
4. Mastoiditis
5. Nasopharyngeal carcinoma
6. Osteoblastic metastasis
7. Osteoma; chondroma
8. Sarcoma of bone (eg, osteosarcoma, chondrosarcoma)
9. Sphenoid sinusitis; mucocele

Reference:

Potter GD: Sclerosis of the base of the skull as a manifestation of naso-pharyngeal carcinoma. *Radiology* 94:35–38, 1970.

GENERALIZED INCREASED DENSITY
OF BASE OF SKULL
(See also Gamut A-11)

COMMON

1. Fibrous dysplasia
2. Paget's disease

UNCOMMON

1. Anemia, severe (eg, thalassemia, sickle cell)
2. Craniometaphyseal dysplasia (Pyle's disease)
3. Cretinism
4. Engelmann's disease (progressive diaphyseal dysplasia)
5. Fluorosis
6. Hyperparathyroidism, primary or secondary (treated)
7. Hypervitaminosis D
8. Idiopathic hypercalcemia
9. Melorheostosis
10. Meningioma
11. Neurofibromatosis
12. Osteodysplasia (Melnick-Needles)
13. Osteopetrosis
14. Ribbing's disease (hereditary multiple diaphyseal sclerosis)
15. Vitamin D resistant rickets (healing)

Reference:

DuBoulay GH: *Principles of X-ray Diagnosis of the Skull.* Washington, Butterworths, 1965, pp 209–222.

THINNING OF THE SKULL, LOCALIZED OR GENERALIZED

LOCALIZED

COMMON

1. Chronic subdural hematoma
2. Intracranial tumor, slow growing
3. Parietal thinning

UNCOMMON

1. Congenital arachnoid cyst
2. Leptomeningeal cyst, traumatic
3. Localized temporal horn hydrocephalus
4. Neurofibromatosis
5. Porencephalic cyst; localized cerebral agenesis or atrophy

GENERALIZED

COMMON

1. Craniolacunia
2. Hydrocephalus
3. Osteogenesis imperfecta

UNCOMMON

1. Aminopterin-induced syndrome
2. Cleidocranial dysplasia; cranial dysplasia
3. Hypophosphatasia
4. Increased intracranial pressure, other causes (see Gamut A-41)
5. Osteodysplasia (Melnick-Needles)
6. Progeria
7. Rickets

Reference:

DuBoulay GH: *Principles of X-Ray Diagnosis of the Skull.* Washington, Butterworths, 1965.

DIFFUSE OR WIDESPREAD DEMINERALIZATION OR DESTRUCTION OF THE SKULL (INCLUDING "SALT AND PEPPER" SKULL)

COMMON

1. Hyperparathyroidism, primary or secondary
2. Metastatic carcinoma or neuroblastoma
3. Multiple myeloma
4. Osteoporosis (eg, senile, postmenopausal) (see Gamut D-22)

UNCOMMON

1. Anemia (eg, sickle cell, thalassemia)
2. Electric burn
3. Idiopathic
4. Leukemia
5. Osteomalacia, rickets (see Gamut D-24)
6. Osteomyelitis, diffuse
7. Paget's disease (osteoporosis circumscripta)
8. Primary neoplasm of skull or meninges (eg, Ewing's sarcoma, meningioma)
9. Radiation necrosis; radium poisoning
10. Steroid therapy, Cushing's syndrome
11. Syphilis

EROSION OF THE INNER TABLE
OF THE SKULL

COMMON

1. Pacchionian granulation
2. Porencephaly
3. Subdural hematoma, chronic

UNCOMMON

1. Arteriovenous malformation of brain surface
2. Cisterna magna anomaly
3. Eosinophilic granuloma
4. Epidermoid
5. Glioma or cyst of superficial brain cortex (eg, oligodendro-glioma, leptomeningeal cyst)
6. Hemangioma of skull
7. Meningioma
8. Metastasis
9. Neoplasm of dura, other (eg, sarcoma, melanoma)
10. Sinus pericranii

BUTTON SEQUESTRUM OF THE SKULL

COMMON

1. Eosinophilic granuloma
2. Metastatic carcinoma (eg, breast)
3. Osteomyelitis

UNCOMMON

1. [Burr hole or bone flap]
2. [Hemangioma]
3. Radiation necrosis
4. Syphilis
5. Tuberculosis

Reference:

Rosen IW, Nadel HI: Button sequestrum of the skull. *Radiology* 92:969–971, 1969.

SOLITARY OSTEOLYTIC SKULL LESION

COMMON

1. Cholesteatoma, epidermoid
2. Dermal sinus, dermoid cyst
3. Fibrous dysplasia
4. Fracture (esp. depressed)
5. Hemangioma
6. Histiocytosis X
7. Meningocele, encephalocele, cranium bifidum
8. Metastasis
9. Normal variant (eg, venous lake, enlarged emissary channel, pacchionian granulation, parietal foramen) (see Gamut A-30)
10. Osteomyelitis
11. Paget's disease (osteoporosis circumscripta)
12. Plasmacytoma, myeloma
13. Surgical defect (eg, burr hole, craniotomy flap)

UNCOMMON

1. Arachnoid cyst
2. Arteriovenous malformation
3. Benign bone tumor, other
4. Benign tumor of scalp (eg, neurofibroma, sebaceous cyst)
5. Bone sarcoma
6. Brown tumor of hyperparathyroidism
7. Calvarial "doughnut," idiopathic
8. Carcinoma of scalp, rodent ulcer

(Continued)

9. Glomus jugulare tumor (base)

10. Hydatid cyst

11. Idiopathic

12. Leptomeningeal cyst (secondary to skull fracture)

13. Lymphoma

14. Meningioma or other brain tumor with bone erosion

15. Mucocele or neoplasm of paranasal sinus

16. Neurofibromatosis (eg, asterion defect)

17. Radiation necrosis

18. Sarcoidosis

19. Syphilis, secondary

20. Tuberculosis, fungus disease

References:

1. DuBoulay GH: *Principles of X-ray Diagnosis of the Skull.* Washington, Butterworths, 1965, pp 57–94.

2. Lane B: Erosions of the skull. *Rad Clin North Am* 12:257–282, 1974.

3. Taveras JM, Wood EH: *Diagnostic Neuroradiology.* Baltimore, Williams & Wilkins, 1964.

LYTIC LESION OR BONE DEFECT IN THE SKULL OF A CHILD, SOLITARY OR MULTIPLE

I. Congenital
   1. Cranium bifidum, meningocele, encephalocele, dermal sinus
   2. Epidermoid
   3. [Lacunar skull]
   4. Neurofibromatosis

II. Physiologic
   1. Fontanelle
   2. Pacchionian depression
   3. Parietal foramina
   4. Venous lake

III. Infection
   1. Hydatid disease
   2. Osteomyelitis, bacterial or fungal
   3. Syphilis
   4. Tuberculosis

IV. Neoplasm
   1. Dermoid
   2. Hemangioma
   3. Metastasis
   4. Sarcoma (eg, Ewing's, osteosarcoma)

V. Trauma
   1. Burr hole
   2. Fracture, depressed
   3. Intraosseous hematoma
   4. Leptomeningeal cyst

(Continued)

VI. Miscellaneous
1. Aneurysmal bone cyst
2. Arteriovenous malformation
3. Fibrous dysplasia
4. Hemophilic pseudotumor
5. Histiocytosis X

References:

1. Jacobson HG: Personal communication.
2. LoPresti JM: Personal communication.

RADIOLUCENT LESION OR BONE DEFECT
IN THE SKULL, SOLITARY OR MULTIPLE
(See also Gamuts A-17 and A-18)

A. Congenital or developmental defect
  *1. [Craniolacunia (lacunar skull)]
  2. Dermoid
  3. Epidermoid (cholesteatoma)
  4. Encephalocele, meningoencephalocele, dermal sinus
  5. Fibrous dysplasia
  6. Fontanelle
  *7. Frontal fenestrae
  8. Hemangioma or arteriovenous malformation of bone or scalp
  *9. Pacchionian depression
  *10. Parietal foramina
  *11. Parietal thinning
  *12. Wide sutures (see Subgamut A-32A)

B. Traumatic
  *1. Burr hole
  2. Fracture
  3. Hematoma (cephalohematoma, intradiploic, subdural)
  4. Leptomeningeal cyst

C. Inflammatory
  1. Cholesteatoma
  2. Fibrosing osteitis
  3. Hydatid cyst
  4. Mucocele of frontal sinus
  *5. Osteomyelitis
  *6. Sarcoidosis
  *7. Syphilis
  *8. Tuberculosis

(Continued)

D. Neoplastic
1. Hemangioma
2. Intracranial tumor with erosion
*3. Lymphoma, leukemia
4. Meningioma
*5. Metastasis
*6. Myeloma, plasmacytoma
7. Neurofibroma of bone or scalp; neurofibromatosis
8. Sarcoma of bone
9. Sinus neoplasm with erosion
10. Skin tumor with invasion (rodent ulcer)

E. Miscellaneous
*1. Brown tumor of hyperparathyroidism
*2. Button sequestrum (see Gamut A-16)
*3. Gaucher's disease; Niemann Pick disease; Weber-Christian disease
*4. Histiocytosis X
5. Paget's disease (osteoporosis circumscripta)
*6. Parietal thinning, senile
*7. Radiation necrosis

*May be multiple

ENLARGED, ERODED, OR DESTROYED SELLA TURCICA (INCLUDES INTRASELLAR OR PARASELLAR MASSES)

COMMON

1. Aneurysm of internal carotid artery (cavernous or suprasellar segment); carotid-cavernous fistula

2. Craniopharyngioma

3. Empty sella syndrome

4. Increased intracranial pressure, chronic (eg, obstructive hydrocephalus, dilated third ventricle, neoplasm)

5. Pituitary tumor (eg, chromophobe adenoma, eosinophilic adenoma, carcinoma or carcinosarcoma)

6. [Osteoporotic states; hyperparathyroidism]

7. Other juxtasellar or suprasellar tumor (eg, parasellar or tuberculum sellae meningioma, hypothalamic tumor)

UNCOMMON

1. Basal (transsphenoid) encephalocele

2. Benign tumor of skull base (eg, ossifying fibroma, osteochondroma, osteoma, chondroma)

3. Chordoma

4. Cretinism

5. Frontal lobe tumor

6. Hurler syndrome (often with suprasellar arachnoid cyst)

7. Hypogonadism

8. Metastasis

9. Mucocele of sphenoid sinus

10. Nasopharyngeal or sphenoid sinus neoplasm (eg, carcinoma, angiofibroma)

(Continued)

11. Neurofibromatosis (dysplastic asymmetric sellar enlargement)

12. Optic chiasm glioma

13. Optic nerve sheath tumor (eg, glioma, neurofibroma, meningioma)

14. Osteomyelitis (eg, syphilis, tuberculosis, fungus disease)

15. Oxycephaly

16. Postoperative change

References:

1. DuBoulay GH: *Principles of X-ray Diagnosis of the Skull.* Washington, Butterworths, 1965, pp 145–164.

2. Newton TH, Potts DG: *Radiology of the Skull and Brain.* St. Louis, Mosby, 1971, vol 1 book 1, pp 372–402.

SMALL SELLA TURCICA

COMMON

1. Hypopituitarism and growth hormone deficiency
2. Normal variant

UNCOMMON

1. Cretinism
2. Cushing's S.
3. Down's S. (mongolism)
4. Dystrophia myotonica
5. Genetic (primordial) dwarfism
6. Prader-Willi S.
7. Radiation therapy during childhood
8. Sheehan's S.
9. Vestigial or dysplastic sella with pituitary insufficiency
10. Werner's S.

Reference:

Newton TH, Potts DG: *Radiology of the Skull and Brain*. St. Louis, Mosby, 1971, vol 1 book 1, pp 371–372.

THE J-SHAPED SELLA TURCICA

COMMON

1. Hydrocephalus, mild arrested
2. Normal variant
3. Optic chiasm glioma

UNCOMMON

1. Cretinism
2. Hurler syndrome (gargoylism)
3. Neurofibroma
4. Pituitary tumor extending anteriorly
5. Suprasellar tumor

EXPANSION OF THE MIDDLE FOSSA

COMMON

1. Chronic subdural hematoma; hygroma
2. Middle fossa tumor, slow growing (eg, temporal glioma)

UNCOMMON

1. Localized temporal horn hydrocephalus
2. Neurofibromatosis
3. Oxycephaly with partial stenosis of sagittal suture
4. Porencephalic cyst
5. Subarachnoid cyst
6. Temporal lobe agenesis with overlying cerebrospinal fluid collection

EROSION OF THE MIDDLE FOSSA FLOOR
(See also Gamut A-47)

COMMON

1. Aneurysm of internal carotid artery (large); carotid-cavernous fistula
2. Chordoma
3. Glomus jugulare or vagale tumor
4. Meningioma
5. Nasopharyngeal or paranasal sinus malignancy

UNCOMMON

1. Chondroma
2. Congenital defect
3. Epidermoid, cholesteatoma
4. Histiocytosis X
5. Increased intracranial pressure, chronic
6. Metastasis
7. Neurofibromatosis
8. Neuroma of fifth nerve (foramen ovale)
9. Subarachnoid cyst
10. Temporal lobe glioma

References:

1. DuBoulay GH: *Principles of X-ray Diagnosis of the Skull.* Washington, Butterworths, 1965, pp 177–180.
2. Newton TH, Potts DG: *Radiology of the Skull and Brain.* St. Louis, Mosby, 1971, vol 1 book 1, pp 311–313.

EROSION OF THE SPHENOID WINGS
(See also Gamut B-6)

COMMON

1. Congenital defect, isolated or with neurofibromatosis
*2. Meningioma

UNCOMMON

1. Chordoma
*2. Craniopharyngioma
3. Expansion of middle fossa (see Gamut A-23)
*4. Glioma
5. Histiocytosis X
6. Increased intracranial pressure, chronic
7. Metastasis
8. Parasellar aneurysm
9. Pituitary adenoma
10. Plexiform neurofibroma

*Lesser wing erosion; other lesions listed involve the greater wing of the sphenoid.

EROSION OR WIDENING
OF THE INTERNAL AUDITORY MEATUS

COMMON

1. Acoustic neuroma

UNCOMMON

1. Aneurysm of internal auditory canal artery
2. Arteriovenous malformation
3. Brain stem glioma
4. Epidermoid
5. Meningioma of cerebellopontine angle or petrous apex
6. Metastasis
7. [Normal patulous canal]
8. Other neuroma (V and VII nerves)

References:

1. DuBoulay GH: *Principles of X-ray Diagnosis of the Skull.* Washington, Butterworths, 1965, pp 183–191.

2. Newton TH, Potts DG: *Radiology of the Skull and Brain.* St. Louis, Mosby, 1971, vol 1 book 1, pp 442–446.

EROSION OF THE PETROUS RIDGE OR APEX

1. Acoustic neuroma
2. Aneurysm of intracavernous or intrapetrous carotid artery
3. Bone tumor, benign or malignant (eg, hemangioma, chordoma, metastasis)
4. Epidermoid, cholesteatoma
5. Fifth nerve neuroma
6. Glomus jugulare tumor
7. Histiocytosis X
8. Leptomeningeal cyst
9. Meningioma (Meckel's cave)
10. Nasopharyngeal malignancy (invasive)
11. Osteomyelitis, petrositis

References:

1. DuBoulay GH: *Principles of X-ray Diagnosis of the Skull*. Washington, Butterworths, 1965, p 191.

2. Newton TH, Potts DG: *Radiology of the Skull and Brain*. St. Louis, Mosby, 1971, vol 1 book 1, pp 424, 447.

EROSION OF TYMPANIC PORTION
OF PETROUS BONE
(See also Gamut B-34)

COMMON

1. Cholesteatoma (postinfection)
2. Mastoiditis, acute or chronic
3. [Postoperative defect]

UNCOMMON

1. Bone tumor, benign or malignant (eg, hemangioma, metastasis)
2. Carcinoma of mastoid, external auditory meatus, or middle ear
3. Dermoid cyst
4. Glomus jugulare tumor
5. Granuloma
6. Histiocytosis X
7. Nasopharyngeal tumor invasion

Reference:

DuBoulay GH: *Principles of X-ray Diagnosis of the Skull.* Washington, Butterworths, 1965, pp 191–199.

SKULL AND FACIAL BONES
OF MEMBRANOUS ORIGIN

1. Facial bones, including mandible
2. Frontal bone
3. Occipital bone, upper squamosa
4. Parietal bone
5. Pterygoid (medial plate)
6. Temporal bone (squamosal and tympanic parts)
7. Vomer

Reference:

Greenfield GB: *Radiology of Bone Diseases*. Philadelphia, JB Lippincott Co, 1969, p 2.

NORMAL SKULL VARIANT

COMMON

1. [Artefact (eg, hair braid, rubber band, skin fold, EEG paste)]
2. Arterial groove (eg, middle meningeal)
3. Convolutional impressions
4. Dural sinus (eg, transverse or sigmoid sinus)
5. Emissary vein
6. Mendosal suture
7. Metopic suture
8. Pacchionian granulation
9. Sutural (Wormian) bones; atypical suture line
10. Torcular Herophili
11. Venous lake or channel

UNCOMMON

1. Cruciate ridge
2. Interparietal bone
3. Parietal foramina
4. Parietal thinning

Reference:

LoPresti JM: Personal communication.

MULTIPLE WORMIAN BONES

COMMON

1. Cleidocranial dysplasia
2. Cretinism, hypothyroidism
3. Normal; idiopathic
4. Osteogenesis imperfecta

UNCOMMON

1. Aminopterin-induced S.
2. Down's S. (mongolism)
3. Hajdu-Cheney S. (idiopathic acro-osteolysis)
4. Hallerman-Streiff S.
5. Hypophosphatasia
6. Kinky hair S.
7. Otopalatodigital S.
8. Pachydermoperiostosis
9. Prader-Willi S.
10. Progeria
11. Pyknodysostosis
12. Rickets

CONGENITAL SYNDROMES WITH OPEN OR DELAYED CLOSURE OF FONTANELLES

COMMON

1. Cleidocranial dysplasia
2. Cretinism, hypothyroidism
3. Down's S. (mongolism)
4. Rubella S.

UNCOMMON

1. Aminopterin-induced S.
2. Cerebrohepatorenal S. (Zellweger)
3. Chondrodysplasia punctata (Conradi's disease)
4. [Congenital scalp defect]
5. Cutis laxa
6. Hypophosphatasia
7. Metaphyseal chondrodysplasia (McKusick)
8. Oculomandibulofacial S. (Hallerman-Streiff)
9. Osteodysplasia (Melnick-Needles)
10. Osteogenesis imperfecta
11. Otopalatodigital S.
12. Pachydermoperiostosis
13. Progeria
14. Pyknodysostosis
15. Rubinstein-Taybi S.
16. Russell-Silver S.
17. Stanesco's dysplasia
18. Trisomy 13 S.

(Continued)

CONGENITAL SYNDROMES WITH OPEN OR DELAYED CLOSURE OF FONTANELLES
(Continued)

19. Trisomy 18 S.
20. Tubular stenosis (Kenny-Caffey)

References:

1. Dorst J: Scientific exhibit, Radiological Society of North America, 1972.

2. Felson B, Editor: Dwarfs and Other Little People. *Semin Roentgenol* 8:258, 1973.

3. Smith DW: *Recognizable Patterns of Human Malformation.* Philadelphia, WB Saunders Co, 1970.

SUBGAMUT A-32A
DELAYED CLOSURE OR
INCOMPLETE OSSIFICATION OF SUTURES

COMMON

1. Cleidocranial dysplasia
2. Cretinism, hypothyroidism
3. Hydrocephalus
4. Osteogenesis imperfecta
5. Rickets

UNCOMMON

1. Aminopterin-induced S.
2. Cranium bifidum
3. Hypophosphatasia
4. Neurofibromatosis
5. Pachydermoperiostosis
6. Prematurity
7. Progeria
8. Pyknodysostosis
9. Renal osteodystrophy

Reference:

Newton TH, Potts DG: *Radiology of the Skull and Brain*. St. Louis, Mosby, 1971, vol 1 book 1, pp 232–236.

DELAYED OR DEFECTIVE CRANIAL OSSIFICATION

I. TRANSIENT — Disappearance of Ossification Defects Before 3 Years of Age

1. Aminopterin-induced S.
2. Cerebrohepatorenal S.
3. Congenital lacunar skull
4. Congenital scalp defect
5. Cutis laxa
6. Down's S. (mongolism)
7. Hypophosphatasia
8. Kinky hair S.
9. Metaphyseal chondrodysplasia (McKusick)
10. Mucopolysaccharidosis (eg, Hunter, Hurler)
11. Osteogenesis imperfecta
12. Rubinstein-Taybi S.
13. Russell-Silver dwarfism
14. Trisomy 13 S.
15. Trisomy 18 S.

II. INTERMEDIATE — Disappearance of Ossification Defects Between 3 and 10 Years

1. Hypothyroidism
2. Otopalatodigital S.
3. Pachydermoperiostosis
4. Progeria
5. Rickets

(Continued)

III. PROTRACTED — Ossification Defects Persist Beyond 10 Years of Age

1. Cleidocranial dysplasia

2. Cranium bifidum occultum

3. Dermal sinus

4. Encephalocele

5. Frontonasal dysplasia

6. Hypertelorism with Sprengel's deformity

7. Oculomandibulofacial S.

8. Parietal foramina; occipital foramina

9. Parietal thinning

10. Pyknodysostosis

11. Stanesco's dysplasia

12. Tubular stenosis (Kenny-Caffey)

Reference:

Dorst JP: Personal communication.

SEPARATION OR INFILTRATION
OF SKULL SUTURES IN AN INFANT OR CHILD

COMMON

1. Brain tumor (eg, pinealoma, medulloblastoma)
2. Hydrocephalus (see Gamut A-42 and Subgamut A-42A)
3. Incomplete ossification adjacent to sutures (see Subgamut A-32A)
4. Increased intracranial pressure, other causes (see Gamut A-41)
5. Lead poisoning
6. Leukemia, lymphoma
7. Meningitis, meningoencephalitis
8. Neuroblastoma, metastatic
9. Subdural hematoma, hygroma

UNCOMMON

1. Hydranencephaly
2. Hypervitaminosis A; hypovitaminosis A

INCREASED SIZE OF THE VASCULAR GROOVES OF THE SKULL

COMMON

1. Arteriovenous malformation
2. Hemangioma of skull
3. Meningioma

UNCOMMON

1. Collateral circulation (eg, thrombosis of a venous sinus, occlusion of internal carotid artery)
2. Fibrous dysplasia
3. Metastasis (eg, thyroid carcinoma, hypernephroma)
4. Pacchionian bodies
5. Paget's disease

"HAIR-ON-END" PATTERN IN THE SKULL

COMMON

1. Congenital hemolytic anemia (eg, thalassemia, sicklemia, hereditary spherocytosis, hereditary elliptocytosis, pyruvate kinase deficiency)

UNCOMMON

1. Cyanotic congenital heart disease with secondary polycythemia
2. Hemangioma
3. Iron deficiency anemia
4. Meningioma
5. Metastases (eg, neuroblastoma, thyroid carcinoma)
6. Myeloma
7. Osteosarcoma
8. Polycythemia vera

Reference:

Greenfield GB: *Radiology of Bone Diseases.* Philadelphia, JB Lippincott Co, 1969, p 49.

SELLAR OR PARASELLAR CALCIFICATION

COMMON

1. Aneurysm of a cerebral artery (esp. internal carotid)
2. Atherosclerosis of internal carotid artery
3. Craniopharyngioma
4. Normal (petroclinoid or interclinoid ligament, diaphragma sellae)

UNCOMMON

1. Angiomatous malformation
2. Chordoma
3. Ectopic pinealoma, teratoma
4. Hyperparathyroidism (vascular calcification)
5. Meningioma
6. Normal pituitary gland ("stone")
7. Optic chiasm glioma
8. [Osteochondroma, osteoma]
9. Pituitary adenoma (chromophobe, eosinophilic)
10. Tuberculous meningitis, healed

Reference:

DuBoulay GH: *Principles of X-ray Diagnosis of the Skull.* Washington, Butterworths, 1965, pp 165–175.

SOLITARY INTRACRANIAL CALCIFICATION
(See also Gamuts A-37, A-39, and A-40)

I. Physiologic
   1. Arachnoid granulation
   *2. Choroid plexus
   *3. Diaphragma sellae
   *4. Dura (falx, tentorium, sagittal sinus)
   *5. Habenular commissure
   6. Hypophysis
   *7. Petroclinoid or interclinoid ligaments
   *8. Pineal

II. Infection
   1. Encephalitis, meningitis, brain abscess (healed)
   2. Cysticercus cyst
   3. Granuloma (torulosis and other fungi)
   4. Hydatid cyst
   5. Paragonimiasis
   6. Rubella
   7. Syphilitic gumma
   *8. Tuberculoma

III. Tumor
   1. Chordoma
   2. Choroid plexus papilloma
   *3. Craniopharyngioma
   4. Ependymoma
   5. Epidermoid, dermoid
   *6. Glioma (eg, astrocytoma, oligodendroglioma)
   7. Lipoma of corpus callosum

(Continued)

8. Meningioma
9. Metastatic neoplasm
10. Neuroma
*11. [Osteoma, chondroma, osteochondroma]
12. Pinealoma
13. Pituitary adenoma (esp. chromophobe)

IV. Vascular

1. Aneurysm, including vein of Galen
*2. Arteriosclerosis (esp. carotid artery at siphon)
3. Hemangioma, arteriovenous malformation, Sturge-Weber syndrome

V. Miscellaneous

1. Hematoma (eg, cerebral, subdural, extradural)
2. [Iatrogenic (eg, contrast media injection into an abscess or cyst)]
*3. Idiopathic
4. Infarct, cerebral
5. Radiation necrosis
6. Scarring; gliosis
7. Tuberous sclerosis

*Common

References:

1. DuBoulay GH: *Principles of X-ray Diagnosis of the Skull.* Washington, Butterworths, 1965, pp 237–273.
2. Newton TH, Potts DG: *Radiology of the Skull and Brain.* St. Louis, Mosby, 1971, vol 1 book 2, pp 823–873.
3. Teplick JG, Haskin ME: *Roentgenologic Diagnosis,* ed 2. Philadelphia, WB Saunders Co, 1971, vol 2, p xxxvi.

MULTIPLE INTRACRANIAL CALCIFICATIONS
(See also Gamuts A-38 and A-40)

COMMON

1. Arterial (eg, atherosclerosis, aneurysms)
2. Idiopathic
3. Physiologic (arachnoid granulations, dura, falx, tentorium, petroclinoid ligament, choroid plexi, pineal, habenula, diaphragma sellae, hypophysis)

UNCOMMON

1. Arteriovenous malformation; hemangiomas; Sturge-Weber S.; von Hippel-Lindau disease
2. Basal cell nevus S. (falx, tentorium)
3. Basal ganglia (eg, hypoparathyroidism; pseudohypoparathyroidism; Fahr's disease) (see Gamut A-40)
4. Brain abscesses (healed)
5. Carbon monoxide intoxication
6. Cockayne's S.
7. Cytomegalic inclusion disease
8. Encephalitis (eg, measles, chickenpox, neonatal herpes simplex)
9. Hematomas, old (eg, intracerebral, subdural)
10. Hyperparathyroidism (vascular calcifications)
11. Hypervitaminosis D (dura)
12. [Iatrogenic (eg, pantopaque or other contrast media residual)]
13. Lipoid proteinosis (hyalinosis cutis)
14. Lissencephaly (congenital agyria)
15. Needle-tracks following ventriculography

(Continued)

16. Neurofibromatosis (choroid plexi)

17. Parasitic disease (eg, cysticercosis, paragonimiasis, trichinosis, hydatid cysts)

18. [Scalp sebaceous cysts, cysticercosis, EEG paste]

19. Scarring; gliosis

20. Torulosis

21. Toxoplasmosis

22. Tuberculomas; tuberculous meningitis (treated)

23. Tuberous sclerosis

24. Tumors, multiple (eg, meningiomas, gliomas, metastases)

25. Wilson's disease

References:

1. Babbitt DP, Tang T, Dobbs J, Berk R: Idiopathic familial cerebro-vascular ferrocalcinosis (Fahr's disease) and review of differential diagnosis of intracranial calcification in children. *Am J Roentgenol* 105:352–358, 1969.

2. DuBoulay GH: *Principles of X-ray Diagnosis of the Skull*. Washington, Butterworths, 1965, pp 237–273.

3. Legré J, Massad A: Radiological study of intracranial calcifications. *Radiology* 70:760, 1958 (abstract).

4. Newton TH, Potts DG: *Radiology of the Skull and Brain*. St. Louis, Mosby, 1971, vol 1 book 2, pp 823–873.

5. Teplick JG, Haskin ME: *Roentgenologic Diagnosis*, ed 2. Philadelphia, WB Saunders Co, 1971, vol 2, p xxxvi.

BASAL GANGLIA CALCIFICATION

COMMON

1. Idiopathic
2. Hypoparathyroidism, pseudohypoparathyroidism

UNCOMMON

1. Birth anoxia
2. Carbon monoxide intoxication
3. Cockayne's syndrome
4. Cytomegalic inclusion disease
5. Encephalitis (eg, measles, chickenpox)
6. Fahr's syndrome (ferrocalcinosis)
7. Familial idiopathic symmetrical basal ganglia calcification
8. Hastings-James syndrome (idiopathic lenticulodentate calcification)
9. Hemorrhage
10. Hyperparathyroidism
11. Hypothyroidism
12. Lead intoxication
13. Lipoid proteinosis (hyalinosis cutis)
14. Parkinsonism
15. Pseudopseudohypoparathyroidism
16. Radiation therapy
17. Toxoplasmosis
18. Tuberous sclerosis
19. Vascular disease

References:

1. Bennett JC, Maffly RH, Steinbach HL: The significance of bilateral basal ganglia calcification. *Radiology* 72:368–378, 1959.
2. Harwood-Nash DCF, Reilly BJ: Calcification of the basal ganglia following radiation therapy. *Am J Roentgenol* 108:392–395, 1970.
3. Newton TH, Potts DG: *Radiology of the Skull and Brain.* St. Louis, Mosby, 1971, vol 1 book 2, p 835.

INCREASED INTRACRANIAL PRESSURE

COMMON

1. Cerebral edema, contusion, hemorrhage, or infarction
2. Hydrocephalus, noncommunicating (see Gamut A-42)
3. Lead encephalopathy
4. Meningitis, meningoencephalitis (eg, tuberculosis, torulosis, toxoplasmosis)
5. Metastatic neoplasm (eg, bronchogenic carcinoma, neuroblastoma)
6. Primary brain tumor

UNCOMMON

1. Aqueduct stenosis
2. Arnold-Chiari malformation
3. Brain abscess
4. Craniostenosis, severe
5. Dandy-Walker syndrome
6. Drug therapy (eg, tetracycline)
7. Hyperthyroidism
8. Hypervitaminosis A; hypovitaminosis A
9. Hypoparathyroidism
10. Leukemia, lymphoma
11. Meningocele
12. Parasitic disease (eg, cysticercosis, hydatid disease, paragonimiasis)
13. Pseudotumor cerebri
14. Subdural hematoma, hygroma

SUBGAMUT A-41A
RADIOLOGIC FEATURES
OF INCREASED INTRACRANIAL PRESSURE

1. Increased craniofacial ratio
2. Increased digital markings of calvarium ("hammered silver" appearance)
3. Sellar changes
    a. Decalcification of floor and dorsum of sella
    b. Pointed anterior clinoids
    c. Sellar enlargement
    d. Thinning or loss of posterior clinoids
4. Sutural diastasis; unusually deep sutural interdigitations
5. Thinning of calvarium

HYDROCEPHALUS

I. Atrophic hydrocephalus

    1. Congenital inflammatory disease (eg, toxoplasmosis, torulosis, cytomegalic inclusion disease)

    2. Arteriovenous malformation, vascular lesion

    3. Cerebral maldevelopment (eg, lissencephaly)

    4. Idiopathic

II. Nonabsorptive hydrocephalus secondary to obstruction of subarachnoid spaces at cerebral convexity, basal cisterns, or foramen magnum

    1. Achondroplasia

    2. Arnold-Chiari malformation

    3. Basilar impression (see Gamut A-7)

    4. Encephalocele

    5. Meningitis

    6. Meningomyelocele

III. Obstructive hydrocephalus secondary to intraventricular, aqueductal, or foramina of Magendie and Luschka obstruction

    1. Abscess

    2. Arachnoid cyst

    3. Basal arachnoiditis

    4. Colloid cyst

    5. Congenital aqueductal stenosis

    6. Cysticercosis

    7. Dandy-Walker syndrome

    8. Hematoma

    9. Neoplasm

(Continued)

HYDROCEPHALUS (Continued)

IV. Overproduction of cerebrospinal fluid (eg, choroid plexus papilloma)

Reference:

Brucher JA, Salmon JH: Hydrocephalus. *Semin Roentgenol* 5:186–195, 1970.

SUBGAMUT A-42A
CONGENITAL SYNDROMES
ASSOCIATED WITH HYDROCEPHALUS

1. Achondroplasia

2. Basal cell nevus S. (Gorlin)

3. Hurler S.

4. Orodigitofacial S.

5. Osteopetrosis, severe

6. Riley-Day S.

7. Trisomy 13 S.

8. Trisomy 18 S.

9. X-linked hydrocephalus

Reference:

Smith DW: *Recognizable Patterns of Human Malformation.* Philadelphia, WB Saunders Co, 1970, p 278.

OBSTRUCTION AT THE
FOURTH VENTRICLE OUTLET

COMMON

1. Arnold-Chiari malformation
2. Atresia of fourth ventricle foramina (eg, Dandy-Walker cyst)
3. Basilar arachnoiditis (eg, tuberculous meningitis)
4. Basilar impression (eg, Paget's disease)
5. Neoplasm (esp. medulloblastoma, ependymoma)
6. Tonsillar herniation

UNCOMMON

1. Congenital arachnoid cyst
2. Cysticercus cyst
3. Fusion deformity of upper cervical spine
4. Meningocele

MASS INVOLVING THE FOURTH VENTRICLE

COMMON

1. Ependymoma
2. Tumor invading from neighboring structure
   a. Astrocytoma
   b. Hemangioblastoma
   c. Medulloblastoma
   d. Metastasis
   e. Pontine glioma

UNCOMMON

1. Choroid papilloma
2. Cysticercus cyst
3. Dermoid, epidermoid
4. Intraventricular meningioma

MASS IN THE CLIVUS OR PREPONTINE AREA

COMMON

1. Aneurysm of basilar or vertebral artery
2. Chordoma
3. Meningioma

UNCOMMON

1. Bone sarcoma (esp. chondrosarcoma, osteosarcoma)
2. Epidermoid
3. Metastasis
4. Nasopharyngeal neoplasm with extension
5. Osteochondroma
6. Parasellar neoplasm with extension (eg, craniopharyngioma, optic glioma, chromophobe adenoma)

CEREBELLOPONTINE ANGLE MASS

COMMON

1. Acoustic neuroma
2. Epidermoid
3. Meningioma
4. Pontine glioma with lateral extension

UNCOMMON

1. Aneurysm, arteriovenous malformation
2. Arachnoid cyst
3. Cerebellar tumor with extension
4. Chordoma
5. Glomus jugulare tumor
6. Other neuroma (V, VII, X, XII nerves)
7. [Parasellar tumor with extension (eg, chromophobe adenoma, optic glioma, craniopharyngioma)]

MASS IN THE MIDDLE FOSSA
(See also Gamut A-24)

COMMON

1. Aneurysm of internal carotid artery (large); carotid-cavernous fistula

2. Intra-axial temporal lobe neoplasm, hematoma, or abscess

3. Meningioma of sphenoid ridge or middle fossa

4. Nasopharyngeal or paranasal sinus carcinoma or other tumor with middle fossa extension

5. Subdural hematoma

UNCOMMON

1. Epidermoid (cholesteatoma)

2. Histiocytosis X

3. Metastasis

4. Midline tumor extending laterally (eg, chordoma, craniopharyngioma, pituitary adenoma)

5. Neuroma (eg, fifth nerve, gasserian ganglion)

6. Subarachnoid cyst

References:

1. DuBoulay GH: *Principles of X-ray Diagnosis of the Skull.* Washington, Butterworths, 1965, pp 177–180.

2. Newton TH, Potts DG: *Radiology of the Skull and Brain.* St. Louis, Mosby, 1971, vol 1 book 1, pp 311–313.

MASS INVOLVING THE POSTERIOR PORTION OF THE THIRD VENTRICLE

COMMON

1. Ependymoma
2. Glioma or other tumor arising from quadrigeminal body
3. Pinealoma, teratoma

UNCOMMON

1. Aneurysm (esp. vein of Galen)
2. Meningioma (eg, intraventricular or incisural)
3. Quadrigeminal cyst

WIDENING OF THE SEPTUM PELLUCIDUM (GREATER THAN 3 MM)

COMMON

1. Cyst or tumor of septum pellucidum
2. Noncommunicating cavum septi pellucidi

UNCOMMON

1. Corpus callosum tumor infiltrating septum pellucidum
2. Intraventricular astrocytoma extending into septum pellucidum
3. Lipoma of corpus callosum
4. Tumor of third ventricle

VENTRICULAR WALL NODULE(S)

COMMON

1. Choroid plexus
2. Nodular caudate nucleus
3. [Ribbing of ventricular walls in hydrocephalus]
4. Tuberous sclerosis

UNCOMMON

1. Coarctation of lateral ventricles with ependymal adhesions
2. Cysticercosis
3. Ependymal seeding from malignant brain tumor (eg, ependymoma, medulloblastoma, glioblastoma)
4. Ependymitis (esp. torulosis)
5. Heterotopic cortical gray matter in lateral ventricles (esp. with absence of corpus callosum)
*6. Intraventricular neoplasm (eg, ependymoma, epidermoid, meningioma, choroid plexus papilloma)

*Solitary; all others may be multiple

Reference:

Bergeron RT: Pneumographic demonstration of subependymal heterotopic cortical gray matter in children. *Am J Roentgenol* 101:168–177, 1967.

CEREBRAL ARTERIAL DISEASE ON ANGIOGRAPHY (NARROWING, IRREGULARITY, OCCLUSION, ANEURYSM)

A. Arteritis

1. Bacterial arteritis, mycotic aneurysm (eg, from abscess, meningitis, osteomyelitis, embolism)

2. Carotid arteritis (infant or child)

3. Collagen disease arteritis (esp. lupus erythematosus)

4. Drug or chemical arteritis (eg, ergot, amphetamine, heroin, arsenic, carbon monoxide)

5. Fungal arteritis (esp. actinomycosis, nocardiosis, torulosis, aspergillosis, phycomycosis)

6. Necrotizing angiitis (eg, polyarteritis nodosa, hypersensitivity angiitis, giant cell arteritis, temporal arteritis)

7. Radiation arteritis

8. Syphilitic arteritis

9. Takayasu's arteritis

10. Tuberculous arteritis

11. Viral arteritis (eg, herpes zoster)

B. Other Causes

1. Arterial spasm (eg, subarachnoid or cerebral hemorrhage; migraine)

2. Arteriosclerosis

3. Arteriovenous malformation

4. Berry aneurysm

5. Cerebral thrombosis (eg, sickle cell anemia, oral contraceptives)

6. Embolism (eg, subacute bacterial endocarditis, atrial myxoma)

(Continued)

7. Fibromuscular dysplasia (usually extracarnial)

8. Idiopathic

9. [Increased intracranial pressure]

10. Inflammatory disease of brain (eg, abscess; purulent or tuberculous meningitis)

11. Multiple progressive intracranial artery occlusions with telangiectasia (Moya-moya)

12. Neoplasm (eg, glioblastoma, lymphoma, metastasis)

13. Neurocutaneous syndromes (eg, neurofibromatosis, Sturge-Weber S., tuberous sclerosis)

14. Trauma

References:

1. Ferris EJ, Levine HL: Cerebral arteritis: classification. *Radiology* 109:327–341, 1973.

2. Hilal SK, Solomon GE, Gold AP, Carter S: Primary cerebral arterial occlusive disease in children. *Radiology* 99:71–94, 1971.

3. Leeds NE, Rosenblatt R: Arterial wall irregularities in intracranial neoplasms. *Radiology* 103:121–124, 1972.

INTRACRANIAL ARTERIOVENOUS SHUNTING AND EARLY VENOUS FILLING ON CEREBRAL ANGIOGRAPHY

COMMON

1. Arteriovenous malformation, congenital or acquired
2. Infarction of brain
3. Malignant brain tumor, primary or metastatic

UNCOMMON

1. Contusion of brain
2. Inflammatory lesion (eg, brain abscess)
3. Intracerebral hematoma

Reference:

Glickman MG, Mainzer F, Gletne JS: Early venous opacification in cerebral contusion. *Radiology* 100:615–622, 1971.

AVASCULAR ZONE NEAR THE BRAIN SURFACE ON CEREBRAL ANGIOGRAPHY

COMMON

1. Cortical atrophy
2. "Cortical steal" by deep arteriovenous shunt
3. Epidural hematoma, hygroma, or empyema
4. Meningeal neoplasm (eg, avascular meningioma; meningeal involvement by carcinoma, lymphoma, leukemia, sarcoma, neuroblastoma, or melanoma)
5. Occlusive vascular disease; brain infarct
6. Subdural hematoma, hygroma, or empyema

UNCOMMON

1. Arachnoid cyst; porencephaly
2. Bone tumor infiltrating dura (eg, metastasis, sarcoma, epidermold, histiocytosis X)
3. Normal large subarachnoid space (infant)
4. Subdural invasion by glioma
5. Syphilitic pachymeningitis
6. Tuberculoma

Reference:

Ferris EJ, Lehrer H, Shapiro JH: Pseudo-subdural hematoma. *Radiology* 88: 75–84, 1967.

EXTRACRANIAL ISCHEMIC LESION SECONDARILY INVOLVING THE BRAIN

COMMON

1. Occlusion or stenosis of brachiocephalic vessels
2. Steal syndromes (eg, subclavian steal)

UNCOMMON

1. Dissecting aneurysm of thoracic aorta
2. Embolization secondary to mitral valve disease or atrial myxoma
3. Takayasu's arteritis
4. Trauma to neck
5. Tumor in neck compromising cervical vessels (eg, thyroid adenoma, neurilemmoma)

Reference:

Mishkin MM: Extracranial ischemic lesions which secondarily involve the brain. *Rad Clin North Am* 5:395–408, 1967.

NOTES

NOTES

NOTES

TABLE OF CONTENTS

B. FACIAL BONES, JAWS, SINUSES AND NECK

ORBIT

TEETH AND JAWS

(Continued)

B

B

B

MALFORMATION OF THE ORBIT

COMMON

1. Craniostenosis
2. Enucleation in childhood
3. Fibrous dysplasia, leontiasis ossea

UNCOMMON

1. Anophthalmos, microphthalmos
2. Encroachment from adjacent mass (eg, frontal sinus mucocele, antral neoplasm or cyst)
3. Hypertelorism (eg, Apert's S., Crouzon's disease, Treacher Collins S.) (see Gamut B-4 and Subgamut B-4A)
4. Hypotelorism (see Gamut B-3)
5. Neurofibromatosis
6. Radiation therapy
7. Tumor (eg, neurofibroma)

B

CONGENITAL SYNDROMES
WITH SHALLOW ORBITAL RIDGES

1. Acrocephalosyndactyly (Apert's S.)

2. Aminopterin-induced S.

3. Cerebrohepatorenal S. (Zellweger S.)

4. Craniofacial dysostosis (Crouzon's disease)

5. Stanesco's dysplasia

6. Trisomy 13 S.

7. Trisomy 18 S.

Reference:

Smith DW: *Recognizable Patterns of Human Malformation*. Philadelphia, WB Saunders Co, 1970, p 279.

B

HYPOTELORISM
(DECREASED INTERORBITAL DISTANCE)

1. Down's S. (mongolism)
2. Glycogen storage disease
3. Holoprosencephaly (arhinencephaly)
4. Oculodentodigital dysplasia
5. Phenylketonuria
6. Trigonocephaly
7. Trisomy 13 S.

CONGENITAL SYNDROMES
WITH HYPERTELORISM

1. Aminopterin-induced S.
2. Acrocephalosyndactyly (Apert's S.)
3. Basal cell nevus S. (Gorlin)
4. Bonnevie-Ullrich S.
5. Cat-cry S.
6. Central facial hyperplasia (Grieg)
7. Cerebral gigantism (Soto's S.)
8. Chondrodysplasia punctata (Conradi's disease)
9. Cleidocranial dysplasia
10. Cornelia de Lange S.
11. Craniofacial dysostosis (Crouzon's disease)
12. Dubowitz S.
13. Facial duplication
14. Fraser S.
15. Hurler S.
16. Hypertelorism-hypospadias S.
17. Larsen's S.
18. Metaphyseal chondrodysplasia (Jansen)
19. Metaphyseal dysplasia (Pyle's disease)
20. Noonan's S.
21. Orodigitofacial S.
22. Osteogenesis imperfecta
23. Otopalatodigital S.
24. Rubinstein-Taybi S.
25. Seckel's bird-headed dwarfism

(Continued)

26. Shawl scrotum S. (Aarskog-Scott)
27. Short arm 18 deletion S.
28. Sjögren-Larsson S.
29. [Thalassemia]
30. Treacher Collins S. (mandibulofacial dysostosis)
31. Turner's S.
32. William's S.
33. XXXXX S.
34. XXXXY S.

Reference:

Smith DW: *Recognizable Patterns of Human Malformation*. Philadelphia, WB Saunders Co, 1970, p 279.

SUBGAMUT B-4A
HYPERTELORISM, LOCAL CAUSES

1. Anterior meningocele or encephalocele; cranium bifidum
2. Craniostenosis of coronal sutures
3. Fibrous dysplasia, leontiasis ossea
4. Idiopathic
5. Midline dermoid or teratoma
6. Severe hydrocephalus in growth period (overgrowth of lesser wing of sphenoid)

UNILATERAL EXOPHTHALMOS (PROPTOSIS)

A. Bone Disease

COMMON

1. Fracture with retro-orbital hematoma or orbital emphysema
2. Metastasis

UNCOMMON

1. Craniostenosis, severe
2. Histiocytosis X
3. Myeloma
4. Neurofibromatosis
5. Ossifying fibroma, fibrous dysplasia
6. Osteoma of a paranasal sinus
7. Osteomyelitis
8. Paget's disease
9. Primary benign or malignant bone neoplasm (eg, osteosarcoma)

B. Paranasal Sinus or Nasopharyngeal Disease with Intra-orbital Extension

COMMON

1. Carcinoma, lymphoepithelioma, or other neoplasm
2. Mucocele

UNCOMMON

1. Sinusitis

(Continued)

UNILATERAL EXOPHTHALMOS (PROPTOSIS)
(Continued)

C. Primary Orbital Soft Tissue Disease (including extension from an intracranial lesion)

COMMON

1. Abscess or cellulitis (retrobulbar or periorbital)
2. Granuloma
3. Hemangioma
4. Lacrimal gland tumor
5. Meningioma (esp. sphenoid ridge)

UNCOMMON

1. Benign or malignant mesenchymal tumor (eg, angioma, lipoma, myoma, fibroma, and their sarcomatous counterparts; rhabdomyosarcoma)
2. Carotid artery aneurysm, carotid-cavernous fistula, cavernous sinus thrombosis, arteriovenous malformation (congenital or traumatic)
3. Dermoid, teratoma
4. Epidermoid (cholesteatoma)
5. Foreign body
6. Hydatid cyst
7. Lymphoma
8. Neurofibroma
9. Optic glioma
10. Orbital meningocele or encephalocele (congenital or traumatic)
11. Orbital varices
12. Pseudotumor of orbit
13. Retinoblastoma; sympathicoblastoma; neuroblastoma

(Continued)

D. Systemic Disease

COMMON

1. Hyperthyroidism, thyrotoxicosis

References:

1. Bullock LJ, Reeves RJ: Unilateral exophthalmos: roentgenographic aspects. *Am J Roentgenol* 82:290–299, 1959.

2. Lee KF, Hodes PJ, Greenberg L, Sinotti A: Three rare causes of unilateral exophthalmos. *Radiology* 90:1009–1015, 1968.

3. Lloyd GAS: The radiological investigation of proptosis. *Br J Radiol* 43:1–18, 1970.

4. Newton TH, Potts DG: *Radiology of the Skull and Brain.* St. Louis, Mosby, 1971, vol 1 book 2, pp 468–469

ENLARGED SUPERIOR ORBITAL (SPHENOIDAL) FISSURE (EROSION AND WIDENING)

COMMON

1. Aneurysm of intracavernous portion of internal carotid artery
2. Normal asymmetry
3. Pituitary tumor (esp. chromophobe adenoma)

UNCOMMON

1. Carotid-cavernous fistula
2. Chordoma
3. Chronic increased intracranial pressure
4. Craniopharyngioma
5. Extension from orbital or infraorbital mass (juvenile xanthogranuloma, lymphoma, Burkitt tumor, neuroblastoma) or from paranasal sinus malignancy
6. Histiocytosis X
7. Meningioma
8. Metastatic carcinoma to sphenoid wing
9. Middle fossa mass (eg, infratemporal chronic subdural hematoma or hygroma; arachnoid cyst with temporal lobe agenesis; temporal lobe astrocytoma)
10. Mucocele of sphenoid sinus
11. Neurofibroma
12. Neurofibromatosis (orbital dysplasia)
13. Orbital varix
14. Posterior orbital encephalocele
15. Pseudotumor of orbit

References:

1. DuBoulay GH: *Principles of X-ray Diagnosis of the Skull.* Washington, Butterworths, 1965, p 204–207.
2. Newton TH, Potts DG: *Radiology of the Skull and Brain.* St. Louis, Mosby, 1971, vol 1 book 2, pp 508–521.

NARROWED SUPERIOR ORBITAL (SPHENOIDAL) FISSURE

COMMON

1. Fibrous dysplasia
2. Paget's disease
3. Normal variant; congenital asymmetry or narrowing

UNCOMMON

1. Bone tumor (eg, osteoma, osteoblastic metastasis)
2. Meningioma with hyperostosis
3. Osteitis secondary to sinusitis
4. Osteopetrosis
5. Thalassemia, severe

References:

1. Newton TH, Potts DG: *Radiology of the Skull and Brain.* St. Louis, Mosby, 1971, vol 1 book 2, pp 521–524.

2. Shapiro R, Robinson F: Alterations of the sphenoidal fissure produced by local and systemic processes. *Am J Roentgenol* 101:814–827, 1967.

SMALL ORBIT AND/OR OPTIC CANAL

COMMON

1. Enucleation in childhood
2. Radiation therapy

UNCOMMON

1. Anophthalmos, microphthalmos (eg, Hallerman-Streiff S., oculovertebral S. — unilateral)
2. Craniostenosis of coronal suture
3. Encroachment from adjacent mass (eg, frontal sinus mucocele or neoplasm; antral neoplasm or cyst)
4. Increased bone density with encroachment on orbit (eg, meningioma, fibrous dysplasia, Paget's disease, osteopetrosis, Pyle's disease, thalassemia)
5. Neurofibromatosis
6. Osteitis (eg, from sphenoid sinusitis)

Reference:

Newton TH, Potts DG: *Radiology of the Skull and Brain.* St. Louis, Mosby, 1971, vol 1 book 2, pp 469–470, 502–506.

LARGE ORBIT

1. Congenital glaucoma (buphthalmos, hydrophthalmos)
2. Congenital serous cyst (often associated with anophthalmos or microphthalmos)
3. Exophthalmos (eg, thyrotoxicosis)
4. Neurofibromatosis (orbital dysplasia)
5. Pseudotumor
6. Tumor within muscle cone (eg, hemangioma, optic nerve glioma, neurofibroma, dermoid cyst, retinoblastoma)
7. Varix of orbital vein

Reference:

Newton TH, Potts DG: *Radiology of the Skull and Brain.* St. Louis, Mosby, 1971, vol 1 book 2, pp 470–473.

OPTIC CANAL ENLARGEMENT
(OVER 6.5 MM IN DIAMETER)

COMMON

1. Glioma of optic nerve
2. Neurofibromatosis with or without optic neurofibroma

UNCOMMON

1. Aneurysm of ophthalmic artery
2. Arteriovenous malformation
3. Hurler syndrome
4. Increased intracranial pressure
5. Inflammatory disease (eg, tuberculous or sarcoid granuloma; chiasmatic arachnoiditis)
6. Meningioma of optic nerve sheath
7. Pituitary adenoma
8. Retinoblastoma with intracranial extension

Reference:

Newton TH, Potts DG: *Radiology of the Skull and Brain.* St. Louis, Mosby, 1971, vol 1 book 2, pp 492–496.

LOCALIZED BONY DEFECT OR
EROSION ABOUT THE OPTIC CANAL

COMMON

1. Aneurysm of internal carotid artery
2. Malignant tumor arising in orbit, sphenoid sinus, or nasal cavity
3. Pituitary tumor
4. Tumor of orbital apex

UNCOMMON

1. Craniopharyngioma
2. Eosinophilic granuloma
3. Granuloma or other infection of sphenoid sinus
4. Metastasis
5. Mucocele of sphenoid sinus
6. Surgical defect
7. Tumor of anterior fossa (eg, meningioma, astrocytoma, glioma)

Reference:

Newton TH, Potts DG: *Radiology of the Skull and Brain*. St. Louis, Mosby, 1971, vol 1 book 2, pp 496–501.

LESIONS INVOLVING THE ORBIT

A. Arising within the orbit

  I. In muscle cone

    1. Meningioma

    2. Neurofibroma

    3. Optic glioma

    4. Retinoblastoma

  II. Between periosteum and muscle cone

    1. Dermoid

    2. Lacrimal gland tumor

    3. Lymphoma

    4. Metastasis

    5. Pseudotumor

    6. Rhabdomyosarcoma

    7. Vascular lesion (eg, hemangioma, hemangioblastoma, varices, hematoma)

B. Arising extraorbitally and extracranially in nasopharynx, paranasal sinuses, or bone

  1. Bone tumor, primary or metastatic

  2. Carcinoma

  3. Fibrous dysplasia

  4. Histiocytosis X

  5. Infection

  6. Lymphoma

  7. Mucocele

  8. Osteoma

  9. Paget's disease

(Continued)

C. Arising intracranially with secondary involvement of orbit
   1. Aneurysm of internal carotid artery
   2. Carotid-cavernous fistula
   3. Encephalocele
   4. Meningioma
   5. Optic glioma

Reference:

Arger PH, Mishkin MM, Nenninger RH: An approach to orbital lesions. *Am J Roentgenol* 115:595–606, 1972.

BONY DEFECT OR
RADIOLUCENT LESION OF THE ORBIT
(See also Gamuts B-11 and B-12)

COMMON

1. Extrinsic tumor invading orbit (eg, meningioma; carcinoma or lymphoma of nasopharynx, nasal cavity or paranasal sinus; carcinoma of skin or eyelid

2. Metastasis (eg, breast, lung, neuroblastoma, Ewing's sarcoma)

3. Mucocele

4. Osteomyelitis secondary to sinusitis

UNCOMMON

1. Encephalocele, meningocele

2. Histiocytosis X

3. Juvenile xanthogranuloma

4. Lymphoma, Burkitt tumor

5. Myeloma

6. Neurofibromatosis (orbital dysplasia)

7. Primary bone tumor

8. Primary orbital tumor (eg, hemangioma, hemangioblastoma, lacrimal gland tumor, dermoid, epidermoid, neurofibroma, melanoma, retinoblastoma, rhabdomyosarcoma)

Reference:

Newton TH, Potts DG: *Radiology of the Skull and Brain.* St. Louis, Mosby, 1971, vol 1 book 2, pp 476–482.

SCLEROSIS AND THICKENING
OF THE ORBITAL ROOF OR WALLS

COMMON

1. Fibrous dysplasia, leontiasis ossea
2. Meningioma
3. Osteitis secondary to chronic sinusitis, mucocele, or pyocele
4. Paget's disease

UNCOMMON

1. Dermoid
2. Histiocytosis X
3. Infantile cortical hyperostosis (Caffey's disease)
4. Lacrimal gland carcinoma
5. Lymphoma
6. Osteoblastic metastasis (eg, breast, prostate)
7. Osteoma
8. Osteopetrosis
9. Osteosarcoma
10. Radiation therapy

Reference:

Newton TH, Potts DG: *Radiology of the Skull and Brain*. St. Louis, Mosby, 1971, vol 1 book 2, pp 482–485.

INTRAORBITAL CALCIFICATION

COMMON

1. Cataract
2. [Foreign body]
3. Phlebolith (eg, orbital varices, hemangioma)
4. Phthisis bulbi (old trauma or infection of choroid or vitreous with shrunken globe)
5. Retinoblastoma

UNCOMMON

1. Aneurysm or atherosclerosis of internal carotid or ophthalmic artery; vascular calcification in sarcoidosis, syphilis, diabetes
2. Collagen disease (eg, band keratopathy of cornea in rheumatoid arthritis)
3. Hematoma; myositis ossificans of extraocular muscles
4. Hypercalcemia (metastatic calcification in conjunctiva and cornea) (eg, hypervitaminosis D, primary and secondary hyperparathyroidism, metastases, multiple myeloma, milk-alkali syndrome)
5. Idiopathic
6. Intraocular infection (eg, abscess, bacterial opthalmitis, tuberculosis, syphilis)
7. Intraorbital neoplasm (eg, meningioma, dermoid cyst, optic glioma, plexiform neurofibroma, lacrimal gland carcinoma, hemangioendothelioma, metastasis)
8. Mucocele invading orbit
9. [Osteoma]
10. Parasitic disease (eg, hydatid cyst, cysticercosis)
11. Retinal disease (eg, detachment, retinitis, fibrosis, retrolental fibroplasia)

References:

1. Ashton N: Calcareous degeneration and ossification. In Duke-Elder S, Editor: *System of Ophthalmology*. St. Louis, Mosby, 1962, vol 7.
2. Newton TH, Potts DG: *Radiology of the Skull and Brain*. St. Louis, Mosby, 1971, vol 1 book 2, pp 525–540.

CONGENITAL SYNDROMES WITH DELAYED AND/OR DEFECTIVE DENTITION
(See also Gamuts B-17 and B-18)

COMMON

1. Basal cell nevus S. (Gorlin) (odontogenic cyst, irregular placement, caries)
2. Chondroectodermal dysplasia (Ellis-Van Creveld S.) (neonatal teeth, conical, peg-shaped teeth, partial anodontia, delayed eruption)
3. Cleidocranial dysplasia (delayed eruption, supernumerary teeth, partial anodontia, malformed roots, enamel hypoplasia)
4. Craniometaphyseal dysplasia (Pyle's disease) (poor teeth)
5. Cretinism
6. Down's S. (mongolism) (hypodontia, microdontia, delayed eruption)
7. [Fibrous dysplasia, cherubism (premature or delayed eruption)]
8. Hypophosphatasia (early loss, poor dentin)
9. [Hypophosphatemic rickets (delayed eruption, enamel hypoplasia, gingival and periapical infection)]
10. Mucopolysaccharidosis (eg, Hurler, Hunter, Morquio) (malaligned teeth, thin enamel)
11. Osteogenesis imperfecta (poor dentin, short roots)
12. Osteopetrosis (delayed eruption)
13. Pseudohypoparathyroidism (delayed eruption, enamel hypoplasia)
14. [Syphilis, congenital (Hutchinson's teeth)]

UNCOMMON

1. Acrocephalosyndactyly (Apert's S.) (delayed eruption)
2. Aglossia-adactylia S. (missing incisors)
3. Amelogenesis imperfecta
4. Aminopterin-induced S.
5. Bird-headed dwarfism (Seckel's S.)
6. Böök's S. (bicuspid hypodontia)

(Continued)

CONGENITAL SYNDROMES WITH
DELAYED AND/OR DEFECTIVE DENTITION
(See also Gamuts B-17 and B-18) (Continued)

7. Cockayne's S. (caries)
8. Craniofacial dysostosis (Crouzon's disease) (partial anodontia, wide spacing)
9. Dentinal dysplasia
10. Dyskeratosis congenita S. (caries, malalignment)
11. Ectodermal dysplasias (eg, hereditary, hypohidrotic, or Robinson type) (partial anodontia, conical teeth)
12. Ehlers-Danlos S. (small, irregular teeth, partial anodontia)
13. Enamel hypoplasia — curly hair S. (enamel hypoplasia, microdontia)
14. [Fluoride intoxication]
15. Gardner's S.
16. Goldenhar's S.
17. Goltz S. (hypodontia, enamel hypoplasia, delayed eruption, malformed teeth, irregular placement)
18. Homocystinuria (irregular, crowded teeth)
19. Incontinentia pigmenti (hypodontia, delayed eruption, conical teeth)
20. Marshall S.
21. Mohr S. (missing central incisors)
22. Oculocerebral-renal S. (cysts)
23. Oculodentodigital dysplasia (hypodontia, microdontia, enamel hypoplasia)
24. Oculomandibulofacial S. (Hallerman-Streiff) (hypodontia, malimplantation, supernumerary teeth, neonatal teeth, delayed eruption)
25. Orodigitofacial S. (missing lateral incisors, supernumerary cuspids and bicuspids)
26. Osteodysplasia (Melnick-Needles) (malaligned teeth)
27. Otopalatodigital S.
28. Pachyonychia congenita

(Continued)

29. Prader-Willi S. (dental caries, enamel hypoplasia)

30. Progeria (delayed eruption, crowded teeth)

31. Pyknodysostosis (delayed eruption, partial anodontia, irregular placement)

32. Rieger's S. (hypodontia, microdontia)

33. Rothmund S.

34. Sjögren-Larsson S.

35. Stanesco's dysplasia (small, crowded teeth, enamel hypoplasia)

36. Treacher Collins S. (mandibulofacial dysostosis)

37. Weill-Marchesani S.

38. Werner's S.

39. William's S.

40. XXXXY S.

References:

1. Berkman MD: Pedodontic radiographic interpretation. *Dental Radiogr Photogr* 44:27–39, 1971.

2. Greenfield GB: *Radiology of Bone Diseases.* Philadelphia, JB Lippincott Co, 1969, p 225.

3. Smith DW: *Recognizable Patterns of Human Malformation.* Philadelphia, WB Saunders Co, 1970, p 284.

DELAYED ERUPTION OR
NONERUPTION OF TEETH

I. Congenital Syndromes (see Gamut B-16)
  1. Acrocephalosyndactyly (Apert's S.)
  2. Chondroectodermal dysplasia (Ellis-Van Creveld S.)
  3. Cleidocranial dysplasia
  4. Down's S. (mongolism)
  5. Goltz S.
  6. [Hypophosphatemic rickets]
  7. Incontinentia pigmenti
  8. Oculomandibulofacial S. (Hallerman-Streiff)
  9. Osteopetrosis
  10. Progeria
  11. Pseudohypoparathyroidism
  12. Pyknodysostosis

II. Endocrinopathies
  1. Hypoparathyroidism
  2. Hypopituitarism
  3. Hypothyroidism

III. Familial Tendency

IV. Idiopathic

V. Local Factors
  1. Developmental
    a. Cleft lip and/or cleft palate
    b. Disorientation of tooth germ
    c. Ectopic eruption
    d. Lack of space
    e. Prolonged retention of deciduous teeth

(Continued)

  f. Submersion and ankylosis

  g. Supernumerary teeth

2. Hereditary (eg, amelogenesis imperfecta)

3. Iatrogenic

  a. Improperly contoured restoration (eg, stainless steel crowns)

  b. Lack of space (eg, premature extraction of deciduous teeth and loss of space for permanent successor)

  c. Over-retained roots of deciduous teeth

4. Inflammatory (eg, Garré's chronic sclerosing osteo-myelitis)

5. Mechanical (eg, fibrosis of alveolar mucosa, dilacera-tion of tooth, impaction)

6. Neoplastic

  a. Obstruction by dentigerous or radicular cyst

  b. Odontogenic tumor
   (1) Adenoameloblastoma
   (2) Ameloblastic fibroma
   (3) Ameloblastic odontoma
   (4) Neuroectodermal tumor of infancy (melanotic progonoma)
   (5) Odontogenic fibroma
   (6) Odontoma

  c. Nonodontogenic jaw tumor
   (1) Central giant cell reparative granuloma
   (2) Ossifying fibroma, fibrous dysplasia, cherubism

7. Traumatic (eg, injury to deciduous teeth early in life; jaw fracture)

Reference:

Berkman MD: Pedodontic radiographic intrepretation. *Dental Radiogr Photogr* 44:27–39, 1971.

CONGENITAL SYNDROMES
WITH MULTIPLE MISSING TEETH
(See also Gamut B-16)

1. Aglossia-adactylia S.
2. Böök's S.
3. Chondroectodermal dysplasia (Ellis-Van Creveld S.)
4. Cleidocranial dysplasia
5. Craniofacial dysostosis (Crouzon's disease)
6. Down's S. (mongolism)
7. Ectodermal dysplasias
8. Ehlers-Danlos S.
9. Focal dermal hypoplasia (Goltz S.)
10. Hereditary
11. Idiopathic, nonfamilial
12. Incontinentia pigmenti
13. Mohr S.
14. Oculodentodigital dysplasia
15. Oculomandibulofacial S. (Hallerman-Streiff)
16. Orodigitofacial S.
17. Pyknodysostosis
18. Rieger's S.

Reference:

Berkman MD: Pedodontic radiographic interpretation. *Dental Radiogr Photogr* 44:27–39, 1971.

PROGNATHISM

COMMON

1. Acromegaly
2. Normal variant (racial); idiopathic

UNCOMMON

1. Basal cell nevus S. (Gorlin)
2. Cerebral gigantism
3. Cherubism (fibrous dysplasia)
4. Cockayne's S.
5. Edentulous mandible
6. Facial hemihypertrophy (unilateral prognathism)
7. Lymphangioma of tongue
8. Paget's disease
9. Wiedemann-Beckwith S.
10. XXXXY S.

MICROGNATHIA

1. Aminopterin-induced S.
2. Bird-headed dwarfism (Seckel's S.)
3. Bloom's S.
4. Cat-cry S.
5. Chondrodysplasia punctata (Conradi's disease)
6. Cornelia de Lange S.
7. Diastrophic dwarfism
8. Dubowitz S.
9. G deletion S.
10. Goldenhar's S.
11. Larsen's S.
12. Long arm 21 deletion S.
13. Mesomelic dwarfism, Langer type
14. Noonan's S.
15. Oculomandibulofacial S. (Hallerman-Streiff)
16. Orodigitofacial S.
17. Osteodysplasia (Melnick-Needles)
18. Pierre-Robin S.
19. Progeria
20. Pyknodysostosis
21. Rubinstein-Taybi S.
22. Russell-Silver S.
23. Short arm 18 deletion S.
24. Smith-Lemli-Opitz S.
25. Stanesco's dysplasia

(Continued)

26. Thrombocytopenia — absent radius S.

27. Treacher Collins S. (mandibulofacial dysostosis)

28. Trisomy 13 S.

29. Trisomy 18 S.

30. Turner's S.

References:

1. Felson B, Editor: Dwarfs and Other Little People. *Semin Roentgenol* 8:258, 1973.

2. Smith DW: *Recognizable Patterns of Human Malformation*. Philadelphia, WB Saunders Co, 1970, p 283.

CONGENITAL SYNDROMES WITH MAXILLARY AND/OR MALAR (ZYGOMATIC) HYPOPLASIA

1. Achondroplasia
2. Acrocephalosyndactyly (Apert's S.)
3. Aminopterin-induced S.
*4. Bird-headed dwarfism (Seckel's S.)
*5. Bloom's S.
*6. Cockayne's S.
7. Cornelia de Lange S.
8. Craniofacial dysostosis (Crouzon's disease)
9. Down's S. (mongolism)
*10. Goldenhar's S.
11. Leprechaunism
12. Long arm 18 deletion S.
*13. Long arm 21 deletion S.
14. Marshall's S.
15. Mietens-Weber S.
16. Oculodentodigital S.
*17. Oculomandibulofacial S. (Hallerman-Streiff)
*18. Orodigitofacial S.
*19. Otopalatodigital S.
20. Progeria
*21. Pyknodysostosis
22. Rubinstein-Taybi S.
23. Russell-Silver S.
*24. Stanesco's dysplasia

(Continued)

*25. Treacher Collins S. (mandibulofacial dysostosis)

*26. Trisomy 13 S.

*27. Trisomy 18 S.

28. Weill-Marchesani S.

*Malar hypoplasia — some have maxillary hypoplasia in addition

Reference:

Smith DW: *Recognizable Patterns of Human Malformation.* Philadelphia, WB Saunders Co, 1970, p 283.

LOSS OF LAMINA DURA OF THE TEETH

COMMON

1. Local inflammatory disease (eg, gingivitis, pyorrhea, dental caries, periapical granuloma, apical periodontal cyst)
2. Senile osteoporosis

UNCOMMON

1. Burkitt's lymphoma
2. Cushing's syndrome
3. Fibrous dysplasia
4. Histiocytosis X
5. Hyperparathyroidism
6. Hyperphosphatasia
7. Leukemia
8. Metastasis
9. Multiple myeloma
10. Neoplasm, primary (eg, benign cementoblastoma)
11. Osteomalacia
12. Paget's disease
13. Removal of opposing tooth
14. Scleroderma
15. Traumatic (hemorrhagic) cyst

References:

1. Greenfield GB: *Radiology of Bone Diseases.* Philadelphia, JB Lippincott Co, 1969, p 26.
2. Krolls SO: Personal communication.

FLOATING TEETH

COMMON

1. Histiocytosis X
2. Periodontitis, severe

UNCOMMON

1. Agranulocytosis and cyclic neutropenia
2. Ameloblastoma
3. Ewing's sarcoma
4. Familial dysproteinemia
5. Fibrous dysplasia
6. Hyperparathyroidism
7. Hypophosphatasia
8. Leukemia, lymphoma, Burkitt's tumor
9. Melanotic progonoma
10. Mercury poisoning (acrodynia)
11. Metastatic neoplasm (esp. neuroblastoma, retinoblastoma)
12. Papillon-LeFevre syndrome (juvenile periodontosis)
13. Plasmacytoma, myeloma

References:

1. Keusch KD, Poole CA, King DR: The significance of "floating teeth" in children. *Radiology* 86:215–219, 1966.

2. Shafer WG, Hine MK, Levy BM: *A Textbook of Oral Pathology*, ed 3. Philadelphia, WB Saunders Co, 1974.

MANDIBULAR PERIOSTITIS

COMMON

1. Histiocytosis X
2. Malignant neoplasm, primary or metastatic
3. Necrosis (thermal, chemical, radiation)
4. Osteomyelitis, pyogenic

UNCOMMON

1. Actinomycosis
2. Hypervitaminosis A
3. Infantile cortical hyperostosis (Caffey's disease)
4. Syphilis
5. Tuberculosis

References:

1. Jayne HE, Hays RA, O'Brien FW: Cysts and tumors of the man-dible—their differential diagnosis. *Am J Roentgenol* 86:292–309, 1961.

2. Kilcoyne RF, Krolls SO, Allman RM: Luetic osteomyelitis of the mandible. RPC of the month from the AFIP. *Radiology* 94:687–691, 1970.

3. Stafne EC: *Oral Roentgenographic Diagnosis*, ed 2. Philadelphia, WB Saunders Co, 1963.

4. Thoma KH: *Oral Surgery*. St. Louis, CV Mosby Co, 1969.

JAW LESION WITH CORTICAL ALTERATION

A. CORTICAL OVERGROWTH
1. Chronic osteomyelitis (eg, Garré's)
2. Ewing's sarcoma
3. Infantile cortical hyperostosis (Caffey's disease)

B. CORTICAL OSTEOPHYTIC REACTION
1. Juxtacortical osteosarcoma
2. Odontogenic cyst or tumor

C. CORTICAL EXPANSION (see Gamut B-28)
1. Fibrous dysplasia, cherubism
2. Malignant neoplasm
3. Odontogenic cyst or tumor
4. Paget's disease

D. CORTICAL EROSION OR DESTRUCTION
1. Underlying bone lesion
   a. Histiocytosis X (esp. eosinophilic granuloma)
   b. Metastasis
   c. Multiple myeloma
   d. Osteomyelitis; actinomycosis
   e. Primary malignant tumor (eg, sarcoma)
2. Overlying soft tissue lesion
   a. Peripheral giant cell granuloma
   b. Salivary adenocarcinoma
   c. Sarcoma
   d. Soft tissue fissural cyst (nasolabial cyst)
   e. Soft tissue odontogenic cyst (gingival or Gorlin cyst)
   f. Squamous cell carcinoma

Reference:

Eversole LR, Rovin S: Differential radiographic diagnosis of lesions of the jawbones. *Radiology* 105:277–284, 1972.

CYST-LIKE LESION OF THE JAW
(See also Gamuts B-26A, B-27, and B-28)

COMMON

1. Ameloblastoma
2. Brown tumor of hyperparathyroidism
3. Dentigerous (follicular) cyst
4. Fibrous dysplasia, cherubism
5. Odontogenic cyst (eg, keratocyst, primordial cyst, Gorlin cyst)
6. Radicular cyst, periapical granuloma
7. Traumatic (hemorrhagic) cyst

UNCOMMON

1. Adenomatoid odontogenic tumor (adenoameloblastoma)
2. Ameloblastic fibroma
3. Aneurysmal bone cyst
4. Bone cyst
5. Cementoma
6. Central giant cell (reparative) granuloma
7. Fissural developmental cyst (eg, globulomaxillary, median palatal, median mandibular, median alveolar, incisive canal)
8. Giant cell tumor
9. Histiocytosis X (esp. eosinophilic granuloma)
10. Hydatid cyst
11. Malignant neoplasm, primary or metastatic
12. Odontogenic fibroma or myxoma
13. Ossifying fibroma; cementifying fibroma
14. Pindborg tumor

SUBGAMUT B-26A
LOCATION OF CYST-LIKE LESION OF THE JAW

A. At apex of root
   1. Apical scar
   2. Cementoma (early)
   3. Periapical (dental) granuloma or abscess
   4. Radicular cyst

B. Midline of maxilla
   1. Cyst of papilla palatina
   2. Incisive canal cyst (nasopalatine duct cyst)
   3. Median alveolar cyst
   4. Median palatal cyst

C. Lateral to midline of maxilla
   1. Globulomaxillary cyst
   2. Nasolabial cyst (soft tissue)
   3. Surgical ciliated cyst of maxillary sinus

D. Around impacted or unerupted tooth
   1. Adenoameloblastoma
   2. Ameloblastoma
   3. Dental follicle
   4. Dentigerous (follicular) cyst
   5. Melanotic progonoma
   6. Odontogenic fibroma or myxoma
   7. Odontogenic keratocyst
   8. Odontoma, compound
   9. Pindborg tumor

Reference:
Krolls SO: Personal communication.

UNILOCULAR RADIOLUCENT LESION OF THE JAW

WELL-DEFINED BORDERS

1. Adenoameloblastoma
2. Ameloblastoma
3. Bone cyst
4. Cementoma (immature)
5. Central cementifying fibroma (immature)
6. Dentigerous (follicular) cyst
7. Fissural cyst (eg, nasopalatine, globulomaxillary, median palatal, median alveolar, median mandibular)
8. Neurofibroma, neurilemmoma
9. Odontogenic cyst (eg, keratocyst, primordial cyst)
10. Radicular cyst, periapical granuloma

ILL-DEFINED BORDERS

1. Cementoma (immature)
2. Giant cell tumor
3. Histiocytosis X
4. Metastasis
5. Myeloma
6. Odontogenic cyst (eg, Gorlin cyst)
7. Osteoporotic bone marrow defect

Reference:

Eversole LR, Rovin S: Differential radiographic diagnosis of lesions of the jawbones. *Radiology* 105:277–284, 1972.

EXPANSILE MULTILOCULAR RADIOLUCENT LESION OF THE JAW

EXPANSILE WITH DISCRETE MARGINS

1. Ameloblastoma
2. Aneurysmal bone cyst
*3. Brown tumor of hyperparathyroidism
4. Calcifying epithelial odontogenic tumor (Pindborg tumor)
*5. Central giant cell (reparative) granuloma
6. Central hemangioma, arteriovenous malformation
*7. Dentigerous (follicular) cyst
8. Eosinophilic granuloma (histiocytosis X)
*9. Fibrous dysplasia, cherubism, ossifying fibroma
10. Giant cell tumor
11. Myeloma, plasmacytoma
*12. Odontogenic cyst (eg, keratocyst, primordial cyst)
13. Odontogenic myxoma or fibroma

EXPANSILE WITH ILL-DEFINED MARGINS

1. Bone sarcoma (eg, chondrosarcoma)
2. Calcifying epithelial odontogenic cyst (Gorlin cyst)
*3. Fibrous dysplasia
4. Giant cell tumor
5. Metastasis
*6. Myeloma

*Common

Reference:

Eversole LR, Rovin S: Differential radiographic diagnosis of lesions of the jawbones. *Radiology* 105:277–284, 1972.

MIXED RADIOLUCENT AND RADIOPAQUE LESION OF THE JAW

COMMON

1. Fibrous dysplasia, cherubism, ossifying fibroma
2. Odontoma, compound or complex
3. Paget's disease

UNCOMMON

1. Adenoameloblastoma
2. Ameloblastic fibro-odontoma
3. Ameloblastic odontoma
4. Calcifying epithelial odontogenic tumor (Pindborg tumor)
5. Cementoma
6. Chondrosarcoma
7. Gorlin cyst
8. Metastasis (eg, from breast or prostate)
9. Osteoblastoma
10. Osteosarcoma

Reference:

Eversole LR, Rovin S: Differential radiographic diagnosis of lesions of the jawbones. *Radiology* 105:277–284, 1972.

SUBGAMUT B-29A
RADIOLUCENT LESION OF THE JAW
WITH CENTRAL OPACITY (TARGET LESION)

COMMON

1. Ameloblastic fibro-odontoma
2. Cementoma (periapical cemental dysplasia)
3. Odontoma

UNCOMMON

1. Adenomatoid odontogenic tumor (adenoameloblastoma)
2. Ameloblastic odontoma
3. Benign cementoblastoma
4. Calcifying epithelial odontogenic cyst (Gorlin cyst)
5. Ossifying fibroma; cementifying fibroma
6. Osteoid osteoma

Reference:

Eversole LR, Rovin S: Differential radiographic diagnosis of lesions of the jawbones. *Radiology* 105:277–284, 1972.

RADIOPAQUE LESION OF THE JAW

COMMON

*1. Condensing osteitis, focal sclerosing osteitis

2. Fibrous dysplasia, ossifying fibroma

*3. Odontoma, compound or complex

4. Paget's disease

*5. Torus palatinus or mandibularis

*6. [Unerupted tooth; retained root]

UNCOMMON

*1. Cementoma (late stage)

*2. Chondrosarcoma

3. Infantile cortical hyperostosis (Caffey's disease)

*4. Osteoblastic metastasis

*5. Osteoma (eg, Gardner's syndrome)

6. Osteopetrosis

*7. Osteosarcoma

8. Sclerosing osteomyelitis (eg, Garré; chronic diffuse sclerosing osteomyelitis)

*9. [Superimposed sialolith, phlebolith, foreign body]

*Localized

Reference:

Eversole LR, Rovin S: Differential radiographic diagnosis of lesions of the jawbones. *Radiology* 105:277–284, 1972.

DEFORMITY, ASYMMETRY, OR OPACIFICATION OF THE NASAL CAVITY

COMMON

1. Congenital deformity of nasal septum
2. Fracture of nasal plates or septum
3. Mucosal swelling (inflammatory, allergic, traumatic)
4. Pseudopolyp
5. Rhinolith, foreign body
6. Turbinate abnormality (eg, enlargement, congenital absence)

UNCOMMON

1. Benign tumor (eg, fibroma, neurofibroma, ossifying fibroma, osteoma)
2. Carcinoma of nose or antrum
3. Choanal atresia or stenosis
4. Dermoid cyst
5. Encephalomeningocele
6. Hypoplasia of nasal bones in various congenital syndromes
7. Rhinoscleroma with granulomatous mass
8. Wegener's granuloma

Reference:

DuBoulay GH: *Principles of X-ray Diagnosis of the Skull.* Washington, Butterworths, 1969, p 307.

NASOPHARYNGEAL MASS

COMMON

1. Abscess
2. Cervical spine lesion, including fracture
3. Enlarged adenoids, tonsils
4. Hematoma
5. Malignant nasopharyngeal neoplasm (eg, carcinoma, lymphoma, lymphoepithelioma, rhabdomyosarcoma, other sarcomas, mixed salivary tumor, plasmacytoma)

UNCOMMON

1. Aneurysm of internal carotid artery
2. Benign nasopharyngeal neoplasm (eg, juvenile angiofibroma, neurilemmoma, dermoid cyst, angioma, adenoma, chondroma, odontoma)
3. Bone sarcoma (eg, chondrosarcoma, osteosarcoma)
4. Chordoma
5. Foreign body
6. Meningioma of skull base
7. [Nasal polyp; enlarged turbinate]
8. Neoplasm extending from sphenoid sinus, nasal fossa, or parotid gland
9. Rhinoscleroma
10. Sarcoidosis
11. Thornwaldt's cyst (notochord remnant)
12. Tuberculosis of nasopharynx or cervical spine

References:

1. Jing B: Tumors of the nasopharynx. *Rad Cl North Am* 8:323–342, 1970.
2. Newton TH, Potts DG: *Radiology of the Skull and Brain.* St. Louis, Mosby, 1971, vol 1 book 1, pp 251–258.

MASS IN A PARANASAL SINUS

COMMON

1. Carcinoma
2. Dental cyst (eg, follicular, globulomaxillary)
3. Encapsulated exudate, pus or blood
4. Extrinsic neoplasm invading sinus (eg, chordoma; pituitary, orbital, oral, or nasopharyngeal tumor; Burkitt's lymphoma)
5. Fracture with hemorrhage (eg, blow-out fracture of orbit)
6. Mucosal edema or inflammation (eg, from sinusitis due to allergy or infection)
7. Mucous or serous retention cyst
8. Pseudopolyp

UNCOMMON

1. Benign neoplasm (eg, chondroma, hemangioma, angiofibroma, dermoid, lipoma, osteoma)
2. Dental tumor (eg, odontoma)
3. Granuloma
4. Malignant neoplasm, other (eg, sarcoma, lymphoma, mixed salivary tumor, melanoma)
5. Mucocele
6. Ossifying fibroma, fibrous dysplasia
7. Surgical ciliated cyst (post-Caldwell-Luc operation)
8. [Thalassemia]

DESTRUCTIVE MASS
IN THE MIDDLE EAR OR MASTOID

COMMON

1. Cholesteatoma
2. Mastoiditis with abscess
3. [Postoperative defect]

UNCOMMON

1. Carcinoma or sarcoma of middle ear or mastoid
2. Glomus tumor
3. Histiocytosis X
4. Inflammatory granuloma
5. Metastasis
6. Neuroma

References:

1. Duggan CA, Hoffman JC, Brylski JR: The efficacy of angiography in the evaluation of glomus tympanicum tumors. *Radiology* 97:45–49, 1970.

2. Newton TH, Potts DG: *Radiology of the Skull and Brain.* St. Louis, Mosby, 1971, vol 1 book 1, pp 424–442.

CALCIFICATION IN EAR CARTILAGE (PINNA)

COMMON

1. Boxing or other trauma
2. Gout

UNCOMMON

1. Acromegaly
2. Addison's disease
3. Collagen diseases
4. Diabetes mellitus
5. Diastrophic dwarfism
6. Familial cold hypersensitivity
7. Frostbite
8. Hypercalcemia
9. Hypercorticism
10. Hyperthyroidism
11. Hypoparathyroidism
12. Hypopituitarism
13. Idiopathic
14. Inflammatory lesions
15. Ochronosis
16. Polychondritis
17. Sarcoidosis
18. Syphilitic perichondritis
19. Von Meyenburg's disease (systemic chondromalacia)

Reference:

Greenfield GB: *Radiology of Bone Diseases.* Philadelphia, JB Lippincott Co, 1969, p 420.

LARGE TONGUE (MACROGLOSSIA)

COMMON

1. Amyloidosis
2. Cretinism
3. Down's syndrome (mongolism)

UNCOMMON

1. Acromegaly
2. Glycogen storage disease
3. Infant of diabetic mother
4. Jaw or dental deformity with increased mouth size
5. Mucopolysaccharidosis (eg, Hurler); mucolipidosis (eg, generalized gangliosidosis)
6. Muscular dystrophy
7. Neoplasm of tongue (eg, lymphangioma, carcinoma)
8. Trauma
9. Wiedemann-Beckwith visceromegaly syndrome

References:

1. Morfit HM: Lymphangioma of the tongue. *Arch Surg* 81:761–767, 1960.
2. Smith DW: *Recognizable Patterns of Human Malformation.* Philadelphia, WB Saunders Co, 1970, p 284.

SALIVARY GLAND ENLARGEMENT

COMMON

1. Mumps
2. Stone in duct (esp. in submandibular gland)
3. Suppurative sialitis
4. Tumor (esp. mixed tumor)

UNCOMMON

1. Alcoholism
2. Hormonal disturbance (eg, diabetes, hypothyroidism, pregnancy)
3. Idiopathic
4. Kwashiorkor
5. Mikulicz's disease
6. Mucoviscidosis
7. Nutritional deficiency, cirrhosis
8. Sarcoidosis
9. Sjögren's syndrome (associated with rheumatoid arthritis, lupus, or scleroderma)
10. Stricture of duct (see Gamut B-38)

References:

1. Kreel L: *Outline of Radiology.* New York, Appleton-Century-Crofts, 1971, p 91.
2. Krolls SO: Salivary gland diseases. *J Oral Med* 27:96–99, 1972.

SALIVARY DUCT STRICTURE ON SIALOGRAPHY

1. Carcinoma
2. Inflammation (scarring)
3. Radiation therapy
4. Stone
5. Trauma, including surgical

Reference:

Kreel L: *Outline of Radiology*. New York, Appleton-Century-Crofts, 1971, p 92.

CERVICAL SOFT TISSUE MASS
IN A NEONATE OR INFANT

COMMON

1. Abscess
2. Cystic hygroma (lymphangioma)
3. Hemangioma
4. Hematoma
5. Lymphadenopathy

UNCOMMON

1. Branchial cleft cyst
2. Cervical aortic arch
3. Dermoid cyst; teratoma
4. Dilated jugular lymph sac
5. Hemangiopericytoma
6. Laryngocele
7. Neuroblastoma
8. Parotid gland tumor
9. Thymus gland, cervical
10. Thyroglossal duct cyst
11. Thyroid adenoma

INCREASED RETROPHARYNGEAL SPACE IN AN INFANT OR CHILD

COMMON

1. Enlarged adenoids or tonsils

2. Retropharyngeal abscess or cellulitis

3. [Technical factors (eg, crying; expiration film; improper positioning with flexion or obliquity of neck; superimposed ear lobe)]

4. Trauma (eg, hematoma, spine fracture)

UNCOMMON

1. Cretinism (myxedema)

2. Cystic hygroma (lymphangioma)

3. Foreign body

4. Hemangioma

5. Retropharyngeal goiter

6. Spinal lesion (eg, tuberculosis, metastasis)

7. Traumatic pseudodiverticulum of pharynx (from finger in infant's mouth during delivery)

8. Tumor (eg, angiofibroma, plexiform neurofibroma, lymphoma)

Reference:

Grünebaum M, Moskowitz G: The retropharyngeal soft tissues in young infants with hypothyroidism. *Am J Roentgenol* 108:543–545, 1970.

SUBGAMUT B-40A
INCREASED RETROPHARYNGEAL SPACE
IN AN ADULT
(See also Gamut B-40)

1. Chordoma
2. Postcricoid carcinoma
3. Retropharyngeal goiter
4. Spine osteophytes, neoplasm, or inflammation
5. Zenker's diverticulum

NOTES

NOTES

TABLE OF CONTENTS

C. SPINE

(Continued)

C

C

C

CONGENITAL SYNDROMES WITH VERTEBRAL ABNORMALITY

COMMON

1. Achondroplasia (narrow spinal canal, scoliosis, lordosis)
2. Cretinism, hypothyroidism (kyphosis, beaked, flat vertebrae)
3. Mucopolysaccharidosis (eg, Hurler, Sanfilippo, Morquio, Maroteaux-Lamy); mucolipidosis (eg, Leroy's I-cell, generalized gangliosidosis) (kyphoscoliosis)
4. Neurofibromatosis (kyphoscoliosis)
5. Osteogenesis imperfecta (scoliosis, fractured vertebrae)

UNCOMMON

1. Achondrogenesis (lumbar vertebrae appear absent)
2. Asphyxiating thoracic dysplasia
3. Basal cell nevus S. (Gorlin)
4. Bird-headed dwarfism (Seckel) (kyphoscoliosis)
5. Campomelic dwarfism
6. Cervico-oculo-acoustic S. (cervical segmentation malformation)
7. Chondrodysplasia punctata (Conradi's disease) (scoliosis, coronal cleft vertebrae)
8. Cleidocranial dysplasia (spina bifida, kyphoscoliosis)
9. Cockayne's S.
10. Diastrophic dwarfism (scoliosis, platyspondyly)
11. Down's S. (mongolism)
12. Ehlers-Danlos S. (scoliosis)
13. Enchondromatosis (Ollier's disease) (kyphoscoliosis)
14. Geroderma osteodysplastica (platyspondyly)
15. Goldenhar's S.

(Continued)

CONGENITAL SYNDROMES WITH VERTEBRAL ABNORMALITY
(Continued)

16. Hajdu-Cheney S. (kyphoscoliosis, osteoporosis)

17. Hereditary arthro-ophthalmopathy (Stickler)

18. Homocystinuria (kyphoscoliosis, osteoporosis)

19. Hyperphosphatasia (scoliosis, biconcave vertebrae)

20. Hypochondroplasia (narrow spinal canal, lordosis)

21. Incontinentia pigmenti S.

22. Kniest's disease (platyspondyly, lordosis, kyphoscoliosis)

23. Larsen's S.

24. Long arm 21 deletion S.

25. Marfan's S. (scoliosis)

26. Metaphyseal chondrodysplasias (Jansen, McKusick)

27. Metaphyseal dysplasia (Pyle's disease) (platyspondyly)

28. Metatropic dwarfism (kyphoscoliosis, platyspondyly, posterior concavity)

29. Multiple epiphyseal dysplasia (Fairbank)

30. Nail-patella S. (Fong's S.) (spina bifida)

31. Oculomandibulofacial S. (Hallerman-Streiff S.) (spina bifida)

32. Oculovertebral S. (hemivertebra, block vertebrae)

33. Osteochondromuscular dystrophy (Schwartz-Jampel S.)

34. Osteodysplasia (Melnick-Needles) (increased vertebral height, anterior concavity)

35. Otopalatodigital S. (posterior spinal defects)

36. Parastremmatic dwarfism (kyphoscoliosis, platyspondyly)

37. Popliteal web S. (spina bifida)

38. Prader-Willi S. (kyphosis)

(Continued)

39. Progeria

40. Radial aplasia-thrombocytopenia S.

41. Rubinstein-Taybi S.

42. Shawl scrotum S. (hypoplasia C1, subluxation C1-C2)

43. Spondylocostal dysostosis (fused, absent, butterfly, or hemivertebrae)

44. Spondyloepiphyseal dysplasia, all forms (scoliosis, platyspondyly)

45. Spondylometaphyseal dysplasia (Kozlowski) (kyphosis)

46. Thanatophoric dwarfism (platyspondyly, narrow spinal canal)

47. Trisomy 13 S.

48. Trisomy 18 S.

References:

1. Felson B, Editor: Dwarfs and Other Little People. *Semin Roentgenol* 8:258–259, 1973.
2. Smith DW: *Recognizable Patterns of Human Malformation.* Philadelphia, WB Saunders Co, 1970.

NONSPINAL CONDITIONS ASSOCIATED WITH VERTEBRAL ANOMALIES
(See also Gamut C-1)

COMMON

1. Cloacal abnormality
2. Congenital heart disease
3. Genitourinary abnormality
4. Neurofibromatosis
5. Sprengel's deformity

UNCOMMON

1. Neurenteric cyst; duplication cyst
2. Venolobar syndrome (eg, scimitar syndrome, lobar agenesis)

CONGENITAL PLATYSPONDYLY

COMMON

1. Achondroplasia, pseudoachondroplasia
2. Mucopolysaccharidosis (eg, Hurler, Hunter, Morquio); mucolipidosis II, III, generalized gangliosidosis
3. Osteogenesis imperfecta

UNCOMMON

1. Cretinism
2. Diastrophic dwarfism
3. Geroderma osteodysplastica
4. Kniest's disease
5. Metaphyseal dysplasia (Pyle's disease)
6. Metatropic dwarfism
7. Parastremmatic dwarfism
8. Spondyloepiphyseal dysplasia, all forms
9. Thanatophoric dwarfism

BEAKED OR HOOK-SHAPED VERTEBRAE AT THORACOLUMBAR JUNCTION IN A CHILD

COMMON

1. Achondroplasia

2. Cretinism

3. Down's syndrome (mongolism)

4. Mucopolysaccharidosis (eg, Hurler, Hunter, Morquio, Maroteaux-Lamy); mucolipidosis II and III (Leroy's I-cell, pseudo-Hurler polydystrophy)

5. Normal variant

6. Trauma, acute; battered child

UNCOMMON

1. Diastrophic dwarfism

2. Neuromuscular disease with generalized hypotonia (eg, Werdnig-Hoffman disease, Niemann-Pick disease, phenyl-ketonuria, mental retardation)

Reference:

Swischuk LE: The beaked, notched, or hooked vertebra; its significance in infants and young children. *Radiology* 95:661–664, 1970.

KYPHOSIS
(See also Gamut C-6)

COMMON

1. Congenital spinal anomaly (eg, fused vertebrae, hemi-vertebra, spina bifida with meningocele)
2. Congenital syndromes (see Gamut C-1)
3. Faulty or occupational posture
4. Fracture, traumatic or pathologic; dislocation
5. Idiopathic
6. Infection (eg, spinal osteomyelitis or tuberculosis — Pott's disease)
7. Neoplasm of spine, primary or metastatic; multiple myeloma
8. Neuromuscular disorder (eg, cerebral palsy, muscular dystrophy, myasthenia gravis)
9. Osteoporosis (esp. senile or postmenopausal) (see Gamut D-22)
10. Paget's disease
11. Paralysis (eg, poliomyelitis, paraplegia)
12. Rheumatoid or ankylosing spondylitis
13. Scheuermann's disease (juvenile kyphosis)

UNCOMMON

1. Acromegaly; excessive endocrine growth
2. Charcot spine
3. Generalized weakness
4. Neurofibromatosis
5. Osteomalacia, rickets
6. Radiation therapy atrophy
7. Syringomyelia

Reference:

Schmorl G, Junghanns H: *The Human Spine in Health and Disease,* ed 2. New York, Grune and Stratton, 1971, pp 344–362.

SCOLIOSIS
(See also Gamut C-5)

COMMON

1. Congenital spinal anomaly (eg, fusion of posterior elements, segmentation, hemivertebra)

2. Congenital syndromes (See also Gamut C-1)

3. Fracture

4. Idiopathic

5. Infection (eg, spinal tuberculosis, osteomyelitis)

6. Leg shortening or amputation; foot deformity

7. Neoplasm, primary or metastatic; multiple myeloma

8. Neuromuscular disorder (eg, cerebral palsy, muscular dystrophy, Friedreich's ataxia)

9. Osteoporosis (see Gamut D-22)

10. Paralysis (eg, poliomyelitis, paraplegia)

11. Spasm (eg, retroperitoneal, psoas or abdominal abscess, inflammation, or hemorrhage; ureteral or renal calculus)

UNCOMMON

1. Chest wall abnormality (eg, congenital rib anomalies)

2. Congenital heart disease (eg, ASD, tetralogy)

3. Intraspinal or extraspinal tumor

4. Neurofibromatosis

5. Osteoid osteoma

6. Postoperative (eg, thoracoplasty)

7. Pulmonary or pleural disease, chronic unilateral (eg, fibrosis, fibrothorax, empyema)

8. Radiation therapy atrophy

9. Rickets

(Continued)

10. Syringomyelia

Reference:

Schmorl G, Junghanns H: *The Human Spine in Health and Disease*, ed 2. New York, Grune and Stratton, 1971, pp 364–374.

ATLANTO-AXIAL SUBLUXATION

COMMON

1. Rheumatoid arthritis; ankylosing spondylitis
2. Trauma (fracture or torn ligaments)

UNCOMMON

1. Absent anterior arch of atlas
2. Absent or separate odontoid process
3. Atlanto-occipital fusion
4. Down's syndrome (mongolism)
5. Lupus erythematosus
6. Morquio's syndrome
7. Psoriatic arthritis
8. Retropharyngeal abscess (child)

Reference:

Wortzman G, Dewar FP: Rotary fixation of the atlantoaxial joint: rotational atlantoaxial subluxation. *Radiology* 90:479–487, 1968.

INCREASE IN SIZE OF ONE OR MORE VERTEBRAE

COMMON

1. Acromegaly
2. Paget's disease

UNCOMMON

1. Benign bone tumor (eg, giant cell tumor, hemangioma, aneurysmal bone cyst)
2. Compensatory enlargement from non-weightbearing (eg, paralysis)
3. Congenital
4. Fibrous dysplasia
5. Hyperphosphatasia

Reference:

Greenfield GB: *Radiology of Bone Diseases.* Philadelphia, JB Lippincott Co, 1969, p 224.

"SQUARING" OF ONE OR MORE VERTEBRAL BODIES

COMMON

1. Ankylosing spondylitis
2. Paget's disease

UNCOMMON

1. Normal variant
2. Psoriatic arthritis
3. Reiter's syndrome
4. Rheumatoid arthritis

Reference:

Jacobson HG: Personal communication.

DENSE SCLEROTIC VERTEBRA, SOLITARY OR MULTIPLE

COMMON

1. Fracture (compression or healing)
2. Idiopathic
*3. Lymphoma
*4. Myelosclerosis (myeloid metaplasia)
*5. Osteoblastic metastasis
6. Osteomyelitis, chronic sclerosing (eg, tuberculosis, syphilis, brucella, typhoid)
*7. Paget's disease
8. Renal osteodystrophy

UNCOMMON

1. Endosteoma
*2. Fluorosis
3. Hemangioma
4. Idiopathic hypercalcemia
5. Mastocytosis
6. Osteoblastoma
*7. Osteopetrosis
8. Osteosarcoma; chrondrosarcoma; Ewing's sarcoma
9. Radiation therapy, radium poisoning
10. Sarcoidosis
11. Sickle cell anemia
12. Tuberous sclerosis

*Can cause ''ivory'' vertebra(e)

Reference:

Jacobson HG, Siegelman SS: Some miscellaneous solitary bone lesions. *Semin Roentgenol* 1:314–335, 1966.

EXAGGERATED CONCAVITY (SCALLOPING) OF POSTERIOR SURFACE OF ONE OR MORE VERTEBRAL BODIES

COMMON

1. Achondroplasia
2. Increased intraspinal pressure
3. Neurofibromatosis with or without neurofibroma ("dural ectasia"); congenital expansion of the subarachnoid space ("intraspinal meningocele")
4. Normal variant (physiologic scalloping)
5. Tumor of spinal canal (eg, ependymoma, dermoid, lipoma, neurofibroma, meningioma)

UNCOMMON

1. Acromegaly
2. Cyst of spinal canal
3. Hydatid disease
4. Other congenital syndromes
   a. Ehlers-Danlos S.
   b. Marfan's S.
   c. Metatropic dwarfism
   d. Mucopolysaccharidosis (eg, Hurler, Morquio)
   e. Osteogenesis imperfecta tarda
5. Severe communicating hydrocephalus
6. Syringomyelia, hydromyelia

(Continued)

References:

1. Greenfield GB: *Radiology of Bone Diseases.* Philadelphia, JB Lippincott Co, 1969, p 224.
2. Heard G, Payne EE: Scalloping of the vertebral bodies in von Recklinghausen's disease of the nervous system (neurofibromatosis). *J Neurol Neurosurg Psychiat* 25:345–351, 1962.
3. Howieson J, Norrell HA, Wilson CB: Expansion of the subarachnoid space in the lumbosacral region. *Radiology* 90:488–492, 1968.
4. Leeds NE, Jacobson HG: Plain film examination of the spinal canal. *Semin Roentgenol* 7:179–196, 1972.
5. Mitchell GE, Lourie H, Berne AS: The various causes of scalloped vertebrae with notes on their pathogenesis. *Radiology* 89:67–74, 1967.
6. Salerno NR, Edeiken J: Vertebral scalloping in neurofibromatosis. *Radiology* 97:509–510, 1970.

ANTERIOR GOUGE DEFECT (SCALLOPING) OF ONE OR MORE VERTEBRAL BODIES

1. Aneurysm of aorta
2. Lymphadenopathy from metastases or inflammation
3. Lymphoma, chronic leukemia
4. Tuberculosis

ENLARGED CERVICAL INTERVERTEBRAL FORAMEN

COMMON

1. Neurofibroma

UNCOMMON

1. Congenital absence of pedicle
2. Dermoid
3. Hydatid disease
4. Lateral meningocele
5. Lipoma
6. Lymphoma
7. Meningioma
8. Neuroblastoma
9. Traumatic avulsion of nerve root with "diverticulum"
10. Vertebral artery aneurysm or tortuosity

Reference:

Anderson RE, Shealy CN: Cervical pedicle erosion and rootlet compression caused by a tortuous vertebral artery. *Radiology* 96:537–538, 1970.

VERTEBRAL PEDICLE EROSION OR DESTRUCTION

COMMON

1. Intraspinal neoplasm or cyst (esp. neurofibroma, meningioma)
2. Metastasis
3. Tuberculosis, fungus, or other granulomatous disease

UNCOMMON

1. Benign bone tumor (eg, aneurysmal bone cyst, giant cell tumor, hemangiopericytoma)
2. [Congenital absence]
3. Histiocytosis X
4. Multiple myeloma
5. Syringomyelia
6. Vertebral artery aneurysm or tortuosity (cervical spine)

CYST-LIKE EXPANSILE LESION OF THE BODY AND/OR APPENDAGES OF A VERTEBRA

COMMON

1. Aneurysmal bone cyst
2. Hemangioma, hemangiopericytoma
3. Osteoblastoma

UNCOMMON

1. Chondroid lesion
2. Fibrous dysplasia
3. Giant cell tumor
4. Hyatid cyst
5. Metastasis
6. Myeloma
7. Nonossifying fibroma

SPINAL OSTEOPENIA (LOSS OF DENSITY)

COMMON

1. Anemia (esp. sickle cell anemia, thalassemia)
2. Carcinomatosis
3. Hyperparathyroidism (primary or secondary)
4. Multiple myeloma
5. Osteomalacia (see Gamut D-24)
6. Osteoporosis (esp. senile or postmenopausal) (see Gamut D-22)
7. Steroid therapy; Cushing's disease

UNCOMMON

1. Acromegaly
2. Amyloidosis
3. Fibrogenesis imperfecta ossium
4. Gaucher's disease; Niemann-Pick disease
5. Hyperthyroidism
6. Hypogonadism (eg, Fröhlich's)
7. Lymphoma, leukemia
8. Osteogenesis imperfecta

Reference:

Greenfield GB: *Radiology of Bone Diseases.* Philadelphia, JB Lippincott Co, 1969, p 11.

SOLITARY COLLAPSED VERTEBRA
(See also Gamut C-18)

COMMON

1. Eosinophilic granuloma (histiocytosis X)
2. Fracture, traumatic or pathologic
3. Hemangioma
4. Hyperparathyroidism, brown tumor
5. Lymphoma
6. Metastasis
7. Myeloma, plasmacytoma
8. Osteomyelitis (eg, tuberculous, fungal, brucellar, typhoid)
9. Osteoporosis (eg, senile, postmenopausal) (see Gamut D-22)
10. Paget's disease
11. Steroid therapy; Cushing's disease

UNCOMMON

1. Amyloidosis
2. Benign tumor (eg, giant cell tumor, aneurysmal bone cyst)
3. Chordoma
4. Hydatid cyst
5. Sarcoidosis
6. Sarcoma (eg, Ewing's, osteosarcoma, chondrosarcoma)
7. Scheuermann's disease
8. Traumatic ischemic necrosis (eg, Kümmell's disease)

MULTIPLE COLLAPSED VERTEBRAE
(See also Gamut C-3)

COMMON

1. Fractures, traumatic or pathologic
2. Hyperparathyroidism
3. Metastases
4. Multiple myeloma
5. Osteomyelitis (eg, tuberculous, fungal, brucellar)
6. Osteoporosis (eg, senile, postmenopausal, idiopathic juvenile; hypogonadism) (see Gamut D-22)
7. Scheuermann's disease
8. Steroid therapy; Cushing's disease

UNCOMMON

1. Amyloidosis
2. Congenital fibromatosis
3. Convulsions (eg, tetanus, tetany, hypoglycemia, shock therapy)
4. Hemangiomatosis (vanishing bone disease)
5. Histiocytosis X
6. Hydatid disease
7. Leukemia, lymphoma
8. Malignant histiocytosis
9. Osteogenesis imperfecta
10. Osteomalacia (see Gamut D-24)
11. Paget's disease

(Continued)

12. [Platyspondyly, esp. dwarf syndromes (eg, Morquio, pseudoachondroplasia, thanatophoric dwarfism) (see Gamut C-3)]

13. Rheumatoid arthritis

14. Sickle cell anemia

SACROILIAC JOINT DISEASE

COMMON

1. Ankylosing spondylitis
2. Infectious arthritis or osteomyelitis (eg, tuberculous, pyogenic)
3. [Osteitis condensans ilii]
4. Osteoarthritis (degenerative joint disease)
5. Rheumatoid arthritis

UNCOMMON

1. [Bone neoplasm, primary (eg, sarcoma) or metastatic]
2. Gout
3. Hyperparathyroidism
4. Leukemia
5. Occupational acro-osteolysis (eg, polyvinylchloride osteolysis)
6. Paraplegia
7. Post-traumatic arthritis
8. Pseudohypoparathyroidism
9. Psoriatic arthritis
10. Regional enteritis
11. Reiter's syndrome
12. Ulcerative colitis arthritis
13. Whipple's disease

Reference:
Cavanagh RC: Personal communication.

PARASPINAL SOFT TISSUE MASS
(See also Gamut F-51)

COMMON

1. Aortic aneurysm; tortuous aorta
2. Hematoma, traumatic or spontaneous
3. Lymphoma
4. Metastatic neoplasm
5. Myeloma
6. Neurogenic tumor (neurofibroma, neurilemmoma, ganglio-neuroma, neuroblastoma)
7. Osteoarthritis (spondylosis deformans)
8. Osteomyelitis of spine with abscess (eg, tuberculous, sarcoid, fungal, brucellar, other bacterial)
9. [Pleural effusion]

UNCOMMON

1. Bronchogenic cyst
2. Chemodectoma
3. Dilated azygos system (eg, superior or inferior vena cava obstruction); mediastinal varices
4. Eosinophilic granuloma of vertebra
5. Extramedullary hematopoiesis (esp. in thalassemia)
6. Intraspinal tumor of hourglass type
7. [Mesothelioma]
8. Neurenteric cyst
9. Paget's disease (uncalcified osteoid)
10. Spine neoplasm, primary (eg, giant cell tumor, chordoma, sarcoma)

Reference:

Greenfield GB: *Radiology of Bone Diseases.* Philadelphia, JB Lippincott Co, 1969, p 435.

SACROCOCCYGEAL OR PRESACRAL MASS

COMMON

1. Abscess (eg, rectal perforation; sinus tract from Crohn's disease, ulcerative colitis, amebiasis, schistosomiasis, tuberculosis, or lymphogranuloma venereum)
2. Bone neoplasm, benign or malignant (see Gamuts D-48, 49, 52)
3. Carcinoma of prostate
4. Chordoma
5. Dermoid cyst; teratoma

UNCOMMON

1. Arachnoid, extradural, or perineural cyst
2. [Ectopic kidney]
3. Hamartoma
4. Hematoma
5. Hydatid cyst
6. Lymphoma
7. Meningocele, anterior sacral
8. Mesenchymal tumor (eg, fibroma, leiomyoma, lipoma, and their sarcomatous counterparts)
9. Metastasis
10. Neurenteric cyst
11. Neurogenic tumor
12. Osteomyelitis of sacrum
13. Other intraspinal tumor (eg, ependymoma, lipoma)
14. Ovarian tumor, tubovarian abscess

(Continued)

References:
1. Caffey JR: *Pediatric X-ray Diagnosis*, ed 6.   Chicago, Year Book Medical Publishers, 1972.
2. Epstein BS: *The Spine,* ed 3. Philadelphia, Lea & Febiger, 1969.
3. Lombardi G, Passerini A: *Spinal Cord Diseases: A Radiologic and Myelographic Analysis.* Baltimore. Williams & Wilkins, 1964.
4. Werner JL, Taybi H: Presacral masses in childhood. *Am J Roentgenol* 109:403–410, 1970.

CALCIFICATION OF ONE OR MORE INTERVERTEBRAL DISCS

COMMON

1. Degenerative
2. Idiopathic (eg, transient calcification in children; persistent type in adults)
3. Post-traumatic

UNCOMMON

1. Ankylosing spondylitis
2. Gout
3. Hemochromatosis
4. Hyperparathyroidism
5. Hypervitaminosis D
6. Ochronosis
7. Pseudogout

References:

1. Edeiken J, Hodes PJ: *Roentgen Diagnosis of Diseases of Bone*, ed 2. Baltimore, Williams & Wilkins Co, 1973.
2. Greenfield GB: *Radiology of Bone Diseases.* Philadelphia, JB Lippincott Co, 1969, p 420.
3. Mainzer F: Herniation of the nucleus pulposus. A rare complication of intervertebral-disk calcification in children. *Radiology* 107:167–170, 1973.
4. Murray RO, Jacobson HG: *The Radiology of Skeletal Disorders.* Baltimore, Williams & Wilkins Co, 1971.

WIDENING OF SPINAL CORD ON MYELOGRAPHY
(See also Gamut C-24)

COMMON

1. [Extrinsic compression (eg, by cervical ridge, herniated disc, large extramedullary or extradural tumor)]
2. Intramedullary tumor (eg, glioma, lipoma, epidermoid, metastasis, melanoma)
3. Syringomyelia, hydromyelia

UNCOMMON

1. Arteriovenous malformation, angioma
2. Diastematomyelia
3. Hematoma, contusion of cord
4. Sarcoidosis

Reference:

Epstein BS: Spinal canal mass lesions. *Radiol Clin North Am* 4:185–202, 1966.

INTRAMEDULLARY LESION ON MYELOGRAPHY
(See also Gamut C-23)

COMMON

1. Glioma (esp. ependymoma)
2. Syringomyelia, hydromyelia

UNCOMMON

1. Dermoid, epidermoid
2. Hematoma, contused cord
3. Lipoma
4. Melanoma
5. Metastasis
6. Sarcoidosis, tuberculoma
7. Vascular malformation, angioma

Reference:

Epstein B S: Spinal canal mass lesions. *Radiol Clin North Am* 4: 185–202, 1966.

INTRADURAL EXTRAMEDULLARY LESION ON MYELOGRAPHY

COMMON

1. Arachnoiditis
2. Meningioma
3. Metastasis ("seeding")
4. Neurofibroma

UNCOMMON

1. Arachnoid cyst
2. Dermoid, epidermoid
3. Ependymoma in lumbar area
4. Infection (eg, tuberculoma, cysticercosis)
5. Lipoma
6. [Tortuosity of nerve roots]
7. Vascular malformation, angioma

EXTRADURAL LESION ON MYELOGRAPHY

COMMON

1. Epidural scar (eg, after disc surgery)
2. Fracture fragment from vertebral trauma
3. Hematoma, traumatic or spontaneous
4. Herniated disc
5. [Iatrogenic (needle point defect, extradural injection of pantopaque)]
6. Ligamentum flavum thickening
7. Lymphoma
8. Meningioma
9. Metastatic neoplasm (esp. carcinoma of lung, breast, GI tract)
10. Neurogenic tumor (eg, neurofibroma)
11. Spondylosis
12. Tuberculous, pyogenic, or parasitic infection (eg, hydatid disease, schistosomiasis)
13. Vertebral neoplasm with intraspinal extension (eg, sarcoma, myeloma, chordoma, hemangioma)

UNCOMMON

1. Abscess, epidural
2. Amyloidosis
3. Arachnoid cyst
4. Extramedullary hematopoiesis
5. Lipoma
6. Paget's disease (uncalcified osteoid)
7. Retroperitoneal neoplasm extending through vertebral foramen (eg, neuroblastoma, lymphoma)

References:

1. Epstein BS: Spinal canal mass lesions. *Rad Cl North Am* 4:185–202, 1966.
2. Taveras JM, Wood EH: *Diagnostic Neuroradiology.* Baltimore, Williams & Wilkins Co, 1964.

NOTES

NOTES

TABLE OF CONTENTS

D. BONE, JOINTS, AND SOFT TISSUES

I. BONE — GENERALIZED OR UNSPECIFIED GROWTH OR MODELING DISORDERS

EPIPHYSEAL OR METAPHYSEAL DISORDERS

(Continued)

D

(Continued)

D

TUMORS

(Continued)

D

PERIOSTEAL OR CORTICAL DISORDERS

D

MISCELLANEOUS

(Continued)

II. BONE — ANATOMICAL

HANDS AND FEET

GAMUT

D-74	Congenital Abnormalities of the Thumbs
D-75	Clinodactyly of the Fifth Finger
D-76	Congenital Syndromes With Short Phalanges (Other Than Fifth Finger)
D-77	Congenital Syndromes With Short Middle Phalanx of Fifth Finger
D-78	Spontaneous Amputation of Fingers or Phalanges in Children
D-79	Clubbing of the Fingers
D-80	Congenital Syndromes With Accessory Carpal Ossicles
D-81	Carpal Fusion
D-82	Syndactyly (Cutaneous or Osseous)
D-83	Polydactyly
D-84	Brachydactyly (See also Gamuts D-76, D-85 and D-86)
D-85	Short Metacarpals or Metatarsals (Excluding Generalized Shortening)
D-86	Congenital Syndromes With Short Hands and Feet (See also Subgamut D-86A)
D-86A	Acquired Diseases Causing Short Hands and Feet
D-87	Abnormal Tapering of Short Tubular Bones of the Hands and Feet
D-88	Neurotrophic Bone Changes (Pointed or Spindled Bones) in the Hands or Feet
D-89	Erosion of Multiple Terminal Phalangeal Tufts (Acro-osteolysis)
D-89A	Acro-osteolysis Confined to One Digit
D-90	Congenital Syndromes Associated With an Abnormal Carpal Angle
D-91	Cyst-like Lesion in a Phalanx (Solitary or Multiple)
D-92	Dactylitis
D-93	Congenital Abnormality of the Great Toe
D-94	Congenital Syndromes Associated With Clubfoot or Other Foot Deformity

D

(Continued)

SHOULDER GIRDLE AND UPPER EXTREMITIES

GAMUT D-95   Hypoplasia of the Radius

D-96   Congenital Syndromes with Elbow Anomaly (See also Gamut D-95)

D-97   Grooved Defect of the Humeral Head

D-98   Lesion of the Scapula in a Child

D-98A   Hypoplasia of the Scapula

D-99   Lesion of the Clavicle in a Child

D-99A   Hypoplasia of the Clavicle

D-100   Erosion, Destruction, or Defect of the Outer End of the Clavicle

PELVIS AND LOWER EXTREMITIES

D-101   Congenital Syndromes With Patellar Dysplasia

D-102   Solitary Circumscribed Lytic Patellar Lesion

D-103   Genu Varum (Bow Legs)

D-104   Genu Valgum (Knock-knee)

D-105   Coxa Vara (Unilateral or Bilateral)

D-106   Coxa Valga

D-107   Fragmented or Irregular Femoral Head

D-108   Slipped Capital Femoral Epiphyses

D-109   Congenital Syndromes With an Abnormal Pelvis (See also Gamut D-110)

D-110   Congenital Syndromes With Decreased Acetabular Angle

D-111   Protrusio Acetabuli (Otto Pelvis), Unilateral or Bilateral

D-112   Bridging of the Pubic Symphysis

D-113   Widening of the Pubic Symphysis

(Continued)

D

RIBS

III. JOINTS

D

(Continued)

IV. SOFT TISSUES

D

Nomenclature for the Constitutional (Intrinsic) Diseases of Bones*

Constitutional Diseases of Bones with Unknown Pathogenesis

Osteochondrodysplasia (Abnormalities of Cartilage and/or Bone Growth and Development)

(1) *Defects of growth of tubular bones and/or spine*

A. *Manifested at birth*

1. Achondrogenesis
2. Thanatophoric dwarfism
3. Achondroplasia
4. Chondrodysplasia punctata (formerly stippled epiphyses) (several forms)
5. Metatropic dwarfism
6. Diastrophic dwarfism
7. Chondroectodermal dysplasia (Ellis-Van Creveld)
8. Asphyxiating thoracic dysplasia (Jeune)
9. Spondyloepiphyseal dysplasia congenita
10. Mesomelic dwarfism: type Nievergelt; type Langer
11. Cleidocranial dysplasia (formerly cleidocranial dysostosis)

B. *Manifested in later life*

1. Hypochondroplasia
2. Dyschondrosteosis
3. Metaphyseal chondrodysplasia type Jansen
4. Metaphyseal chondrodysplasia type Schmid
5. Metaphyseal chondrodysplasia type McKusick (formerly cartilage-hair hypoplasia)
6. Metaphyseal chondrodysplasia with malabsorption and neutropenia
7. Metaphyseal chondrodysplasia with thymolymphopenia
8. Spondylometaphyseal dysplasia (Kozlowski)

9. Multiple epiphyseal dysplasia (several forms)
10. Hereditary arthro-ophthalmopathy
11. Pseudoachondroplastic dysplasia (formerly spondyloepiphyseal pseudoachondroplastic dysplasia)
12. Spondyloepiphyseal dysplasia tarda
13. Acrodysplasia
Rhinotrichophalangeal syndrome (Giedion)
Epiphyseal (Thiemann)
Epiphysometaphyseal (Brailsford)

(2) *Disorganized development of cartilage and fibrous components of the skeleton*

1. Dysplasia epiphysealis hemimelica
2. Multiple cartilaginous exostoses
3. Enchondromatosis (Ollier's disease)
4. Enchondromatosis with hemangioma (Maffucci's syndrome)
5. Fibrous dysplasia (Jaffe-Lichtenstein)
6. Fibrous dysplasia with skin pigmentation and precocious puberty (McCune-Albright)
7. Cherubism
8. Multiple fibromatosis

(3) *Abnormalities of density, of cortical diaphyseal structure, and/or of metaphyseal modeling*

1. Osteogenesis imperfecta congenita (Vrolik, Porak-Durante)
2. Osteogenesis imperfecta tarda (Lobstein)
3. Juvenile idiopathic osteoporosis
4. Osteopetrosis with precocious manifestations
5. Osteopetrosis with delayed manifestations
6. Pyknodysostosis
7. Osteopoikilosis
8. Melorheostosis

*Established by the Society for Pediatric Radiology. Radiology 99:699, 1971.

9. Diaphyseal dysplasia
   (Camurati-Engelmann)
10. Craniodiaphyseal dysplasia
11. Endosteal hyperostosis
    (Van Buchem and other forms)
12. Tubular stenosis (Kenny-Caffey)
13. Osteodysplasia (Melnick-Needles)
14. Pachydermoperiostosis
15. Osteoectasia with hyperphosphatasia
16. Metaphyseal dysplasia (Pyle's disease)
17. Craniometaphyseal dysplasia
    (several forms)
18. Frontometaphyseal dysplasia
19. Oculo-dental-osseous dysplasia
    (formerly oculo-dento-digital
    syndrome)

Dysostosis (Malformation of Individual Bones, Single or in Combination)

(1) *Dysostosis with cranial and facial involvement*

1. Craniosynostosis, several forms
2. Craniofacial dysostosis (Crouzon)
3. Acrocephalosyndactylia (Apert)
4. Acrocephalopolysyndactylia
   (Carpenter)
5. Mandibulofacial dysostosis (Treacher-Collins, Franceschetti, and others)
6. Mandibular hypoplasia (includes Pierre Robin syndrome)
7. Oculomandibulofacial syndrome
   (Hallermann-Streiff-François)
8. Nevoid basal-cell carcinoma syndrome

(2) *Dysostosis with predominant axial involvement*

1. Vertebral segmentation defects
   (including Klippel-Feil)
2. Cervico-oculo-acoustic syndrome
   (Wildervanck)
3. Sprengel's deformity
4. Spondylocostal dysostosis (several forms)
5. Oculovertebral syndrome (Weyers)
6. Osteo-onychodysostosis
   (formerly nail-patella-syndrome)

(3) *Dysostosis with predominant involvement of extremities*

1. Amelia
2. Hemimelia (several types)
3. Acheiria
4. Apodia
5. Adactylia and oligodactylia
6. Phocomelia
7. Aglossia-adactylia syndrome
8. Congenital bowing of long bones
   (several types)
9. Familial radioulnar synostosis
10. Brachydactylia (several types)
11. Symphalangism
12. Polydactylia (several types)
13. Syndactylia (several types)
14. Polysyndactylia (several types)
15. Camptodactylia
16. Clinodactylia
17. Laurence-Moon syndrome
18. Popliteal pterygium syndrome
19. Pectoral aplasia—dysdactylia
    syndrome (Poland)
20. Rubinstein-Taybi syndrome
21. Pancytopenia—dysmelia syndrome
    (Fanconi)
22. Thrombocytopenia—radial aplasia
    syndrome
23. Orodigitofacial syndrome
    (Papillon-Leage)
24. Cardiomelic syndrome (Holt - Oram, and others)

Idiopathic Osteolysis

Acro-osteolysis:
   Phalangeal type
   Tarso-carpal form with or without
   nephropathy
Multicentric osteolysis

Primary Disturbances of Growth

1. Primordial dwarfism (without associated malformation)
2. Cornelia de Lange's syndrome
3. Bird-headed dwarfism (Virchow, Seckel)
4. Leprechaunism
5. Russell-Silver syndrome
6. Progeria
7. Cockayne's syndrome

8. Bloom's syndrome
9. Geroderma osteodysplastica
10. Spherophakia—brachymorphia syndrome (Weill-Marchesani)
11. Marfan's syndrome

Constitutional Diseases of Bones With Known Pathogenesis

Chromosomal Aberrations
Primary, Metabolic Abnormalities

(1) *Calcium-phosphorus metabolism*

1. Hypophosphatemic familial rickets
2. Pseudodeficiency rickets (type Royer, Prader)
3. Late rickets (type McCance)
4. Idiopathic hypercalciuria
5. Hypophosphatasia (several forms)
6. Idiopathic hypercalcemia
7. Pseudohypoparathyroidism (normo- and hypercalcemic forms)

(2) *Mucopolysaccharidosis*

1. Mucopolysaccharidosis I (Hurler)
2. Mucopolysaccharidosis II (Hunter)
3. Mucopolysaccharidosis III (Sanfilippo)
4. Mucopolysaccharidosis IV (Morquio)
5. Mucopolysaccharidosis V (Ullrich-Scheie)
6. Mucopolysaccharidosis VI (Maroteaux-Lamy)

(3) *Mucolipidosis and lipidosis*

1. Mucolipidosis I (Spranger-Wiedemann)
2. Mucolipidosis II (Leroy)
3. Mucolipidosis III (pseudopolydystrophy)
4. Fucosidosis
5. Mannosidosis
6. Generalized GM$_1$ gangliosidosis (several forms)
7. Sulfatidosis with mucopolysacchariduria (Austin, Thieffry)
8. Cerebrosidosis including Gaucher's disease

(4) *Other metabolic extraosseous disorders*

Bone Abnormalities Secondary to Disturbances of Extraskeletal Systems

1. Endocrine
2. Hematologic
3. Neurologic
4. Renal
5. Gastrointestinal
6. Cardiopulmonary

CONGENITAL SYNDROMES WITH SHORT LIMBS

COMMON

1. Achondroplasia
2. Chondrodysplasia punctata (Conradi's disease)
3. Enchondromatosis (Ollier's disease)
4. Mucopolysaccharidosis (eg, Hurler); mucolipidosis
5. Osteogenesis imperfecta congenita

UNCOMMON

1. Achondrogenesis
2. Asphyxiating thoracic dysplasia
3. Bloom's S.
4. Campomelic dwarfism
5. Chondroectodermal dysplasia (Ellis-Van Creveld S.)
6. Cornelia de Lange S.
7. Diastrophic dwarfism
8. Dyschondrosteosis
9. Hypochondroplasia
10. Hypophosphatasia
11. Kniest's disease
12. Mesomelic dwarfism
13. Metaphyseal chondrodysplasias (Jansen, McKusick)
14. Metatropic dwarfism
15. Mietens-Weber S.
16. Multiple epiphyseal dysplasia (Fairbank)
17. Phocomelia, including maternal thalidamide ingestion or diabetes

(Continued)

18. Spondyloepiphyseal dysplasias
19. Stanesco's dysplasia
20. Thanatophoric dwarfism
21. Weill-Marchesani S.

Reference:

   Felson B, Editor: Dwarfs and Other Little People. *Semin Roentgenol* 8:255, 1973.

EPIPHYSEAL OR METAPHYSEAL INSULT RESULTING IN A SHORTENED BONE (LOCALIZED RETARDED SKELETAL MATURATION)

COMMON

1. Osteomyelitis (eg, bacterial, yaws, smallpox)
2. Trauma

UNCOMMON

1. Enchondromatosis (Ollier's disease)
2. Hypervitaminosis A
3. Infarction (eg, sickle cell anemia)
4. Neoplasm
5. Radiation injury
6. Rickets
7. Scurvy
8. Thermal injury

Reference:

Greenfield GB: *Radiology of Bone Diseases*. Philadelphia, JB Lippin-cott Co, 1969, pp 99 and 223.

DISCREPANCY IN LENGTH OF A LONG BONE COMPARED TO ITS CONTRALATERAL COUNTERPART
(See also Gamuts D-3, D-5, and D-6)

COMMON

1. Hyperemia (secondary to chronic infection, rheumatoid arthritis, hemophilia, etc.)
2. Neurologic disorder (eg, poliomyelitis, Erb's palsy)
3. Osteomyelitis (eg, bacterial, yaws, smallpox)
4. Trauma (eg, burn, epiphyseal injury, impacted or distracted fracture, surgical procedure)

UNCOMMON

1. Arteriovenous fistula, hemangioma (Klippel-Trenaunay-Weber S.)
1. Arteriovenous fistula, hemangioma, lipoma (Klippel-Trenaunay-Weber S.)
2. Congenital hemihypertrophy
3. Fibrous dysplasia
4. Macrodystrophia lipomatosa
5. Neurofibromatosis
6. Osteochondrodysplasias
   a. Chondrodysplasia punctata (Conradi's disease)
   b. Dysplasia epiphysealis hemimelica (Trevor's disease)
   c. Enchondromatosis (Ollier's disease)
7. Osteogenesis imperfecta
8. Phocomelia (eg, thalidomide poisoning); other congenital limb hypoplasia
9. Radiation therapy
10. Scurvy (following epiphyseal trauma)

CONDITIONS ASSOCIATED WITH
HEMIHYPERTROPHY

COMMON

1. Tumor (gonadal, Wilms', adrenocortical carcinoma, hepatoblastoma, neuroblastoma)

UNCOMMON

1. Endocrine disorders (eg, adrenogenital syndrome)
2. Hemangioma
3. Hypospadias; cryptorchidism
4. Lymphangiectasia (intestinal, pulmonary, extremity)
5. Medullary sponge kidney
6. Neurocutaneous syndromes (esp. von Hippel-Lindau disease)
7. Renal hypertrophy, unilateral or bilateral
8. Russell-Silver syndrome
9. Wiedemann-Beckwith fetal visceromegaly syndrome

LOCALIZED ELONGATION OR OVERGROWTH OF BONE

COMMON

1. Arteriovenous fistula
2. Chronic arthritis (eg, tuberculous, juvenile rheumatoid)
3. Hemangioma, lymphangioma
4. Hyperemia, any cause
5. Neurofibromatosis

UNCOMMON

1. Chronic osteomyelitis (eg, tuberculous, tropical ulcer)
2. Dysplasia epiphysialis hemimelica (Trevor's disease)
3. Healing fracture
4. Hemihypertrophy (see Gamut D-5)
5. Hemophilic hemarthrosis
6. Idiopathic
7. Macrodystrophia lipomatosa; congenital macrodactyly

Reference:

Greenfield GB: *Radiology of Bone Diseases.* Philadelphia, JB Lippincott Co, 1969, pp 99 and 223.

GENERALIZED OR WIDESPREAD ELONGATION OF BONE

1. Cerebral gigantism (hypothalamic)
2. Hemihypertrophy
3. Homocystinuria
4. Hyperpituitarism
5. Klinefelter's S.
6. Marfan's S.
7. Total lipodystrophy

Reference:

Greenfield GB: *Radiology of Bone Diseases.*   Philadelphia, JB Lippincott Co, 1969, p 223.

GENERALIZED RETARDED SKELETAL MATURATION (DECREASED BONE AGE)

COMMON

1. Congenital heart disease (esp. cyanotic)
2. Congenital syndromes of dwarfism or mental retardation (see Subgamut D-8A)
3. Constitutional delay of growth and adolescence
4. Diabetes mellitus, juvenile
5. Hypogonadism (eg, Turner's syndrome)
6. Hypopituitarism with growth hormone deficiency (idiopathic or secondary to craniopharyngioma or other neoplasm)
7. Hypothyroidism, congenital or acquired
8. Malnutrition
9. Nephrosis or other renal disease
10. Severe constitutional disease (eg, celiac disease, ulcerative colitis)

UNCOMMON

1. Addison's disease
2. Anemia, chronic (eg, sickle cell anemia, thalassemia)
3. Cerebral hypoplasia
4. Congenital hyperuricosuria
5. Idiopathic
6. Intrauterine growth retardation
7. Phenylketonuria
8. Rickets, all types
9. Steroid therapy; Cushing's syndrome

(Continued)

GENERALIZED RETARDED SKELETAL MATURATION (DECREASED BONE AGE) (Continued)

References:

1. Dorst J: Personal communication.

2. Greenfield GB: *Radiology of Bone Diseases.* Philadelphia, JB Lippincott Co, 1969, p 99.

3. Teplick JG, Haskin ME: *Roentgenologic Diagnosis,* ed 2. Philadelphia, WB Saunders Co, 1971, vol 2, p xxxv.

SUBGAMUT D-8A
CONGENITAL SYNDROMES WITH RETARDED
SKELETAL MATURATION

1. Aarskog-Scott S. (shawl-scrotum S.)
2. Celiac disease (gluten-induced enteropathy)
3. Fanconi's S. (pancytopenia-dysmelia S.)
4. Geroderma osteodysplastica
5. Hypothyroidism (cretinism)
6. Metaphyseal chondrodysplasia (McKusick)
7. Mietens-Weber S.
8. Mucopolysaccharidosis; mucolipidosis
9. Oculocerebral-renal S. (Lowe)
10. Osteochondromuscular dystrophy (Schwartz-Jampel)
11. Osteodysplasia (Melnick-Needles)
12. Primordial dwarfism
13. Rhinotrichophalangeal S.
14. Rubinstein-Taybi S.
15. Russell-Silver S.
16. Spondylometaphyseal dysplasia (Kozlowski)

Reference:

Felson B, Editor: Dwarfs and Other Little People. *Semin Roentgenol* 8:255, 1973.

GENERALIZED ACCELERATED SKELETAL MATURATION (INCREASED BONE AGE)

COMMON

1. Adrenogenital syndrome (adrenocortical tumor or hyperplasia)
2. Constitutional (congenital tall stature)
3. Excessive androgen or estrogen administration or production (virilizing adrenal tumor or hyperplasia, androgen- or estrogen-secreting gonadal tumor, hypergonadism)
4. Pituitary or cerebral gigantism
5. Polyostotic fibrous dysplasia (esp. Albright's S.)

UNCOMMON

1. Chondroectodermal dysplasia (Ellis-Van Creveld S.)
2. Congenital brain defect
3. Ectopic gonadotropin production (hepatoma, choriocarcinoma, teratoma)
4. Encephalitis
5. Exogenous obesity with overgrowth and tall stature
6. Homocystinuria
7. Hydrocephalus
8. Hyperthyroidism (maternal or acquired)
9. Hypothalamic or parahypothalamic neoplasm or inflammation with sexual precocity (eg, craniopharyngioma, tuberculosis)
10. Idiopathic isosexual precocious puberty
11. Neurofibromatosis
12. Pinealoma, primary or ectopic
13. Primary hyperaldosteronism

(Continued)

14. Total lipodystrophy
15. Tuberous sclerosis

References:

1. Dorst J, Thompson R, Penny R, Kuhn J: Personal communication.

2. Wesenberg RL, Gwinn JL, Barnes GR Jr: The roentgenographic findings in total lipodystrophy. *Am J Roentgenol* 103:154–164, 1968.

UNDERCONSTRICTION OR UNDERTUBULATION
(WIDE DIAMETAPHYSIS)

COMMON

1. Anemia (eg, thalassemia, sickle cell anemia)
2. Fibrous dysplasia
3. Gaucher's disease; Niemann-Pick disease
4. Healing fracture; metaphyseal injury

UNCOMMON

1. Biliary atresia; biliary cirrhosis
2. Cleidocranial dysplasia
3. Enchondromatosis (Ollier's disease)
4. Engelmann's disease
5. Healing rickets or scurvy
6. Hypervitaminosis D
7. Hypophosphatasia (adult)
8. Infantile cortical hyperostosis (Caffey's disease)
9. Lead poisoning (late)
10. Metaphyseal dysplasia (Pyle's disease)
11. Mucopolysaccharidosis (eg, Hurler, Hunter, Morquio)
12. Multiple cartilaginous exostoses
13. Neoplasm, benign expansile
14. Osteopetrosis
15. Other chondrodysplasias (see Gamut D-1)
16. Peripheral dysostosis
17. Pyknodysostosis
18. Rubella, congenital

(Continued)

19. Total lipodystrophy

Reference:

Greenfield GB: *Radiology of Bone Diseases.* Philadelphia, JB Lippincott Co, 1969, p 223.

OVERCONSTRICTION OR OVERTUBULATION (NARROW DIAMETAPHYSIS)

COMMON

1. Atrophy of disuse
2. Neuromuscular and paralytic states (eg, poliomyelitis, arthrogryposis, progressive muscular dystrophy)

UNCOMMON

1. Acromegaly (phalanges)
2. Congenital pseudarthrosis
3. Dermatomyositis
4. Epidermolysis bullosa dystrophica
5. Hallermann-Streiff syndrome
6. Hereditary arthro-opthalmopathy (Stickler syndrome)
7. Homocystinuria
8. Hypopituitarism (eg, primordial dwarfism)
9. Marfan's syndrome
10. Medullary stenosis (idiopathic or hypocalcemic); tubular stenosis (Kenny-Caffey)
11. Neurofibromatosis
12. Osteogenesis imperfecta
13. Progeria
14. Rheumatoid arthritis, juvenile

Reference:

Greenfield GB: *Radiology of Bone Diseases.* Philadelphia, JB Lippincott Co, 1969, p 223.

SUPERNUMERARY EPIPHYSEAL OSSIFICATION CENTERS

1. Cleidocranial dysplasia
2. Down's S. (mongolism)
3. Hand-foot-uterus S.
4. Hypothyroidism
5. Idiopathic
6. Larsen's S.
7. Otopalatodigital S.
8. Peripheral dysostosis

Reference:

Greenfield GB: *Radiology of Bone Diseases.* Philadelphia, JB Lippincott Co, 1969, p 224.

IRREGULARITY, FRAGMENTATION, OR STIPPLING OF MULTIPLE EPIPHYSEAL OSSIFICATION CENTERS

COMMON

1. Aseptic necroses; osteochondroses
2. Cretinism
3. Normal (at certain ages)

UNCOMMON

1. Cerebrohepatorenal S.
2. Chondrodysplasia punctata (congenital stippled epiphyses, Conradi's disease)
3. Cockayne's S.
4. Down's S. (mongolism)
5. Dysplasia epiphysealis hemimelica (Trevor's disease) (unilateral knee and ankle)
6. Enchondromatosis (Ollier's disease); Maffucci's S.
7. Hereditary arthro-ophthalmopathy (Stickler S.)
8. Hereditary multiple epiphyseal disturbances (Ribbing)
9. Homocystinuria (stippled physeal plates)
10. Kniest's disease
11. Metatropic dwarfism
12. Mucopolysaccharidosis (eg, Morquio)
13. Multiple epiphyseal dysplasia (Fairbank)
14. Osteopetrosis
15. Osteopoikilosis; osteopathia striata
16. Parastremmatic dwarfism
17. Pituitary gigantism

(Continued)

18. Rhinotrichophalangeal S. (hips)
19. Smith-Lemli-Opitz S.
20. Spondyloepiphyseal dysplasia (congenita and pseudo-achondroplastic types)

References:

1. Felson B, Editor: Dwarfs and Other Little People. *Semin Roentgenol* 8:256, 1973.

2. Greenfield GB: *Radiology of Bone Diseases.* Philadelphia, JB Lippincott Co, 1969, p 120.

ALTERATION IN SIZE OR APPEARANCE OF MULTIPLE EPIPHYSES
(See also Gamut D-13)

COMMON

1. Achondroplasia
2. Arthritis (eg, rheumatoid, psoriatic)
3. Aseptic necrosis (eg, sicklemia, steroid therapy) (see Gamut D-28)
4. Cone-shaped epiphyses (see Gamut D-15)
5. Hemophilia
6. Hypothyroidism

UNCOMMON

1. Chondrodysplasia punctata (congenital stippled epiphyses, Conradi's disease)
2. Chondroectodermal dysplasia (Ellis-Van Creveld S.)
3. Diastrophic dwarfism
4. Dysplasia epiphysealis hemimelica (Trevor's disease) (unilateral knee and ankle)
5. Enchondromatosis (Ollier's disease)
6. Hereditary arthro-ophthalmopathy (Stickler S.)
7. Hypochondroplasia
8. Hypophosphatasia
9. Infection (eg, smallpox, tuberculosis)
10. Kniest's disease
11. Metaphyseal chondrodysplasia
12. Metatropic dwarfism
13. Mucopolysaccharidosis (eg, Hurler, Hunter, Morquio)
14. Multiple epiphyseal dysplasia (Fairbank)

(Continued)

15. Normal variant

16. Osteogenesis imperfecta

17. Parastremmatic dwarfism

18. Rickets

19. Scurvy

20. Spondyloepiphyseal dysplasia (congenita or pseudo-achondroplastic types)

21. Thermal injury

22. Thiemann's disease

23. Trauma, including battered child

CONE-SHAPED EPIPHYSES

COMMON

1. Idiopathic or normal

UNCOMMON

1. Achondroplasia
2. Acrocephalosyndactyly (Apert's S.)
3. Asphyxiating thoracic dysplasia
4. Chondroectodermal dysplasia (Ellis-Van Creveld S.)
5. Cleidocranial dysplasia
6. Dactylitis (esp. sickle cell, smallpox)
7. Epiphyseal dysplasia
8. Hypervitaminosis A
9. Neonatal hyperthyroidism
10. Orodigitofacial S.
11. Osteopetrosis
12. Otopalatodigital S.
13. Peripheral dysostosis (acrodysostosis)
14. Phalangeal giantism
15. Pseudohypoparathyroidism, pseudopseudohypopara-thyroidism
16. Rhinotrichophalangeal S.

References:

1. Giedion A: Cone-shaped epiphyses of the hands and their diagnostic value. The tricho-rhino-phalangeal syndrome. *Ann Radiol* 10:322–329, 1967.
2. Newcombe DS, Keats TE: Roentgenographic manifestations of hereditary peripheral dysostosis. *Am J Roentgenol* 106:178–189, 1969.
3. Poznanski AK: *The Hand in Radiologic Diagnosis.* Philadelphia, WB Saunders Co, 1974, pp 110–116.
4. Saldino RM, Mainzer F: Cone-shaped epiphyses (CSE) in siblings with hereditary renal disease and retinitis pigmentosa. *Radiology* 98:39–45, 1971.

RADIOLUCENT METAPHYSEAL BANDS

COMMON

1. Leukemia
2. Metastatic neoplasm (esp. neuroblastoma)
3. Normal variant (esp. in neonate)
4. Systemic illness or stress in infancy or in utero
5. Transplacental infection (eg, toxoplasmosis, rubella, cytomegalic inclusion disease, herpes, syphilis)

UNCOMMON

1. Cushing's syndrome
2. Hypervitaminosis D
3. Osteogenesis imperfecta
4. Osteopetrosis
5. Postnatal infection (eg, brucellosis)
6. Scurvy

TRANSVERSE LINES OR ZONES OF INCREASED DENSITY IN THE METAPHYSES

COMMON

1. Lead poisoning
2. Leukemia, treated
3. Normal variant (esp. in the neonate)
4. Protracted anemia (eg, sicklemia, thalassemia)
5. Rickets, renal osteodystrophy (healing)
6. Systemic illness or stress in infancy (growth lines)

UNCOMMON

1. Aminopterin-induced syndrome
2. Cretinism, hypothyroidism
3. Estrogen in high doses or heavy metal therapy to mother during pregnancy
4. Heavy metal or chemical absorption (eg, bismuth, arsenic, phosphorus, fluoride, mercury, lithium, radium)
5. Hypervitaminosis D
6. Idiopathic hypercalcemia
7. Metaphyseal chondrodysplasia (Schmid)
8. Methotrexate therapy
9. Osteopetrosis
10. Parathormone therapy
11. Radiation from bone seeking isotopes (SR^{90}, Y^{90}, P^{32})
12. Scurvy, healing
13. Steroids (in high doses)
14. Transplacental infection (eg, toxoplasmosis, rubella, cytomegalic inclusion disease, herpes, syphilis)

Reference:

Follis RH Jr, Park EA: Some observations on bone growth, with particular respect to zones and transverse lines of increased density in the metaphysis. *Am J Roentgenol* 68:709–724, 1952.

SPLAYING OR FLARING OF THE METAPHYSES

COMMON

1. Chronic hemolytic anemia (eg, sicklemia, thalassemia)
2. Fracture
3. Lipid storage disorders (esp. Gaucher's disease, Niemann-Pick disease)
4. Normal variant
5. Rickets, including renal osteodystrophy and biliary rickets

UNCOMMON

1. Congenital syndromes
   a. Enchondromatosis (Ollier's disease)
   b. Hypophosphatasia
   c. Kniest's disease
   d. Metaphyseal chondrodysplasia (types Jansen, McKusick, Schmid)
   e. Metaphyseal dysplasia (Pyle's disease)
   f. Metatropic dwarfism
   g. Multiple cartilaginous exostoses
   h. Osteodysplasia (Melnick-Needles)
   i. Osteopetrosis
   j. Spondyloepiphyseal dysplasia (congenita or pseudo-achondroplastic types)
   k. Thanatophoric dwarfism
2. Histiocytosis X
3. Lead poisoning
4. Mucoviscidosis

METAPHYSEAL CUPPING

COMMON

1. Cone-shaped epiphyses (see Gamut D-15)

2. Normal variant (eg, distal ulna and fibula; triangular shaped toe phalanges)

3. Prolonged immobilization of joints causing distal metaphyseal cupping (eg, poliomyelitis; tuberculosis or pyarthrosis of hip; slipped femoral epiphysis; congenital hip dislocation)

4. Rickets, all types

UNCOMMON

1. Copper deficiency; kinky-hair syndrome

2. Homocystinuria

3. Hypervitaminosis A

4. Hypophosphatasia

5. Infarction; hypovascularity

6. Leukemia

7. Osteochondrodysplasias (eg, achondroplasia; hypochondroplasia; chondroectodermal dysplasia; peripheral dysostosis; thanatophoric dwarfism; pseudoachondroplastic dysplasia; metaphyseal chondrodysplasia; rhinotrichophalangeal S.)

8. Osteomyelitis (eg, bacterial, syphilis, yaws, smallpox)

9. Osteopetrosis

10. Phenylketonuria

11. Scurvy, after a compression fracture

12. Sickle cell anemia

13. Thermal injury

14. Trauma (to cartilage)

(Continued)

References:

1. Caffey J: Traumatic cupping of the metaphyses of growing bones. *Am J Roentgenol* 108:451-460, 1970.

2. Greenfield GB: *Radiology of Bone Diseases.* Philadelphia, JB Lippincott Co, 1969, p 224.

REGIONAL OSTEOPOROSIS, BONE ATROPHY

COMMON

1. Acro-osteolysis
2. Arthritis (esp. rheumatoid) (see Gamut D-130)
3. Burn, frostbite, electroshock
4. Disuse atrophy, immobilization (eg, fracture, cast)
5. Infection (eg, osteomyelitis, tuberculosis)
6. Local hemorrhage (eg, trauma, hemophilia)
7. Paralysis, neural or muscular
8. Sudeck's atrophy (see Gamut D-21)

UNCOMMON

1. Arteriovenous malformation, hemangioma
2. Congenital pseudarthrosis
3. Diabetes mellitus (diabetic osteopathy)
4. Osteoporosis circumscripta (Paget's disease)
5. Regional transitory osteoporosis
6. Shoulder-hand syndrome (eg, myocardial infarction, scalenus anticus syndrome)
7. Tumor, benign or malignant, primary or metastatic

SUDECK'S ATROPHY
(SPOTTY OSTEOPOROSIS)
(See also Gamut D-20)

COMMON

1. Burn, frostbite, electroshock
2. Immobilization
3. Infection (eg, suppurative arthritis, human bite)
4. Rheumatoid arthritis
5. Shoulder-hand syndrome (eg, myocardial infarction, cervical rib, scalenus anticus syndrome)
6. Trauma with or without fracture; fracture complications (eg, nonunion, malposition, infection)

UNCOMMON

1. Idiopathic
2. Vascular insufficiency, arterial or venous (eg, arteriosclerosis obliterans, Buerger's disease, Raynaud's disease)

GENERALIZED OSTEOPOROSIS

I. Congenital

   1. Ehlers-Danlos S.

   2. Familial osteoectasia (hyperphosphatasia)

   3. Fanconi's S. (pancytopenia-dysmelia S.)

   4. Gonadal dysgenesis (Turner's S.)

   5. Hajdu-Cheney S. (idiopathic osteolysis)

   6. Hypophosphatasia

   7. Mucopolysaccharidosis (eg, Hurler, Hunter)

  *8. Neuromuscular diseases and dystrophies

   9. Osteochondrodysplasias, several types (see Gamut D-1)

*10. Osteogenesis imperfecta, fibrogenesis imperfecta

 11. Progeria; Werner's S.

 12. Pseudohypoparathyroidism, pseudopseudohypoparathyroidism

 13. Trisomy 13 S.

 14. Trisomy 18 S.

II. Deficiency due to malassimilation

  *1. Calcium and phosphorus deficiency

   2. Copper deficiency (in infants)

  *3. Malabsorption (see Gamut G-34)

  *4. Malnutrition

  *5. Protein deficiency

   6. Vitamin C deficiency (scurvy)

  *7. Vitamin D deficiency (rickets)

(Continued)

III. Disuse atrophy (muscle weakness; lack of stress stimulus or weight bearing)

    *1. Cerebral palsy; spinal cord disease

    *2. Immobilization (eg, chronic disease, major fracture)

    *3. Muscular dystrophy

IV. Endocrine

    1. Adrenocortical abnormality (eg, Addison's disease, Cushing's S.)

    *2. Hypogonadism
       a. Ovarian (eg, menopause, Turner's S.)
       b. Testicular (eg, eunuchoidism, prepubertal castration S.)

    3. Non-endocrine steroid-producing tumor (eg, oat cell carcinoma)

    4. Pancreatic abnormality (eg, poorly controlled diabetes mellitus, pancreatic insufficiency)

    5. [Parathyroid abnormality (eg, hyperparathyroidism, hypoparathyroidism with steatorrhea)]

    6. Pituitary abnormality (eg, acromegaly, Cushing's syndrome due to basophilic adenoma, hypopituitarism)

    7. Thyroid abnormality (eg, hyperthyroidism, thyrotoxicosis, hypothyroidism, cretinism)

V. Miscellaneous

    *1. Anemia (eg, sickle cell, thalassemia, severe iron deficiency)

    *2. Collagen disease (eg, rheumatoid arthritis, ankylosing spondylitis, lupus erythematosus, scleroderma, dermatomyositis)

    3. Familial Mediterranean fever

    4. Gaucher's disease; Niemann-Pick disease

    5. Hemochromatosis

(Continued)

GENERALIZED OSTEOPOROSIS
(Continued)

6. Hemophilia

7. Hypoxia (eg, chronic pulmonary disease, congenital heart disease)

*8. Iatrogenic, drug therapy (eg, excessive steroid therapy, heparin)

9. Idiopathic (eg, idiopathic osteoporosis in young people)

10. Idiopathic hypercalcemia (late)

11. Leukemia (acute)

12. Liver disease (eg, jaundice; hepatolenticular degeneration; liver tumor or cyst with protein disturbance; biliary atresia)

13. Mastocytosis

14. Metabolic error (eg, homocystinuria; phenylketonuria)

*15. Metastatic disease (carcinomatosis)

*16. Multiple myeloma

17. Ochronosis

18. [Osteomalacia]

*19. Renal loss of protein (eg, oxalosis, renal osteodystrophy, renal tubular acidosis)

*20. Senile osteoporosis

21. Waldenstrom's macroglobulinemia

*Common

References:

1. Greenfield GB: *Radiology of Bone Diseases.* Philadelphia, JB Lippincott Co, 1969, p 10.

2. Teplick JG, Haskin ME: *Roentgenologic Diagnosis*, ed 2. Philadelphia, WB Saunders Co, 1971, vol 2, p xxxiii.

SITES OF SUBPERIOSTEAL RESORPTION IN
PRIMARY HYPERPARATHYROIDISM
(IN DECREASING FREQUENCY)

1. Middle phalanges of 2nd and 3rd fingers, radial aspects
2. Clavicle, outer end
3. Femur, tibia, and humerus, upper inner aspects
4. Lamina dura of teeth
5. Ischial tuberosity
6. Pubic symphysis
7. Sacroiliac joint
8. Calcaneal borders
9. Radius and ulna, distal ends
10. Sesamoid bones
11. Rib, esp. upper border
12. Sella turcica
13. Tuft of terminal phalanx

Reference:
Jacobson HG: Personal communication.

OSTEOMALACIA AND RICKETS

I. Deficient absorption of calcium or phosphorus
  A. Malabsorption states
    1. Cathartic abuse (esp. oily cathartics or magnesium sulfate)
    2. Mesenteric disease
    3. Pancreatic insufficiency (exocrine), pancreatitis
    4. Postoperative gastric or small bowel resection
    5. Primary small bowel disease (celiac disease, sprue, amyloidosis, regional enteritis, lymphoma, small bowel fistula)
    6. Steatorrhea, idiopathic
  B. Obstructive jaundice
    1. Acquired chronic biliary obstruction
    2. Biliary atresia
  C. Vitamin D deficient rickets
II. Dietary calcium deficiency
III. Enzyme abnormality (eg, hypophosphatasia)
IV. Excessive excretion of calcium or phosphorus via breast or placenta (puerperal osteomalacia)
V. Excessive renal excretion of calcium or phosphorus
  A. Glomerular (hyperphosphatemic)
    1. Renal osteodystrophy
    2. Renal osteomalacia
  B. Tubular (hypophosphatemic)
    1. Fanconi syndromes (glycosuria, aminoaciduria, and proteinuria), primary or acquired
    2. Hypophosphatemic familial rickets (Vitamin D resistant rickets)
    3. Inborn metabolic disturbances (eg, galactosemia, oxalosis, tyrosinosis, Wilson's disease)
    4. Pseudodeficiency rickets (Vitamin D dependency rickets)

(Continued)

VI. Excessive utilization of calcium as fixed base

   A. Chronic obstructive renal disease

   B. Idiopathic hypercalciuria

   C. Renal tubular acidosis

   D. Rickets following ureterosigmoidostomy (hyperchloremia)

VII. Miscellaneous

   A. Anticonvulsant drug (eg, dilantin)

   B. Autoimmune disorders

   C. Cadmium intoxication

   D. Congenital rickets (mother with osteomalacia)

   E. Fibrogenesis imperfecta ossium

   F. Idiopathic axial osteomalacia

   G. Pernicious anemia

   H. Phosphate deficiency from aluminum hydroxide therapy

References:

1. Greenfield GB: *Radiology of Bone Diseases.* Philadelphia, JB Lippincott Co, 1969, p 16.

2. Jacobson HG: Personal communication.

CAUSES OF ALTERED CALCIUM AND PHOSPHORUS CONCENTRATIONS

HYPERCALCEMIA

1. Adrenal insufficiency
2. Hyperparathyroidism
3. Hyperthyroidism, hypothyroidism
4. Hypervitaminosis D
5. Hypophosphatasia
6. Idiopathic hypercalcemia
7. Leukemia, lymphoma
8. Metaphyseal chondrodysplasia (Jansen)
9. Milk-alkali syndrome
10. Myelomatosis
11. Rapid deossification of bone
12. Reticuloses
13. Sarcoidosis
14. Secretion of parathormone-like substance from malignant tumors
15. Skeletal metastases
16. Wermer's syndrome (familial multiple endocrine adenomas)

HYPERPHOSPHATEMIA

1. Acromegaly
2. Glomerular failure
3. Hypervitaminosis D
4. Hypoparathyroidism; pseudohypoparathyroidism
5. Skeletal metastases

HYPOCALCEMIA

1. Acidosis
2. Hypoalbuminemic states
3. Hypoparathyroidism; pseudohypoparathyroidism
4. Malabsorption states
5. Neonate
6. Pancreatitis
7. Uremia; uremic osteodystrophy
8. Vitamin D deficiency

HYPOPHOSPHATEMIA

1. Dietary deficiency
2. Hyperparathyroidism
3. Hypovitaminosis D (eg, Vitamin D deficiency rickets, osteomalacia)
4. Increased carbohydrate metabolism
5. Malabsorption states
6. Pregnancy
7. Renal tubular dysfunction (eg, Fanconi syndrome, Vitamin D resistant rickets)
8. Skeletal metastases

(Continued)

HYPERCALCIURIA

1. Acidosis
2. Active osteoporosis
3. Hypercalcemia
4. Hypervitaminosis D
5. Hyperparathyroidism, primary
6. Renal tubular disease
7. Sarcoidosis
8. Widespread bone destruction

HYPOCALCIURIA

1. Active reconstruction of bone
2. Alkalosis
3. Decreased glomerular filtration rate
4. Hypocalcemia
5. Reduced calcium absorption from intestine
6. Vitamin D deficiency

Reference:

Greenfield GB: *Radiology of Bone Diseases*. Philadelphia, JB Lippincott Co, 1969, p 21.

WIDESPREAD OR GENERALIZED DEMINERALIZATION WITH COARSE TRABECULATION

COMMON

1. Anemia (eg, sickle cell anemia, thalassemia)
2. Hyperparathyroidism, primary or secondary
3. Myelomatosis; carcinomatosis
4. Osteomalacia, rickets (eg, biliary atresia, alimentary tract disorder)
5. Osteoporosis (see Gamut D-22)
6. Paget's disease
7. Paralysis

UNCOMMON

1. Acromegaly
2. Fibrogenesis imperfecta; atypical axial osteomalacia
3. Gaucher's disease
4. Hemophilia
5. Leukemia
6. Recalcification after disuse osteoporosis (eg, after tuberculous arthritis)

BONE INFARCT (DIAMETAPHYSEAL ISCHEMIA)
(See also Gamut D-28)

COMMON

1. Idiopathic
2. Occlusive vascular disease (arteriosclerosis, Buerger's disease, thromboembolic disease)
3. Sickle cell or other primary anemia

UNCOMMON

1. Caisson disease
2. Fat embolism (eg, alcoholism)
3. Gaucher's disease
4. Infection, osteomyelitis
5. Pancreatitis
6. Polyarteritis nodosa (vasculitis)
7. Radiation therapy; radium poisoning

Reference:

Edeiken J, Hodes PJ, Libshitz HI, Weller MH: Bone ischemia. *Radiol Clin North Am* 5:515–529, 1967.

ASEPTIC NECROSIS OF THE HIP OR OTHER JOINTS (EPIPHYSEAL ISCHEMIA)
(See also Gamut D-27)

COMMON

1. Idiopathic (eg, Legg-Perthes disease)
2. Occlusive vascular disease (eg, arteriosclerosis, thromboembolic disease)
3. Osteochondritis dissecans
4. Sickle cell or other primary anemia
5. Steroid therapy; Cushing's syndrome
6. Trauma (eg, fracture, dislocation, surgical correction of congenital hip dislocation or slipped capital epiphysis)

UNCOMMON

1. Caisson disease
2. Charcot joint, atrophic
3. Collagen disease (eg, lupus erythematosus, polyarteritis nodosa, rheumatoid arthritis)
4. Fat embolism (eg, alcoholism)
5. Gaucher's disease
6. Gout
7. Hemophilia
8. Histiocytosis X
9. Methotrexate therapy
10. Osteomyelitis
11. Pancreatitis
12. Radiation therapy; radium poisoning
(Continued)

References:

1. Edeiken J, Hodes PJ, Libshitz HI, Weller MH: Bone ischemia. *Radiol Clin North Am* 5:515–529, 1967.

2. Jacobson HG, Siegelman SS: Some miscellaneous solitary bone lesions. *Semin Roentgenol* 1:314–335, 1966.

3. Jaffe HL: Ischemic necrosis of bone. *Med Radiogr Photogr* 45:58–86, 1969.

4. Martel W, Sitterley BH: Roentgenologic manifestations of osteonecrosis. *Am J Roentgenol* 106:509–522, 1969.

SITES OF PREDILECTION AND EPONYMS
FOR ASEPTIC NECROSIS

COMMON

1. Carpal lunate — Kienböck 1910
2. Femoral capital epiphysis — Legg-Calvé-Perthes 1910
3. Medial tibial condyle — Blount 1937
4. Second metatarsal head (occasionally third or fourth) — Freiberg 1914
5. Secondary patellar center — Sinding-Larsen 1921
6. Tarsal navicular — Köhler 1908
7. Tibial tubercle — Osgood-Schlatter 1903
8. Vertebral body — Calvé 1925
   Kümmell-Verneuil disease
9. Vertebral epiphyses — Scheuermann 1921

UNCOMMON

1. Astragalus — Diaz 1928
2. Basal phalanges — Thiemann 1909
3. Calcaneal apophysis — Sever 1912
4. Capitulum of humerus — Panner 1927
5. Carpal navicular — Preiser 1911
6. Distal tibial center — Liffert and Arkin 1950
7. Entire carpus bilaterally — Caffey 1945
8. Fifth metatarsal base — Iselin 1912
9. Greater trochanter — Mandl 1922
10. Head of humerus — Hass 1921
11. Heads of metacarpals — Mauclaire 1927
    Dietrich 1932

(Continued)

12. Iliac crest	Buchman 1927
13. Intercondylar spines of tibia	Caffey 1956
14. Ischial apophysis	Milch 1953
15. Ischiopubic synchondrosis	Van Neck 1924
16. Lower ulna	Burns 1921
17. Os tibiale externum	Haglund 1908
18. Osteochondritis dissecans	König 1887
19. Primary patellar center	Köhler 1908
20. Symphysis pubis	Pierson 1929

Reference:

Greenfield GB: *Radiology of Bone Diseases.* Philadelphia, JB Lippincott Co, 1969, p 106.

"BONE WITHIN BONE" APPEARANCE

COMMON

1. Osteopetrosis
2. Paget's disease

UNCOMMON

1. Delay of growth (eg, due to disease, stress, chemotherapy)
2. Hypervitaminosis D
3. Normal neonate
4. Phosphorus ingestion
5. Sickle cell anemia
6. Thorotrast

LOCALIZED BONE SCLEROSIS WITH RADIOLUCENT NIDUS AND/OR SEQUESTRUM

COMMON

1. Brodie's abscess, osteomyelitis
2. Osteoid osteoma

UNCOMMON

1. Eosinophilic granuloma
2. Osteoblastoma
3. Syphilis, yaws
4. Tropical ulcer
5. Tuberculosis

SOLITARY OSTEOSCLEROTIC BONE LESION
(See also Gamut D-33)

COMMON

1. Avascular necrosis
2. Bone infarct
3. Bone island
4. Callus (healed or healing fracture)
5. Chondroid lesion (eg, enchondroma, osteochondroma)
6. Healed or healing benign bone lesion (eg, bone cyst, nonossifying fibroma, fibrous cortical defect, brown tumor)
7. Osteoblastic metastasis (see Gamut D-55)
8. Osteoid osteoma
9. Osteoma, endosteoma
10. Sclerosing osteomyelitis (eg, Garré's; Brodie's abscess; granuloma)

UNCOMMON

1. Bone sarcoma (eg, osteosarcoma, chondrosarcoma, Ewing's)
2. Fibrous dysplasia; ossifying fibroma
3. Lymphoma; reticulum cell sarcoma
4. Mastocytosis
5. Osteoblastoma
6. Paget's disease
7. Syphilis; yaws

MULTIPLE OSTEOSCLEROTIC BONE LESIONS

COMMON

1. Bone infarcts
2. Bone islands
3. Callus (eg, healed rib fractures)
4. Osteoblastic metastases (see Gamut D-55)
5. Osteomyelitis, chronic or healed (eg, tuberculous, fungal)
6. Paget's disease

UNCOMMON

1. Avascular necroses
2. Chondrodysplasia punctata (congenital stippled epiphyses, Conradi's disease)
3. Enchondromatosis (Ollier's disease)
4. Fibrous dysplasia
5. Lymphoma
6. Mastocytosis
7. Multiple enchondromas, osteochondromas
8. Multiple healed or healing benign bone lesions (eg, nonossifying fibromas, fibrous cortical defects, brown tumors, bone cysts, Gaucher's disease)
9. Multiple myeloma
10. Multiple osteocartilaginous exostoses
11. Osteomas (eg, Gardner's syndrome)
12. Osteopathia striata
13. Osteopoikilosis
14. Osteosarcomatosis
15. Plasma cell granulomas
16. Syphilis; yaws
17. Tuberous sclerosis

GENERALIZED OR WIDESPREAD OSTEOSCLEROSIS

COMMON

1. Myelosclerosis, myeloid metaplasia
2. Osteoblastic metastases (esp. breast, prostate)
3. Paget's disease
4. Physiologic osteosclerosis of newborn
5. Sickle cell anemia

UNCOMMON

1. Congenital cyanotic heart disease
2. Engelmann's disease
3. Erythroblastosis fetalis
4. Fibrous dysplasia
5. Fluorosis
6. Gaucher's disease
7. Hyperparathyroidism, primary or secondary (esp. treated or in young)
8. Hyperphosphatasia
9. Hypervitaminosis D
10. Hypoparathyroidism, pseudohypoparathyroidism
11. Hypothyroidism, cretinism
12. Idiopathic hypercalcemia (eg, William's syndrome)
13. Idiopathic osteosclerosis
14. Infantile cortical hyperostosis (Caffey's disease)
15. Lymphoma
16. Mastocytosis
17. Melorheostosis

(Continued)

18. Metaphyseal dysplasia (Pyle's disease); craniometaphyseal dysplasia; frontometaphyseal dysplasia

19. Multiple myeloma

20. Osteodysplasia (Melnick-Needles)

21. Osteomalacia, rickets (healing)

22. Osteopathia striata

23. Osteopetrosis

24. Osteopoikilosis

25. Osteosarcomatosis

26. Pachydermoperiostosis

27. Phosphorus or bismuth poisoning

28. Pyknodysostosis

29. Renal osteodystrophy

30. Syphilis

31. Tuberous sclerosis

32. Tubular stenosis (Kenny-Caffey)

33. Van Buchem's disease

References:

1. Greenfield GB: *Radiology of Bone Diseases.* Philadelphia, JB Lippincott Co, 1969, p 227.

2. Teplick JG, Haskin ME: *Roentgenologic Diagnosis*, ed 2. Philadelphia, WB Saunders Co, 1971, vol 2, p xxxiii.

SOLITARY CYST-LIKE LESION OF BONE

COMMON

1. Arthritic or synovial lesion (eg, gout, hemophilia, osteo-arthritis, villonodular synovitis)
2. Bone cyst
3. Enchondroma
4. Fibrous dysplasia (monostotic; cortical)
5. Nonossifying fibroma

UNCOMMON

1. Aneurysmal bone cyst
2. Angiomatous lesions
3. Brown tumor of hyperparathyroidism
4. Chondroblastoma
5. Chondromyxoid fibroma
6. Cystic osteomyelitis (esp. tuberculous)
7. Desmoplastic fibroma
8. Epidermoid inclusion cyst
9. Fibrosarcoma, chondrosarcoma (slow growing)
10. Gaucher's disease
11. Giant cell tumor
12. Hemophilic pseudotumor
13. Histiocytosis X
14. Hydatid cyst
15. Intraosseous ganglion
16. Lipoma

(Continued)

17. Metastatic carcinoma (esp. hypernephroma, thyroid)
18. Ossifying fibroma
19. Osteoblastoma
20. Periosteal chondroma or fibroma
21. Plasmacytoma, myeloma

SOLITARY EXPANSILE LESION OF BONE

Benign Neoplasm of Bone

1. Angioma
2. Chondroblastoma
3. Chondromyxoid fibroma
4. Desmoplastic fibroma
*5. Enchondroma
6. Giant cell tumor
7. Lipoma
*8. Nonossifying fibroma
9. Osteoblastoma
10. Periosteal chondroma
11. Periosteal fibroma

Malignant Neoplasm of Bone

1. Adamantinoma
*2. Chondrosarcoma
3. Fibrosarcoma
4. Hemangiopericytoma; angiosarcoma
5. Malignant giant cell tumor
*6. Metastasis (esp. carcinoma of kidney, thyroid, lung)
*7. Plasmacytoma, myeloma

Tumor-Like Process

1. Aneurysmal bone cyst
*2. Bone cyst
*3. Brown tumor of hyperparathyroidism

(Continued)

4. Epidermoid inclusion cyst

*5. Fibrous dysplasia; cortical fibrous dysplasia (tibia)

6. Gaucher's disease

7. Hemophilic pseudotumor

8. Histiocytosis X

9. Hydatid cyst

*Common

Reference:

Greenfield GB: *Radiology of Bone Diseases.* Philadelphia, JB Lippincott Co, 1969, p 334.

BONE BLISTER
(SOLITARY CYST-LIKE LESION EXPANDING BONE ECCENTRICALLY)

COMMON

1. Giant cell tumor
2. Nonossifying fibroma

UNCOMMON

1. Aneurysmal bone cyst
2. Brown tumor of hyperparathyroidism
3. Chondroid lesion (eg, enchondroma, osteochondroma)
4. Chondromyxoid fibroma
5. Fibrosarcoma (eg, arising in benign fibrous lesion)
6. Fibrous dysplasia (skull); cortical fibrous dysplasia (tibia)
7. Hemangioma
8. Osteoblastoma
9. Periosteal fibroma or chondroma

BLOW-OUT LESION OF BONE
(SOLITARY GROSSLY EXPANSILE CYST-LIKE LYTIC LESION)

COMMON

1. Chondrosarcoma
2. Giant cell tumor
3. Metastatic carcinoma (esp. kidney, thyroid, lung)
4. Plasmacytoma, myeloma

UNCOMMON

1. Aneurysmal bone cyst
2. Brown tumor of hyperparathyroidism
3. Chondromyxoid fibroma
4. Fibrosarcoma
5. Fibrous dysplasia
6. Hemophilic pseudotumor
7. Hydatid cyst

LARGE DESTRUCTIVE BONE LESION
(OVER 5 CM IN DIAMETER)

COMMON

1. Aneurysmal bone cyst
2. Angiomatous lesion; hemangiopericytoma; Gorham's vanishing bone disease
3. Bone cyst
4. Enchondroma
5. Fibrous dysplasia
6. Giant cell tumor
7. Histiocytosis X
8. Metastasis
9. Osteomyelitis; mycetoma
10. Paget's disease (osteoporosis circumscripta)
11. Plasmacytoma, myeloma
12. Primary sarcoma (eg, osteosarcoma, chondrosarcoma, fibrosarcoma, Ewing's, angiosarcoma, reticulum cell sarcoma)

UNCOMMON

1. Adamantinoma
2. Brown tumor of hyperparathyroidism
3. Chondromyxoid fibroma
4. Chordoma
5. Desmoplastic fibroma
6. Gaucher's disease
7. Hemophilic pseudotumor
8. Hydatid disease
9. [Lesion arising in spinal canal (eg, meningocele, ependymoma, neurofibroma)]

(Continued)

10. Lymphoma; Burkitt's tumor

11. [Soft tissue tumor destroying bone (eg, synovioma)]

12. Syphilis, yaws

13. Tropical ulcer, malignant

SOLITARY LYTIC WELL-DEFINED EPIPHYSEAL OR EPIPHYSEAL-METAPHYSEAL LESION OF BONE

COMMON

1. Arthritic lesion (eg, gout, rheumatoid, hemophilia, osteo-arthritis)
2. Chondroblastoma (Codman tumor)
3. Cystic osteomyelitis
*4. Giant cell tumor (originates in metaphysis, invades into epiphysis)
5. Synovial lesion (eg, villonodular synovitis)

UNCOMMON

*1. Angioma
*2. Bone cyst
*3. Enchondroma
4. Eosinophilic granuloma (Histiocytosis X)
5. Intraosseous ganglion
*6. Lipoma
7. Metastasis

*Epiphyseal-metaphyseal location

SOLITARY LYTIC DIAPHYSEAL LESION

COMMON

1. Bone cyst
2. Diametaphyseal lesion extending into diaphysis (eg, non-ossifying fibroma, fibrosarcoma) (see Gamut D-47)
3. Enchondroma
4. Eosinophilic granuloma (Histiocytosis X)
5. Fibrous dysplasia
6. Metastasis
7. Myeloma, plasmacytoma
8. Osteomyelitis
9. Round cell sarcoma (Ewing's tumor, reticulum cell sarcoma, lymphosarcoma)

UNCOMMON

1. Adamantinoma
2. Brown tumor of hyperparathyroidism
3. Cortical fibrous dysplasia (tibia)
4. Hemophilic pseudotumor
5. Hydatid disease
6. Osteosarcoma (25% are diaphyseal)
7. Paget's disease (osteoporosis circumscripta)
8. Syphilis, yaws

SOLITARY WELL-DEMARCATED LYTIC LESION
OF BONE

COMMON

1. Arthritic or synovial lesion (eg, gouty tophus, rheumatoid nodule or synovial cyst, villonodular synovitis, osteo-arthritic cyst, intraosseous ganglion)
*2. Bone cyst
3. Brown tumor of hyperparathyroidism
*4. Enchondroma
*5. Fibrous dysplasia
6. Giant cell tumor
*7. Histiocytosis X
*8. Nonossifying fibroma
*9. Osteomyelitis, cystic; Brodie's abscess

UNCOMMON

1. Adamantinoma
2. Aneurysmal bone cyst
*3. Chondroblastoma
*4. Chondromyxoid fibroma
*5. Granuloma (esp. tuberculous, fungal)
6. Hamartoma
7. Hemangioma, lymphangioma
8. Hemophilic pseudotumor
9. Hydatid cyst
*10. Lipoma
11. Neurofibroma
12. Osteoblastoma

(Continued)

13. Paget's disease (osteoporosis circumscripta)
14. Plasmacytoma, myeloma

*Often has sclerotic rim

SOLITARY POORLY DEMARCATED LYTIC LESION OF BONE

COMMON

1. Histiocytosis X
2. Lymphoma
3. Metastasis
4. Osteomyelitis (eg, tuberculous, fungal, bacterial)
5. Plasmacytoma, myeloma
6. Sarcoma (esp, Ewing's, osteosarcoma, chondrosarcoma) (see Gamut D-52)

UNCOMMON

1. Adamantinoma
2. Angioma
3. Chordoma
4. Fibrous dysplasia
5. Fibrous histiocytoma
6. Giant cell tumor
7. Hemangiopericytoma, hemangioendothelioma
8. Hydatid cyst
9. Paget's disease (osteoporosis circumscripta)
10. Syphilis, yaws

MOTHEATEN OSTEOLYTIC LESION OF BONE, SOLITARY OR MULTIPLE (USUALLY SMALL ROUND CELL LESION)

COMMON

1. Ewing's sarcoma
2. Metastasis, including neuroblastoma
3. Multiple myeloma
4. Osteomyelitis

UNCOMMON

1. Fibrosarcoma
2. Giant cell tumor (at margins)
3. Histiocytosis X (esp. eosinophilic granuloma)
4. Leukemia, lymphoma (eg, Hodgkin's disease, lymphosarcoma, reticulum cell sarcoma, primary or disseminated)
5. Osteosarcoma

MULTIPLE PUNCHED-OUT LYTIC LESIONS OF BONE WITH NONSCLEROTIC MARGINS

COMMON

1. Arthritis (eg, gout, rheumatoid, osteoarthritis)
2. Brown tumors of hyperparathyroidism
3. Histiocytosis X
4. Metastases
5. Multiple myeloma

UNCOMMON

1. Enchondromatosis (Ollier's disease)
2. Fungus disease (esp. blastomycosis, coccidioidomycosis)
3. Gaucher's disease; Niemann-Pick disease
4. Hemangiomatosis, lymphangiomatosis
5. Hemophilia
6. Jackhammer operator disease (driller's disease of wrists)
7. Leprosy
8. Lymphoma
9. Polyvinyl chloride osteolysis
10. Radium poisoning
11. Sarcoidosis
12. Tuberculosis (cystic form)
13. Tuberous sclerosis

AGE OF MAXIMUM INCIDENCE OF VARIOUS BONE TUMORS AND TUMOR-LIKE LESIONS

Tumor	Age (Years)
1. Aneurysmal bone cyst	10–30
2. Bone cyst	5–20
3. Chondroblastoma	10–25
4. Chondromyxoid fibroma	10–30
5. Chondrosarcoma	30–60
6. Ewing's sarcoma	5–20
7. Fibrosarcoma	30–45
8. Giant cell tumor	20–45
9. Metastasis	40–80
10. Multiple myeloma	40–80
11. Neuroblastoma	0–5
12. Nonossifying fibroma	5–20
13. Osteoid osteoma	5–30
14. Osteosarcoma	10–25, 60–75
15. Parosteal sarcoma	30–50
16. Reticulum cell sarcoma of bone	25–40

Reference:

Greenfield GB: *Radiology of Bone Diseases.* Philadelphia, JB Lippincott Co, 1969, p 340.

PREFERENTIAL SITE WITHIN BONE OF VARIOUS OSSEOUS TUMORS
(See also Gamuts D-40 and D-41)

1. Epiphysis
   a. Chondroblastoma
   b. Giant cell tumor (after fusion of epiphyseal plate; originates in metaphysis)

2. Metaphysis
   a. [Bone cyst]
   b. Chondrosarcoma
   c. Giant cell tumor
   d. Osteosarcoma (75%)
   e. [Parosteal sarcoma]

3. Diametaphysis
   a. Chondromyxoid fibroma
   b. Desmoplastic fibroma
   c. Fibrosarcoma
   d. Nonossifying fibroma

4. Diaphysis
   a. Adamantinoma
   b. Ewing's tumor
   c. Myeloma
   d. Osteosarcoma (25%)
   e. Reticulum cell sarcoma, lymphosarcoma

BENIGN BONE TUMOR
(See also Gamuts D-49 and D-49A)

COMMON

1. Enchondroma
2. Nonossifying fibroma
3. Osteochondroma
4. [Osteoid osteoma]
5. Osteoma

UNCOMMON

1. [Aneurysmal bone cyst]
2. Chondroblastoma
3. Chondromyxoid fibroma
4. Desmoplastic fibroma
5. Fibrous osteoma; ossifying fibroma
6. Giant cell tumor
7. Glomus tumor; hemangiopericytoma; hemangioendothelioma
8. Hemangioma
9. Lipoma
10. Neurofibroma
11. Osteoblastoma
12. Parosteal osteoma
13. Periosteal chondroma or fibroma

BENIGN TUMOR-LIKE LESION OF BONE
(See also Subgamut D-49A)

COMMON

1. Arthritic or synovial lesion (eg, gouty tophus, osteoarthritic cyst, intraosseous ganglion, villonodular synovitis)
2. Bone cyst
3. Brown tumor of hyperparathyroidism
4. Fibrous cortical defect
5. Fibrous dysplasia
6. Histiocytosis X
7. Myositis ossificans (parosteal)
8. Osteoid osteoma
9. Osteomyelitis (eg, bacterial, tuberculous, fungal)
10. Paget's disease (esp. osteoporosis circumscripta)
11. Stress fracture, healing (esp. metatarsal)

UNCOMMON

1. Aneurysmal bone cyst
2. Congenital fibromatosis
3. Cortical (subperiosteal) desmoid
4. Epidermoid inclusion cyst; foreign body or "thorn" granuloma
5. Hemophilic pseudotumor
6. Hydatid cyst
7. Sarcoidosis
8. [Soft tissue lesion involving bone (eg, glomus tumor, giant cell tumor of tendon sheath)]

SUBGAMUT D-49A
TYPES OF FIBROCYSTIC BONE LESIONS

1. Bone cyst
2. Cherubism
3. Chondromyxoid fibroma
4. Cortical fibrous dysplasia
5. Desmoplastic fibroma
6. Fibrous cortical defect
7. Fibrous dysplasia
8. Fibrous osteoma (esp. in facial bones)
9. Intraosseous ganglion; fibrocystic changes of degenerative arthritis (esp. in hip)
10. Nonossifying fibroma (fibroxanthoma)
11. Ossifying fibroma

PERIOSTEAL OR PAROSTEAL TUMOR

COMMON

1. [Cortical desmoid]
2. [Osteoid osteoma]
3. [Parosteal myositis ossificans]

UNCOMMON

1. Parosteal lipoma
2. Parosteal osteoma
3. Parosteal sarcoma (osteosarcoma, chondrosarcoma, fibrosarcoma)
4. Periosteal fibroma
5. Periosteal (juxtacortical) chondroma
6. [Soft tissue tumor in a parosteal location (eg, synovioma, giant cell tumor of tendon sheath, glomus tumor)]

Reference:

Greenfield GB: *Radiology of Bone Diseases.* Philadelphia, JB Lippincott Co, 1969, p 321.

EXOSTOSIS

COMMON

1. Bunion
2. [Fracture fragment, healed]
3. [Hypertrophic spur]
4. Multiple cartilaginous exostoses
5. Myositis ossificans (post-traumatic exostosis)
6. Osteochondroma (metaphyseal)

UNCOMMON

1. Blount's disease (tibia vara)
2. Chondroectodermal dysplasia (Ellis-Van Creveld S.) (tibial)
3. Dyschondrosteosis (tibial)
4. Intracapsular chondroma; dysplasia epiphysealis hemimelica (Trevor's disease) (esp. knee and ankle epiphyses)
5. Myositis ossificans progressiva
6. Postradiation therapy
7. Pseudohypoparathyroidism
8. Subungual exostosis
9. [Supracondylar process of humerus]
10. Turner's syndrome (medial tibial condyle)
11. Turret exostosis (phalanx)

Reference:

Greenfield GB: *Radiology of Bone Diseases*. Philadelphia, JB Lippincott Co, 1969, p 224.

TYPES OF PRIMARY MALIGNANT BONE TUMOR

COMMON

1. Chondrosarcoma (central, peripheral, parosteal)
2. Ewing's sarcoma
3. Fibrosarcoma
4. Giant cell tumor, malignant
5. Lymphoma (reticulum cell sarcoma, Hodgkin's disease, lymphosarcoma, Burkitt's tumor)
6. Myeloma
7. Osteosarcoma (conventional, parosteal)
8. Undifferentiated sarcoma

UNCOMMON

1. Adamantinoma
2. Angiosarcoma
3. Chordoma
4. Fibrous histiocytoma, malignant
5. Liposarcoma
6. Malignant hemangiopericytoma, hemangioendothelioma, perithelioma, Kaposi's sarcoma
7. Osteoblastoma, malignant

SUBGAMUT D-52A
RADIOLOGIC CRITERIA SUGGESTING BONE
MALIGNANCY

1. Bone destruction (geographic, motheaten, or permeative)
2. Irregular ill-defined margins of lesion ("wide transition zone" between normal and abnormal bone)
3. Cortical erosion or destruction
4. Codman triangle
5. Periosteal lamellation ("onion skin")
6. Periosteal right angle spiculation ("sunburst" or "hair-on-end")
7. Soft tissue mass adjacent to bone destruction
8. Chondroid or osteoid matrix (esp. in extraosseous tissues)
9. Evidence of metastasis

Reference:

Nelson SW: Some fundamentals in the radiologic differential diagnosis of solitary bone lesions. *Semin Roentgenol* 1:244–267, 1966.

MALIGNANT BONE TUMOR WITH GROSS DESTRUCTION AND MINIMAL OR NO PERIOSTEAL REACTION

COMMON

1. Chondrosarcoma
2. Fibrosarcoma
3. Lymphoma; leukemia in an adult
4. Metastasis
5. Myeloma
6. Osteosarcoma (osteolytic type)

UNCOMMON

1. Adamantinoma
2. Angiosarcoma
3. Chordoma
4. Ewing's sarcoma (occasionally)
5. Fibrous histiocytoma, malignant
6. Giant cell tumor, malignant
7. Liposarcoma
8. Malignant hemangioendothelioma or hemangiopericytoma
9. Reticulum cell sarcoma

MALIGNANT BONE TUMOR WITH MARKED PERIOSTEAL REACTION[1]

1. Burkitt's tumor
*2. Ewing's sarcoma
3. Leukemia in a child
4. Neuroblastoma metastasis
*5. Osteosarcoma

*Often onion-skin periosteal reaction.
[1]May be confused with osteomyelitis.

SUBGAMUT D-54A
MALIGNANT BONE TUMOR WITH MARKED
MINERALIZATION AS COMPARED TO
DESTRUCTION

1. Chondrosarcoma arising in benign cartilaginous lesion
2. Osteoblastic metastasis
3. Osteosarcoma (mature)
4. Parosteal osteosarcoma or chondrosarcoma

OSTEOBLASTIC METASTASES

COMMON

1. Breast carcinoma
2. Lymphoma
3. Prostate carcinoma

UNCOMMON

1. Carcinoid
2. Cerebellar medulloblastoma or sarcoma
3. Meningiosarcoma
4. [Osteosarcomatosis]
5. Other carcinoma (esp. carcinoma of lung, colon, pancreas, urinary bladder, ureter)

LOCALIZED PERIOSTEAL REACTION
(See also Gamuts D-58 and D-60)

COMMON

1. Arthritis (see Gamut D-133)
2. Fracture (traumatic, stress)
3. Histiocytosis X (esp. eosinophilic granuloma)
4. Malignant bone tumor (see Gamut D-52)
5. Osteoid osteoma
6. Osteomyelitis
7. Subperiosteal hemorrhage (eg, trauma, hemophilia)
8. Vascular stasis (eg, chronic venous or lymphatic insufficiency or obstruction)

UNCOMMON

1. Benign bone cyst or neoplasm with expansion or pathologic fracture
2. Chondroblastoma invading metaphysis
3. Infantile cortical hyperostosis (Caffey's disease)
4. Soft tissue ulcer
5. Syphilis; yaws
6. Vasculitis (eg, polyarteritis nodosa)

CODMAN TRIANGLE

COMMON

1. Malignant bone neoplasm, primary

UNCOMMON

1. Aneurysmal bone cyst
2. Healing fracture
3. Metastasis
4. Osteomyelitis
5. Subperiosteal hemorrhage (eg, hemophilia)

Reference:

Nelson SW: Some fundamentals in the radiologic differential diagnosis of solitary bone lesions. *Semin Roentgenol* 1:244–267, 1966.

WIDESPREAD OR GENERALIZED PERIOSTEAL REACTION

COMMON

1. Arthritis (eg, rheumatoid, Reiter's syndrome, psoriatic) (see Gamut D-133)
2. Battered child syndrome; other multiple trauma
3. Idiopathic
4. Hypertrophic osteoarthropathy (see Gamut D-61)
5. Prematurity; physiologic periostitis of newborn
6. Venous or lymphatic stasis

UNCOMMON

1. Caffey's disease
2. Cornelia de Lange syndrome
3. Cushing's syndrome with excess callus
4. Fluorosis
5. Gardner's syndrome
6. Gaucher's disease
7. Hemophilia
8. Histiocytosis X
9. Hypervitaminosis A
10. Osteomyelitis, multiple
11. Pachydermoperiostosis
12. Rickets, healing
13. Rubella syndrome
14. Scurvy
15. Syphilis; yaws

(Continued)

16. Thermal injury

17. Thyroid acropachy

18. Tuberous sclerosis

19. Widespread bone infarcts (esp. hand-foot syndrome in sickle cell anemia)

Reference:

Greenfield GB: *Radiology of Bone Diseases.* Philadelphia, JB Lippincott Co, 1969, p 312.

SYMMETRICAL PERIOSTITIS

COMMON

1. Hypertrophic osteoarthropathy (see Gamut D-61)
2. Leukemia, acute
3. Neuroblastoma metastases
4. Normal infant up to 4 months (physiologic periostitis of newborn)
5. Rheumatoid arthritis (esp. juvenile)
6. Trauma, symmetrical, including battered child
7. Venous or lymphatic stasis; varicose ulcers

UNCOMMON

1. Acromegaly (hands and feet)
2. Engelmann's disease
3. Histiocytosis X
4. Hypervitaminosis A
5. Hypervitaminosis D
6. Infantile cortical hyperostosis (Caffey's disease)
7. Osteomalacia (Milkman syndrome)
8. Pachydermoperiostosis
9. Reiter's syndrome
10. Rickets, healing
11. Rubella syndrome
12. Scurvy
13. Symmetrical osteomyelitis (eg, pyogenic, tuberculous, fungal)
14. Syphilis, congenital
15. Thyroid acropachy
16. Tuberous sclerosis

PERIOSTITIS IN A CHILD

COMMON

1. Histiocytosis X
2. Leukemia
3. Metastasis (eg, neuroblastoma, retinoblastoma, embryonal rhabdomyosarcoma)
4. Osteomyelitis (pyogenic, tuberculous, fungal)
5. Physiologic in early infancy
6. Rickets, all types
7. Sickle cell anemia (hand-foot syndrome)
8. Trauma (eg, callus, traumatic periostitis, battered child syndrome, stress fracture, osteogenesis imperfecta)

UNCOMMON

1. Engelmann's disease
2. Gaucher's disease; Niemann-Pick disease
3. Hemophilia, Christmas disease
4. Hypertrophic osteoarthropathy
5. Hypervitaminosis A
6. Infantile cortical hyperostosis (Caffey's disease)
7. Melorheostosis
8. Sarcoma of bone (eg, Ewing's, osteosarcoma)
9. Scurvy
10. Syphilis, congenital
11. Yaws

SUBGAMUT D-60A
CLUES TO THE BATTERED CHILD

1. "Bucket-handle" sign of metaphyseal fracture
2. Excessive callus formation
3. Intramural hematoma of intestine
4. Multiple fractures at different stages of healing
5. Subdural hematoma
6. Thoracic findings consistent with contusion (eg, local alveolar infiltrate without fever, pneumothorax, pneumo-mediastinum)
7. Underdevelopment, failure to thrive
8. Unsuspected or inadequately explained fractures

Reference:

LoPresti JM: Personal communication.

HYPERTROPHIC OSTEOARTHROPATHY

COMMON

1. Carcinoma of lung

UNCOMMON

1. Benign lung tumor (eg, bronchial adenoma)
2. Celiac disease
3. Chronic liver disease, cirrhosis
4. Chronic pulmonary infection (eg, tuberculosis, fungus disease, bronchiectasis, empyema)
5. Chronic ulcerative colitis
6. Cyanotic congenital heart disease
7. Familial
8. Gastrointestinal malignancy
9. Idiopathic
10. Lung abscess
11. Mesothelioma of pleura
12. Nasopharyngeal carcinoma (Schmincke tumor)
13. Pachydermoperiostosis
14. Polyarteritis nodosa
15. Pulmonary arteriovenous fistula
16. Pulmonary emphysema
17. Pulmonary metastases (esp. from osteosarcoma)
18. Thyroid acropachy

Reference:

Greenfield GB: *Radiology of Bone Diseases.* Philadelphia, JB Lippincott Co, 1969, p 440.

EXCESS CALLUS FORMATION

COMMON

1. Charcot joint
2. Cushing's syndrome; steroid therapy
3. Unrecognized trauma; battered child syndrome

UNCOMMON

1. Congenital insensitivity to pain
2. Familial
3. Paralytic states
4. Osteogenesis imperfecta
5. Renal osteodystrophy

SCLEROSIS OF BONE WITH PERIOSTEAL REACTION

COMMON

1. Healing fracture with callus
2. Malignant neoplasm (eg, Ewing's, osteosarcoma, chondro-sarcoma, lymphoma)
3. Osteoid osteoma
4. Osteomyelitis, including Garre's sclerosing osteomyelitis, Brodie's abscess

UNCOMMON

1. Infantile cortical hyperostosis (Caffey's disease)
2. Mycetoma, fungus disease
3. Syphilis
4. Tuberculosis
5. Yaws

MARKED CORTICAL HYPEROSTOSIS AND THICK PERIOSTEAL REACTION INVOLVING THE SHAFT OF A BONE

COMMON

1. Healing stress or march fracture
2. Osteoid osteoma
3. Reactive periostitis (idiopathic — usually due to trauma)
4. Subperiosteal osteomyelitis
5. Syphilis

UNCOMMON

1. [Cortical fibrous dysplasia (tibia only)]
2. Infantile cortical hyperostosis (Caffey's disease)
3. Melorheostosis
4. Pachydermoperiostosis
5. Yaws

EXTERNAL CORTICAL THICKENING
OF ONE OR MORE BONES
(See also Gamut D-66)

COMMON

1. Bowed bones (see Gamut D-71)
2. Fracture, healing or healed; traumatic periostitis
3. Hypertrophic osteoarthropathy (see Gamut D-61)
4. Osteoid osteoma
5. Osteomyelitis with involucrum; Garre's sclerosing osteo-myelitis; mycetoma
6. Paget's disease
7. Venous or lymphatic stasis

UNCOMMON

1. Bone tumor (esp. enchondroma)
2. Fibrous dysplasia
3. Hypervitaminosis A
4. Infantile cortical hyperostosis (Caffey's disease)
5. Melorheostosis
6. Pachydermoperiostosis
7. Scurvy or rickets, healing
8. Sickle cell anemia
9. Subperiosteal hemorrhage, old (trauma, hemophilia)
10. Syphilis, yaws (healed)
11. Thyroid acropachy
12. Tropical ulcer osteoma

WIDESPREAD CORTICAL THICKENING

COMMON

1. Diseases in which periosteal new bone has blended with the cortex (see Gamut D-63)
2. Fibrous dysplasia
3. Paget's disease

UNCOMMON

1. Acromegaly
2. Engelmann's disease
3. Hyperphosphatasia
4. Melorheostosis
5. Pyknodysostosis
6. Ribbing's disease (hereditary multiple diaphyseal sclerosis)
7. Tuberous sclerosis
8. Tubular stenosis (Kenny-Caffey)
9. Van Buchem's disease

Reference:

Greenfield GB: *Radiology of Bone Diseases.* Philadelphia, JB Lippincott Co, 1969, p 326.

"SPLIT" OR DOUBLE LAYER CORTEX

COMMON

1. Bone infarct (eg, sickle cell anemia)
2. Osteomyelitis

UNCOMMON

1. Battered child syndrome
2. Bone graft (local)
3. Gaucher's disease
4. Hyperphosphatasia
5. Osteopetrosis
6. Osteoporosis (esp. disuse, immobilization)
7. Scurvy

Reference:

Greenfield GB: *Radiology of Bone Diseases.* Philadelphia, JB Lippincott Co, 1969, p 327.

SCALLOPING, EROSION, OR RESORPTION
OF THE INNER CORTICAL MARGIN

COMMON

1. Chondroid lesion (eg, enchondroma, chondrosarcoma)
2. Histiocytosis X
3. Metastasis
4. Multiple myeloma
5. Nonossifying fibroma

UNCOMMON

1. Anemia (esp. thalassemia, sickle cell anemia)
2. Chondroblastoma
3. Chondromyxoid fibroma
4. Fibroma
5. Fibrous dysplasia
6. Gaucher's disease
7. Hyperparathyroidism
8. Lymphoma
9. Metaphyseal chondrodysplasia (Jansen)

Reference:

    Greenfield GB: *Radiology of Bone Diseases.*   Philadelphia, JB Lippin-
cott Co, 1969, p 327.

DESTRUCTION OR EROSION OF EXTERNAL SURFACE OF A BONE

COMMON

1. Absorption of terminal phalanx (see Gamuts D-89 and D-89A)
2. Benign soft tissue tumor (eg, hemangioma, neurofibroma)
3. Cortical desmoid (esp. lower posterior femur)
4. Fibrous cortical defect
5. Gouty tophus
6. Synovial lesion (eg, giant cell tumor of tendon sheath, pigmented villonodular synovitis, synovioma)

UNCOMMON

1. Aneurysm adjacent to bone
2. Glomus tumor
3. Metastasis
4. Other parosteal or periosteal tumor (see Gamut D-50)
5. Periosteal chondroma or fibroma
6. Primary bone neoplasm
7. Squamous cell carcinoma of skin; malignant tropical ulcer
8. Subperiosteal hematoma
9. Subperiosteal osteomyelitis
10. Tuberculosis of soft tissues

POLYOSTOTIC BONE LESIONS*

ADULTS

COMMON

1. Arthritic or synovial cystic lesions
2. Brown tumors of hyperparathyroidism
3. Metastases
4. Multiple myeloma
5. Osteomyelitis (bacterial, tuberculous, fungal)
6. Paget's disease

UNCOMMON

1. Amyloidosis
2. Anemia
3. Gaucher's disease, Niemann-Pick disease
4. Hydatid disease
5. Leprosy
6. Lymphoma
7. Mastocytosis
8. Polyvinyl chloride poisoning
9. Sarcoidosis
10. Syphilis, yaws
11. Tuberous sclerosis

CHILDREN 5–15 YEARS

COMMON

1. Anemia
2. Enchondromatosis (Ollier's disease); Maffucci's syndrome
3. Fibrocystic lesions (eg, polyostotic fibrous dysplasia, nonossifying fibromas)

(Continued)

4. Histiocytosis X
5. Osteochondrodysplasias (see Gamut D-1)
6. Osteomyelitis (bacterial, tuberculous, fungal)

UNCOMMON

1. Ewing's sarcoma metastases
2. Gaucher's disease, Niemann-Pick disease
3. Granulomatous disease of children (leukocyte abnormality)
4. Hemangiomatosis, lymphangiomatosis
5. Hemophilia
6. Leprosy
7. Leukemia, lymphoma
8. Mastocytosis
9. Melorheostosis
10. Metastases
11. Mucopolysaccharidoses; mucolipidoses
12. Multiple cartilaginous exostoses
13. Osteosarcomatosis
14. Syphilis, yaws

INFANTS AND CHILDREN UP TO 5 YEARS

COMMON

1. Anemia
2. Battered child syndrome
3. Histiocytosis X
4. Leukemia
5. Metastases (esp. neuroblastoma)
6. Osteochondrodysplasias (see Gamut D-1)
7. Osteomyelitis

(Continued)

POLYOSTOTIC BONE LESIONS*
(Continued)

8. Physiologic periostitis (up to 6 months)
9. Rickets
10. Transplacental infection (toxoplasmosis, rubella, cytomegalic inclusion disease, herpes, syphilis)

UNCOMMON

1. Congenital fibromatosis
2. Hypervitaminosis A
3. Infantile cortical hyperostosis (Caffey's disease)
4. Mucopolysaccharidoses; mucolipidoses
5. Osteogenesis imperfecta
6. Osteopetrosis
7. Scurvy
8. Yaws

*There may be overlap of entities among these three age groups.

BOWED BONES, SINGLE OR MULTIPLE

COMMON

*1. Congenital (prenatal) bowing of long bones

2. Fibrous dysplasia

3. Osteomalacia (see Gamut D-24)

4. Paget's disease

*5. Physiologic bowing

6. Poliomyelitis

7. Rickets, all types

8. Tibia vara (Blount's disease)

UNCOMMON

*1. Achondroplasia

*2. Campomelic dwarfism

*3. Congenital pseudarthrosis

*4. Cornelia de Lange S.

5. Dyschondrosteosis (radius and tibia)

6. Enchondromatosis (Ollier's disease); Maffucci's S.

*7. Hemihypertrophy

8. Hydatid disease

9. Hyperphosphatasia

10. Hyperparathyroidism, osteitis fibrosa cystica

*11. Hypophosphatasia

12. Klippel-Trenaunay-Weber S. (eg, arteriovenous fistula, hemangioma, lipomatosis)

13. Madelung's deformity

*14. Metaphyseal chondrodysplasias, all types

(Continued)

BOWED BONES, SINGLE OR MULTIPLE
(Continued)

15. Neurofibromatosis
*16. Osteogenesis imperfecta
17. Osteomyelitis, severe (eg, bacterial, yaws, smallpox)
*18. Parastremmatic dwarfism
*19. Pseudohypoparathyroidism
*20. Spondylometaphyseal dysplasia (Kozlowski)
21. Syphilis (sabre shin)
*22. Thanatophoric dwarfism
23. Weismann-Netter S.

*Bowed limbs in infancy.

PSEUDOFRACTURES (LOOSER'S ZONES)

COMMON

1. Osteomalacia (see Gamut D-24)
2. Paget's disease
3. Rickets
4. [Stress fracture; spondylolysis]

UNCOMMON

1. Fibrous dysplasia, including Albright's syndrome
2. Hyperphosphatasia
3. Hypophosphatasia
4. Osteogenesis imperfecta tarda
5. Renal osteodystrophy

Reference:

Greenfield GB: *Radiology of Bone Diseases.* Philadelphia, JB Lippincott Co, 1969, p 19.

PSEUDARTHROSIS

1. Congenital
2. Fibrous dysplasia
3. Neurofibromatosis
4. Nonunion of a fracture
5. Osteogenesis imperfecta

Reference:

Greenfield GB: *Radiology of Bone Diseases.*   Philadelphia, JB Lippincott Co, 1969, p 223.

CONGENITAL ABNORMALITIES OF THE THUMBS

I. ABSENT THUMB

1. Bird-headed dwarfism (Seckel's S.)
2. Fanconi's S. (pancytopenia-dysmelia S.)
3. Francischetti's S.
4. Holt-Oram S.
5. Phocomelia (eg, thalidomide poisoning)
6. Ring D chromosome S.
7. Rothmund's S.
8. Trisomy 18 S.

II. HYPOPLASTIC OR SHORT THUMB

1. Aminopterin-induced S.
2. Basal cell nevus S. (Gorlin)
3. Brachydactyly C or D; hereditary shortness of thumbs
4. Cornelia de Lange S.
5. Diastrophic dwarfism
6. Ectodermal dysplasia
7. Fanconi's S. (pancytopenia-dysmelia S.)
8. Hand-foot-uterus S.
9. Holt-Oram S.
10. Isolated anomaly
11. Long arm 18 deletion S.
12. Myositis (fibrodysplasia) ossificans progressiva
13. Otopalatodigital S.
14. Phocomelia (eg, thalidomide poisoning)
15. Rubinstein-Taybi S.

(Continued)

CONGENITAL ABNORMALITIES OF THE THUMBS
(Continued)

16. Thrombocytopenia — absent radius (TAR) S.
17. Trisomy 18 S.

III. WIDE THUMB

1. Acrocephalopolysyndactyly (Carpenter's S.)
2. Acrocephalosyndactyly (Apert's S.)
3. Larsen's S.
4. Leri's pleonosteosis
5. Otopalatodigital S.
6. Rubinstein-Taybi S.
7. Trisomy 13 S.

IV. ENLARGED THUMB

1. Angioma
2. Isolated anomaly
3. Neurofibromatosis
4. Triphalangeal thumb (eg, Blackfan-Diamond anemia)

V. "ECTOPIC" THUMB (ABNORMAL POSITION)

1. Cornelia de Lange S. (proximally placed thumb)
2. Diastrophic dwarfism ("hitchhiker thumb")
3. Rubinstein-Taybi S. (radially curved thumb)
4. Whistling face S. (flexed thumb overlaps palm)

(Continued)

References:

1. Caffey J: *Pediatric X-ray Diagnosis*, ed 6. Chicago, Year Book Medical Publishers, 1972.

2. Poznanski AK: *The Hand in Radiologic Diagnosis*. Philadelphia, WB Saunders Co, 1974, pp 157–159, 166–167.

3. Smith DW: *Recognizable Patterns of Human Malformation*. Philadelphia, WB Saunders Co, 1970.

CLINODACTYLY OF THE FIFTH FINGER

COMMON

1. Cornelia de Lange S.
2. Down's S. (mongolism)
3. Familial brachydactyly types A-1, A-3, C
4. Holt-Oram S.
5. Local disorder (eg, trauma, arthritis, contracture)
6. Normal variant, isolated anomaly
7. Oculodentodigital S.
8. Orodigitofacial S.
9. Otopalatodigital S.
10. Symphalangism

UNCOMMON

1. Aarskog-Scott S. (shawl scrotum S.)
2. Acrocephalopolysyndactyly (Carpenter's S.)
3. Bird-headed dwarfism (Seckel's S.)
4. Bloom's S.
5. Cat-cry S.
6. Cerebrohepatorenal S.
7. Fanconi's S. (pancytopenia-dysmelia S.)
8. Focal dermal hypoplasia (Goltz S.)
9. G deletion S. II
10. Hand-foot-uterus S.
11. [Kirner's deformity (distal phalanx)]
12. Laurence-Moon-Biedl S.
13. Marfan's S.

(Continued)

14. Myositis (fibrodysplasia) ossificans progressiva

15. Myotonic dystrophy

16. Noonan's S.

17. Osteo-onychodysplasia (nail-patella S.)

18. Pectoral aplasia-syndactyly S. (Poland's S.)

19. Popliteal pterygium S.

20. Prader-Willi S.

21. Rhinotrichophalangeal S.

22. Rubinstein-Taybi S.

23. Russell-Silver S.

24. Thrombocytopenia — absent radius (TAR) S.

25. Treacher Collins S.

26. Trisomy 18 S.

27. Turner's S.

28. XXXXX S.

29. XXXXY S.

References:

1. Edeiken J, Hodes PJ: *Roentgen Diagnosis of Diseases of Bone*, ed 2. Baltimore, Williams & Wilkins Co, 1973, pp 61–65.

2. Poznanski AK: *The Hand in Radiologic Diagnosis.* Philadelphia, WB Saunders Co, 1974, pp 208–216.

3. Poznanski AK, Pratt GB, Manson G, Weiss L: Clinodactyly, camptodactyly, Kirner's deformity, and other crooked fingers. *Radiology 93:573–582, 1969.*

4. Smith DW: *Recognizable Patterns of Human Malformation.* Philadelphia, WB Saunders Co, 1970.

CONGENITAL SYNDROMES WITH SHORT PHALANGES (OTHER THAN FIFTH FINGER)

1. Acrocephalopolysyndactyly (Carpenter's S.)
2. Acrocephalosyndactyly (Apert's S.)
3. Asphyxiating thoracic dysplasia
4. Basal cell nevus S. (Gorlin)
5. Cleidocranial dysplasia
6. Cornelia de Lange S.
7. Diastrophic dwarfism
8. Dilantin therapy to mother
9. Familial brachydactylies
10. Fanconi's S. (pancytopenia-dysmelia S.)
11. Holt-Oram S.
12. Myositis (fibrodysplasia) ossificans progressiva
13. Otopalatodigital S.
14. Poland's S.
15. Rhinotrichophalangeal S.
16. Rubinstein-Taybi S.
17. Trisomy 13 S.
18. Trisomy 18 S.

Reference:

Poznanski AK: *The Hand in Radiologic Diagnosis.* Philadelphia, WB Saunders Co, 1974, pp 155–167.

CONGENITAL SYNDROMES WITH SHORT MIDDLE PHALANX OF FIFTH FINGER

1. Bloom's S.

2. Cornelia de Lange S.

3. Down's S. (mongolism)

4. Familial brachydactyly A-3

5. Focal dermal hypoplasia (Goltz S.)

6. Hand-foot-uterus S.

7. Holt-Oram S.

8. Myositis (fibrodysplasia) ossificans progressiva

9. Noonan's S.

10. Oculodentodigital S.

11. Otopalatodigital S.

12. Poland's S.

13. Popliteal pterygium S.

14. Russell-Silver S.

15. Symphalangism

16. Thrombocytopenia — absent radius (TAR) S.

17. Treacher Collins S.

18. Trisomy 18 S.

19. XXXXY S.

Reference:

Poznanski AK: *The Hand in Radiologic Diagnosis.* Philadelphia, WB Saunders Co, 1974, p 159.

SPONTANEOUS AMPUTATION OF FINGERS OR PHALANGES IN CHILDREN

COMMON

1. Frostbite, burn, electroshock, other trauma

UNCOMMON

1. Ainhum
2. Congenital indifference to pain
3. Familial dysautonomia
4. Familial hyperuricosemia
5. Intravascular coagulation states (eg, meningococcemia)
6. Leprosy
7. Lesch-Nyhan S.
8. Psychotic states
9. Streeter's bands (congenital amniotic bands)
10. Vascular insufficiency

CLUBBING OF THE FINGERS

COMMON

1. Bronchogenic carcinoma
2. Cirrhosis of liver
3. Congenital heart disease
4. Pulmonary hypertrophic osteoarthropathy (see Gamut D-61)
5. Pulmonary interstitial fibrosis; pneumoconiosis (see Gamuts F-13 and F-43)

UNCOMMON

1. Acromegaly
2. Colitis, chronic (eg, ulcerative, amebic)
3. [Hyperparathyroidism]
4. Idiopathic
5. [Metastases to fingers]
6. Myxedema; thyroid acropachy
7. Pachydermoperiostosis
8. Polycythemia
9. Sprue
10. Subacute bacterial endocarditis
11. Urinary tract infection, chronic

Reference:

Greenfield GB: *Radiology of Bone Diseases.* Philadelphia, JB Lippincott Co, 1969, p 440.

CONGENITAL SYNDROMES WITH ACCESSORY CARPAL OSSICLES

1. Brachydactyly A-1
2. Chondroectodermal dysplasia (Ellis-Van Creveld S.)
3. Diastrophic dwarfism
4. Hand-foot-uterus S.
5. Holt-Oram S.
6. Larsen's S.
7. Otopalatodigital S.
8. Ulnar dimelia

Reference:

Poznanski AK: *The Hand in Radiologic Diagnosis.* Philadelphia, WB Saunders Co, 1974, pp 140–145.

CARPAL FUSION

COMMON

1. Arthritis (esp. rheumatoid, pyogenic)
2. Normal variant, isolated anomaly (esp. triquetrum-lunate fusion)
3. Symphalangism

UNCOMMON

1. Acrocephalosyndactyly (Apert's S.)
2. Aminopterin-induced S.
3. Arthrogryposis multiplex congenita
4. Bird-headed dwarfism (Seckel's S.)
5. Carpal-tarsal fusion
6. Chondroectodermal dysplasia (Ellis-Van Creveld S.)
7. Cornelia de Lange S.
8. Dermatomyositis
9. Diastrophic dwarfism
10. Dyschondrosteosis
11. Hand-foot-uterus S.
12. Holt-Oram S.
13. Osteomyelitis
14. Otopalatodigital S.
15. Polydactyly
16. Post-traumatic; postsurgical
17. Turner's S.
18. Ulnar dimelia

Reference:

Poznanski AK: *The Hand in Radiologic Diagnosis.* Philadelphia, WB Saunders Co, 1974, pp 145–152.

SYNDACTYLY (CUTANEOUS OR OSSEOUS)

COMMON

1. Acrocephalopolysyndactyly (Carpenter's S.)
2. Acrocephalosyndactyly (Apert's S.)
3. Oculodentodigital S.

UNCOMMON

1. Aarskog-Scott S. (shawl scrotum S.)
2. Aminopterin-induced S.
3. Bloom's S.
4. Brachydactyly B
5. Chondrodysplasia punctata (Conradi's disease)
6. Cornelia de Lange S.
7. Down's S. (mongolism) (toes)
8. Ectodermal dysplasia, Robinson type
9. Fanconi's S. (pancytopenia-dysmelia S.)
10. Focal dermal hypoplasia (Goltz S.)
11. Hallerman-Streiff S.
12. Incontinentia pigmenti S.
13. Laurence-Moon-Biedl S.
14. Neurofibromatosis
15. Orodigitofacial S.
16. Otopalatodigital S.
17. Pectoral aplasia-syndactyly S. (Poland's S.)
18. Pierre-Robin S.
19. Polydactyly-syndactyly S.
20. Popliteal pterygium S.

(Continued)

21. Prader-Willi S.

22. Pseudohypoparathyroidism

23. Russell-Silver S.

24. Smith-Lemli-Opitz S.

25. Thrombocytopenia — absent radius (TAR) S.

26. Trisomy 13 S.

27. Trisomy 18 S.

References:

1. Edeiken J, Hodes PJ: *Roentgen Diagnosis of Diseases of Bone*, ed 2. Baltimore, Williams & Wilkins Co, 1973, p 61.

2. Poznanski AK: *The Hand in Radiologic Diagnosis.* Philadelphia, WB Saunders Co, 1974, pp 204–207.

POLYDACTYLY

COMMON

1. Acrocephalopolysyndactyly (Carpenter's S.)
2. Chondroectodermal dysplasia (Ellis-Van Creveld S.)
3. Isolated anomaly

UNCOMMON

1. Asphyxiating thoracic dysplasia
2. Biemond's S.
3. Blackfan-Diamond anemia
4. Bloom's S.
5. Brachydactyly B
6. Chondrodysplasia punctata (Conradi's disease)
7. Ectodermal dysplasia, Robinson type
8. Fanconi's S. (pancytopenia-dysmelia S.)
9. Focal dermal hypoplasia (Goltz S.)
10. Holt-Oram S.
11. Laurence-Moon-Biedl S.
12. Mesomelic dwarfism variant
13. Orodigitofacial S. I and II
14. Polydactyly-syndactyly S.
15. Rubinstein-Taybi S.
16. Short-rib polysyndactyly S.
17. Smith-Lemli-Opitz S.
18. Trisomy 13 S.
19. Ulnar dimelia

(Continued)

References:

1. Edeiken J, Hodes PJ: *Roentgen Diagnosis of Diseases of Bone*, ed 2. Baltimore, Williams & Wilkins Co, 1973, p 61.

2. Poznanski AK: *The Hand in Radiologic Diagnosis.* Philadelphia, WB Saunders Co, 1974, pp 197–204.

3. Smith, DW: *Recognizable Patterns of Human Malformation.* Philadelphia, WB Saunders Co, 1970.

BRACHYDACTYLY
(See also Gamuts D-76, D-85, and D-86)

COMMON

1. Acro-osteolysis (eg, congenital, leprosy) (see Gamut D-89)
2. Congenital syndromes with short hands and feet (esp. chondrodysplasias, mucopolysaccharidoses) (see Gamut D-86)
3. Congenital syndromes with short metacarpals or metatarsals (see Gamut D-85)
4. Congenital syndromes with short phalanges (see Gamut D-76)
5. Osteomyelitis (eg, bacterial, yaws, smallpox)
6. Sickle cell anemia (hand-foot syndrome)
7. Trauma (eg, thermal, electrical, epiphyseal cartilage injury, fracture)

UNCOMMON

1. Arthritis
2. Basal cell nevus S. (Gorlin)
3. Cone-shaped epiphyses (see Gamut D-15)
4. Enchondromatosis (Ollier's disease)
5. Familial brachydactylies
6. Idiopathic
7. Kaschin-Beck disease (in Manchuria, Russia)
8. Myositis (fibrodysplasia) ossificans progressiva
9. Oculodentodigital S.
10. Orodigitofacial S.
11. Pseudohypoparathyroidism, pseudopseudohypoparathyroidism
12. Smith-Lemli-Opitz S.
13. Turner's S.
14. Weill-Marchesani S.

(Continued)

References:

1. Greenfield GB: *Radiology of Bone Diseases.* Philadelphia, JB Lippincott Co, 1969, p 223.

2. Poznanski AK: *The Hand in Radiologic Diagnosis.* Philadelphia, WB Saunders Co, 1974, pp 153–176.

SHORT METACARPALS OR METATARSALS (EXCLUDING GENERALIZED SHORTENING)

COMMON

1. Idiopathic (isolated anomaly)
2. Osteomyelitis (eg, bacterial, yaws, smallpox)
3. Post-infarction (eg, sickle cell anemia)
4. Trauma (eg, thermal, electrical, epiphyseal cartilage injury, fracture)

UNCOMMON

1. Basal cell nevus S. (Gorlin)
2. Beckwith-Wiedemann visceromegaly S.
3. Biemond's S. (4th metacarpal)
4. Brachydactylies, familial
5. Cat-cry S. (5th metacarpal)
6. Chondrodysplasia punctata (Conradi's disease)
7. Cockayne's S.
8. Cornelia de Lange S. (thumb)
9. Diastrophic dwarfism (hitchhiker thumb)
10. Dyschondrosteosis (4th metacarpal)
11. Epiphyseal dysplasia
12. Fanconi's S. (pancytopenia-dysmelia S.) (thumb)
13. Hand-foot-uterus S. (thumb)
14. Holt-Oram S.
15. Klinefelter's S.
16. Larsen's S.
17. Leri's pleonosteosis

(Continued)

18. Long arm 18 deletion S. (thumb)

19. Multiple hereditary osteocartilaginous exostoses

20. Myositis (fibrodysplasia) ossificans progressiva (thumb and great toe)

21. Neonatal hyperthyroidism

22. Orodigitofacial S.

23. Peripheral dysostosis

24. Pseudohypoparathyroidism, pseudopseudohypoparathyroidism

25. Radial hypoplasias (thumb)

26. Radiation or radium injury

27. Rhinotrichophalangeal S.

28. Rubinstein-Taybi S. (thumb and great toe)

29. Russell-Silver S. (5th metacarpal)

30. Turner's S. (4th metacarpal)

References:

1. Edeiken J, Hodes PJ: *Roentgen Diagnosis of Diseases of Bone*, ed 2. Baltimore, Williams & Wilkins Co, 1973, p 61.

2. Jacobson HG, Siegelman SS: Refresher course syllabus.

3. Poznanski AK: *The Hand in Radiologic Diagnosis*. Philadelphia, WB Saunders Co, 1974, pp 166–169.

CONGENITAL SYNDROMES WITH SHORT HANDS AND FEET
(See also Subgamut D-86A)

COMMON

1. Achondroplasia
2. Enchondromatosis (Ollier's disease)
3. Mucopolysaccharidosis (eg, Hurler, Hunter, Morquio)

UNCOMMON

1. Aarskog-Scott S. (shawl scrotum S.)
2. Chondroectodermal dysplasia (Ellis-Van Creveld S.)
3. Cockayne's S.
4. Diastrophic dwarfism
5. Hypochondroplasia
6. Metaphyseal chondrodysplasia
7. Metatropic dwarfism
8. Multiple cartilaginous exostoses
9. Multiple epiphyseal dysplasia (Fairbank)
10. Noonan's S.
11. Orodigitofacial S.
12. Peripheral dysostosis
13. Prader-Willi S.
14. Progeria
15. Pseudohypoparathyroidism, pseudopseudohypoparathyroidism
16. Rhinotrichophalangeal S.
17. Smith-Lemli-Opitz S.

(Continued)

18. Spondyloepiphyseal dysplasia, pseudoachondroplastic type

19. Spondylometaphyseal dysplasia

20. Thanatophoric dwarfism

21. Weill-Marchesani S.

References:

1. Dorst J: Personal communication.

2. Felson B: Dwarfs and Other Little People. *Semin Roentgenol* **8:257,** 1973.

SUBGAMUT D-86A
ACQUIRED DISEASES CAUSING SHORT
HANDS AND FEET

1. Acro-osteolysis (see Gamut D-89)
2. Leprosy
3. Lipoid dermatoarthritis
4. Osteomyelitis, severe (eg, bacterial, yaws, smallpox)
5. Rheumatoid arthritis, arthritis mutilans ("opera glass hands")
6. Sickle cell anemia

ABNORMAL TAPERING OF SHORT TUBULAR BONES OF THE HANDS AND FEET

I. PROXIMAL TAPERING

1. Cornelia de Lange syndrome
2. Mucopolysaccharidosis (eg, Hurler, Hunter, Morquio); mucolipidosis

II. DISTAL TAPERING

1. Acro-osteolysis (see Gamut D-89)
2. Diabetes mellitus
3. Epidermolysis bullosa
4. Hyperparathyroidism
5. Leprosy
6. Other neurotrophic diseases
7. Raynaud's disease
8. Scleroderma
9. Thermal injury

Reference:

Greenfield GB: *Radiology of Bone Diseases.* Philadelphia, JB Lippincott Co, 1969, p 223.

NEUROTROPHIC BONE CHANGES
(POINTED OR SPINDLED BONES)
IN THE HANDS OR FEET

COMMON

1. [Amputation (congenital, traumatic, or surgical)]
2. Arteriosclerosis obliterans
3. Burn, thermal or electric; frostbite
4. Diabetes
5. Psoriatic arthritis
6. Rheumatoid arthritis
7. Scleroderma, dermatomyositis
8. Spinal cord trauma or disease (eg, pernicious anemia, syringomyelia, spina bifida, meningomyelocele, neoplasm)
9. Trophic ulcer of soft tissue with underlying destruction

UNCOMMON

1. [Acro-osteolysis (eg, polyvinyl chloride)] (see Gamut D-89)
2. [Ainhum]
3. [Clubbing of fingers]
4. Congenital acro-osteolysis
5. Congenital indifference to pain
6. Congenital pseudarthrosis
7. Ergot intoxication
8. Hicks' syndrome (familial sensory neural radiculopathy)
9. Idiopathic (eg, sensory neuropathy in alcoholism?)
10. Leprosy
11. Peripheral nerve injury

(Continued)

12. Porphyria

13. [Pyknodysostosis]

14. Raynaud's disease; Buerger's disease

15. Tabes dorsalis

16. Trench foot

References:

1. Gondos B: The pointed tubular bone. *Radiology* 105:541–545, 1972.

2. Hodgson JR, Pugh DG, Young HH: Roentgenologic aspect of certain lesions of bone: neurotrophic or infectious? *Radiology* 50:65–70, 1948.

EROSION OF MULTIPLE TERMINAL PHALANGEAL TUFTS (ACRO-OSTEOLYSIS)

COMMON

1. Arteriosclerosis obliterans
2. Burn, thermal or electrical
3. Diabetic gangrene
4. Frostbite
5. Hyperparathyroidism, primary or secondary
6. Neurotrophic disease (see Gamut D-88)
7. Psoriasis
8. Raynaud's disease
9. Rheumatoid arthritis
*10. Scleroderma, dermatomyositis
11. Trauma

UNCOMMON

1. Brachydactyly B
2. Buerger's disease
3. Clubbing of fingers (see Gamut D-79)
4. Congenital (familial) acro-osteolysis (eg, Hajdu–Cheney S.)
5. Congenital indifference to pain
6. Disseminated lipogranulomatosis
7. Drug therapy (eg, dilantin, phenobarbital, ergot)
8. Ectodermal dysplasia
*9. Epidermolysis bullosa
*10. Gout
11. Leprosy

(Continued)

12. Lesch-Nyhan S. (mental defective finger biting)

13. Osteomalacia (eg, malabsorption syndromes)

14. Osteopetrosis

15. Pachydermoperiostosis

16. Pityriasis rubra

17. Plantar warts

18. Polyvinyl chloride osteolysis

19. Porphyria

20. Progeria; Werner's S.

21. Pseudoxanthoma elasticum

22. Pyknodysostosis

23. Reticulohistiocytoma (lipoid dermatoarthritis)

*24. Rothmund's S.

25. Sarcoidosis

26. Sjögren's syndrome

27. Streeter's congenital amniotic bands

28. Syringomyelia

29. Tabes dorsalis

*30. Thromboangiitis obliterans

*May be associated with calcification.

References:

1. Greenfield GB: *Radiology of Bone Diseases*. Philadelphia, JB Lippincott Co, 1969, p 304.
2. Moss AA, Mainzer F: Osteopetrosis: an unusual cause of terminal-tuft erosion. *Radiology* 97:631-632, 1970.

SUBGAMUT D-89A
ACRO-OSTEOLYSIS CONFINED TO ONE DIGIT

1. Angiomatous malformation
2. Carcinoma of nail bed
3. Epidermoid cyst
4. Fibroma
5. Giant cell tumor of tendon sheath
6. Glomus tumor
7. Infection (eg, whitlow, osteomyelitis)
8. Metastasis; lymphoma
9. Neurofibroma

CONGENITAL SYNDROMES ASSOCIATED WITH AN ABNORMAL CARPAL ANGLE*

DECREASED ANGLE (LESS THAN 124°)

1. Dyschondrosteosis
2. Hurler S.
3. Madelung's deformity
4. Morquio S.
5. Turner's S.

INCREASED ANGLE (GREATER THAN 139°)

1. Arthrogryposis
2. Diastrophic dwarfism
3. Down's S. (mongolism)
4. Epiphyseal dysplasias
5. Frontometaphyseal dysplasia
6. Otopalatodigital S.
7. Spondyloepiphyseal dysplasia

*Normal carpal angle according to Kosowicz is 131.5° ($\pm$ 7.2°)

Reference:

Poznanski AK: *The Hand in Radiologic Diagnosis.* Philadelphia, WB Saunders Co, 1974, pp 138–140.

CYST-LIKE LESION IN A PHALANX
(SOLITARY OR MULTIPLE)

COMMON

*1. Arthritis (esp. gout, rheumatoid arthritis, osteoarthritis)

2. Bone cyst

*3. Enchondroma

UNCOMMON

1. Angioma

2. [Carcinoma of nail bed]

3. Chondromyxoid fibroma; chondroblastoma; chondro-sarcoma

4. Cystic osteomyelitis

5. Epidermoid inclusion cyst (distal phalanx)

6. Giant cell tumor

7. [Glomus tumor (distal phalanx)]

8. Hemophilic pseudotumor

*9. Leprosy (leproma)

*10. Metastasis (esp. lung, breast)

*11. Myeloma

*12. Sarcoidosis

*13. [Synovial lesion (eg, villonodular synovitis, giant cell tumor of tendon sheath)]

14. Thorn granuloma

15. Tuberculosis ("spina ventosa")

*16. Tuberous sclerosis

*17. Wilson's disease

*May be multiple

DACTYLITIS

COMMON

1. Pyogenic osteomyelitis (esp. salmonella)
2. Sickle cell anemia ("hand-foot syndrome" — infarction with or without osteomyelitis)
3. Tuberculosis ("spina ventosa")

UNCOMMON

1. Atypical mycobacteria infection
2. Fungus disease (eg, mycetoma, coccidioidomycosis, blastomycosis, sporotrichosis, Histoplasmosis duboisii)
3. Leprosy
4. [Leukemia]
5. Sarcoidosis
6. Smallpox
7. Syphilis
8. Yaws

CONGENITAL ABNORMALITY OF THE GREAT TOE

COMMON

1. Acrocephalosyndactyly (Apert's S.)
2. Myositis (fibrodysplasia) ossificans progressiva
3. Otopalatodigital S.
4. Rubinstein-Taybi S.

UNCOMMON

1. Acrocephalopolysyndactyly (Carpenter's S.)
2. Cleidocranial dysplasia
3. Cornelia de Lange S.
4. Diastrophic dwarfism
5. Hand-foot-uterus S.
6. Larsen's S.
7. Leri's pleonosteosis
8. Orodigitofacial S.
9. Popliteal pterygium S.
10. Trisomy 13 S.
11. Trisomy 18 S.
12. Whistling face S. (Freeman-Sheldon S.)

Reference:

Poznanski AK: Foot manifestations of the congenital malformation syndromes. *Semin Roentgenol* 5:354–366, 1970.

CONGENITAL SYNDROMES ASSOCIATED WITH CLUBFOOT OR OTHER FOOT DEFORMITY

1. Aminopterin-induced S. (varus)
2. Arthrogryposis multiplex congenita
3. Bloom's S.
4. Cerebrohepatorenal S. (Zellweger)
5. Chondrodysplasia punctata (Conradi's disease)
6. Chondroectodermal dysplasia (Ellis-Van Creveld S.) (valgus)
7. Cornelia de Lange S.
8. Diastrophic dwarfism
9. Ehlers-Danlos S.
10. Homocystinuria (pes planus or cavus, everted feet)
11. Larsen's S.
12. Long arm 18 deletion S.
13. Marfan's S. (long great toes, hammertoes)
14. Mietens-Weber S. (pes valgus planus)
15. Mucopolysaccharidosis (eg, Hurler, Hunter, Morquio) (pes cavus or planus; misshapen tarsals)
16. Mytonic dystrophy
17. Nail-patella S. (hereditary osteo-onychodysplasia)
18. Neurofibromatosis
19. Otopalatodigital S. (tarsal fusion)
20. Popliteal pterygium S.
21. Short arm 4 deletion S.
22. Smith-Lemli-Opitz S.
23. Thrombocytopenia — absent radius (TAR) S.
24. Trisomy 13 S.

(Continued)

CONGENITAL SYNDROMES ASSOCIATED WITH CLUBFOOT OR OTHER FOOT DEFORMITY
(Continued)

25. Trisomy 18 S.

26. Whistling face S. (Freeman-Sheldon S.)

27. XXXXX S.

28. XXXXY S.

References:

1. Poznanski AK: Foot manifestations of the congenital malformation syndromes. *Semin Roentgenol* 5:354–366, 1970.

2. Smith DW: *Recognizable Patterns of Human Malformation*. Philadelphia, WB Saunders Co, 1970.

HYPOPLASIA OF THE RADIUS*

COMMON

1. Isolated anomaly

UNCOMMON

1. Bird-headed dwarfism (Seckel's S.)
2. Cornelia de Lange S.
3. Dyschondrosteosis
4. Ectodermal dysplasia
5. Fanconi's S. (pancytopenia-dysmelia S.)
6. Holt-Oram S.
7. Mesomelic dwarfism
8. Phocomelia (eg, thalidomide poisoning)
9. Ring D chromosome S.
10. Thrombocytopenia — absent radius (TAR) S.
11. Trisomy 13 S.
12. Trisomy 18 S.

*Radial hypoplasia may be seen with certain congenital heart diseases, renal anomalies, esophageal, duodenal, or anal atresia, rib anomalies, Klippel-Feil syndrome, kyphoscoliosis, and hypoplasia or spina bifida of the lumbosacral spine.

References:

1. Edeiken J, Hodes PJ: *Roentgen Diagnosis of Diseases of Bone,* ed 2. Baltimore, Williams & Wilkins Co, 1973, p 61.
2. Poznanski AK. *The Hand in Radiologic Diagnosis.* Philadelphia, WB Saunders Co, 1974, pp 176–180.
3. Smith DW: *Recognizable Patterns of Human Malformation.* Philadelphia, WB Saunders Co, 1970.

CONGENITAL SYNDROMES WITH ELBOW ANOMALY[1]
(See also Gamut D-95)

COMMON

1. Enchondromatosis (Ollier's disease)
*2. Multiple cartilaginous exostoses
*3. Osteo-onychodysplasia (nail-patella S.)
4. Turner's S.

UNCOMMON

1. Cerebrohepatorenal S.
2. Chondroectodermal dysplasia (Ellis-Van Creveld S.)
3. Cleidocranial dysplasia
*4. Cornelia de Lange S.
5. Diastrophic dwarfism
*6. Dyschondrosteosis
*7. Familial idiopathic acro-osteolysis
*8. Fanconi's S. (pancytopenia-dysmelia S.)
9. Holt-Oram S.
10. Idiopathic; isolated anomaly
11. Klinefelter S.
12. Larsen's S.
*13. Mietens-Weber S.
*14. Noonan's S.
15. Oculodentodigital S.
*16. Otopalatodigital S.

(Continued)

17. Pseudohypoparathyroidism

18. Thrombocytopenia — absent radius (TAR) S.

19. Trisomy 18 S.

20. XXXXY S.

¹Usually absence or dysplasia of radial head.

*Radioulnar dislocation (proximal)

References:

1. Greenfield GB: *Radiology of Bone Diseases*. Philadelphia, JB Lippincott Co, 1969, p 224.

2. Smith DW: *Recognizable Patterns of Human Malformation*. Philadelphia, WB Saunders Co, 1970.

GROOVED DEFECT OF THE HUMERAL HEAD

COMMON

1. Chronic dislocation (Hill-Sachs defect)
2. Rheumatoid arthritis

UNCOMMON

1. Atrophy from rotator cuff tear
2. Fracture of greater tuberosity
3. Hemophilia
4. [Humerus varus]
5. [Neuropathic (Charcot) joint]
6. Rickets
7. Tuberculosis

Reference:

Hill HA, Sachs MD: The grooved defect of the humeral head. *Radiology* 35:690–700, 1940.

LESION OF THE SCAPULA IN A CHILD

COMMON

1. Benign bone tumor (eg, osteochondroma, enchondroma)
2. Fracture

UNCOMMON

1. Erb's paralysis
2. Histiocytosis X
3. Hypoplasia (see Subgamut D-98A)
4. Infantile cortical hyperostosis (Caffey's disease)
5. Metastasis
6. Osteomyelitis
7. Sarcoma (esp. Ewing's)
8. Sprengel's deformity

SUBGAMUT D-98A
HYPOPLASIA OF THE SCAPULA

1. Achondrogenesis
2. Achondroplasia
3. Asphyxiating thoracic dysplasia
4. Campomelic dwarfism
5. Hypochondroplasia
6. Sprengel's deformity
7. Short-rib polydactyly syndrome
8. Thanatophoric dwarfism

Reference:

Dorst J: Personal communication.

LESION OF THE CLAVICLE IN A CHILD

COMMON

1. Osteomyelitis
2. Trauma (fracture, dislocation, battered child)

UNCOMMON

1. Achondroplasia
2. Benign bone tumor
3. Congenital hypoplasia or absence (See Subgamut D-99A)
4. Fibrous dysplasia; other fibrocystic lesion
5. Histiocytosis X
6. Hyperparathyroidism (esp. secondary)
7. Infantile cortical hyperostosis (Caffey's disease)
8. Lymphoma (esp. leukemia)
9. Malignant bone tumor (osteosarcoma, Ewing's sarcoma, metastasis)
10. Mucopolysaccharidosis (eg, Hurler)
11. Osteopetrosis
12. Pseudarthrosis, congenital or traumatic
13. Rheumatoid arthritis
14. Syphilis
15. Tuberculosis

SUBGAMUT D-99A
HYPOPLASIA OF THE CLAVICLE

1. Cleidocranial dysplasia
2. Focal dermal hypoplasia (Goltz S.)
3. Holt-Oram S.
4. Progeria
5. Trisomy 13 S.
6. Trisomy 18 S.

Reference:

Smith DW: *Recognizable Patterns of Human Malformation.* Philadelphia, WB Saunders Co, 1970.

EROSION, DESTRUCTION, OR DEFECT OF THE OUTER END OF THE CLAVICLE

COMMON

1. Hyperparathyroidism
2. Myeloma
3. Rheumatoid arthritis
4. Rickets

UNCOMMON

1. Cleidocranial dysplasia
2. Eosinophilic granuloma
3. Gout
4. Hodgkin's disease
5. Lipoid dermatoarthritis (reticulohistiocytoma)
6. Metastasis
7. Mucopolysaccharidosis (eg, Hurler)
8. Osteomyelitis
9. Post-traumatic osteolysis
10. Progeria
11. Pyknodysostosis
12. Scleroderma
13. Tuberculosis

References:

1. Greenfield GB: *Radiology of Bone Diseases.* Philadelphia, JB Lippincott Co, 1969, p 304.
2. Jacobson HG, Siegelman SS: Refresher course syllabus.

CONGENITAL SYNDROMES WITH PATELLAR DYSPLASIA

COMMON

1. Nail-patella S. (hereditary osteo-onychodysplasia)

UNCOMMON

1. Acrocephalopolysyndactyly (Carpenter's S.)
2. Cerebrohepatorenal S. (calcific flecks in patella)
3. Diastrophic dwarfism
4. Familial absence of patella; Seckel's bird-headed dwarfism
5. Hereditary arthro-ophthalmopathy (dislocated patella)
6. Neurofibromatosis (absence)
7. Popliteal pterygium S.

Reference:

Smith DW: *Recognizable Patterns of Human Malformation.* Philadelphia, WB Saunders Co, 1970.

SOLITARY CIRCUMSCRIBED LYTIC PATELLAR LESION

COMMON

1. Chondroma
2. Chondromalacia
3. Cystic osteomyelitis
4. Gout

UNCOMMON

1. Aneurysmal bone cyst
2. Bone cyst
3. Brown tumor of hyperparathyroidism
4. Chondroblastoma
5. Giant cell tumor
6. Hemangioma
7. Osteoblastoma

GENU VARUM (BOW LEGS)

COMMON

1. Idiopathic
2. Physiologic; prenatal bowing
3. Tibia vara (Blount's disease)

UNCOMMON

1. Campomelic dwarfism
2. Dysplasia epiphysealis hemimelica (Trevor's disease) (unilateral)
3. Localized neoplasm (eg, osteochondroma, juxta-articular chondroma)
4. Metaphyseal chondrodysplasia
5. Rickets
6. Spondyloepiphyseal dysplasia (congenita or pseudoachondroplastic types)
7. Trauma
8. Turner's syndrome

GENU VALGUM (KNOCK-KNEE)

COMMON

1. Flatfeet
2. Physiologic
3. Regional muscular weakness

UNCOMMON

1. Achondroplasia
2. Dysplasia epiphysealis hemimelica (Trevor's disease) (unilateral)
3. Hajdu-Cheney S. (idiopathic acro-osteolysis)
4. Hypophosphatasia
5. Localized neoplasm (eg, osteochondroma, juxta-articular chondroma)
6. Metaphyseal chondrodysplasia
7. Metaphyseal dysplasia (Pyle's disease)
8. Mucopolysaccharidosis (eg, Hurler, Morquio)
9. Nail-patella S. (hereditary osteo-onychodysplasia)
10. Rickets

COXA VARA (UNILATERAL OR BILATERAL)

COMMON

1. Idiopathic coxa vara of childhood
2. Legg-Perthes disease, old
3. Malunited fracture
4. Paget's disease
5. Rheumatoid arthritis
6. Rickets; osteomalacia

UNCOMMON

1. Congenital hypoplasia of the femur
2. Diastrophic dwarfism
3. Enchondromatosis (Ollier's disease)
4. Fibrous dysplasia
5. Hyperparathyroidism, secondary
6. Hyperphosphatasia
7. Hypothyroidism
8. Kniest's disease
9. Metaphyseal chondrodysplasia (Schmid)
10. Multiple epiphyseal dysplasia (Fairbank)
11. Osteogenesis imperfecta
12. Osteopetrosis
13. Slipped capital femoral epiphysis
14. Spondyloepiphyseal dysplasia (congenita or pseudo-achondroplastic types)

COXA VALGA

COMMON

1. Paralytic disorder (eg, meningomyelocele, cerebral palsy, muscular dystrophy, poliomyelitis)
2. Rheumatoid arthritis

UNCOMMON

1. Chronic leg injury
2. Cleidocranial dysplasia
3. Dysplasia epiphysealis hemimelica (Trevor's disease)
4. Gonadal dysgenesis (Turner's S.)
5. Hereditary arthro-ophthalmopathy (Stickler S.)
6. Hypoplasia of sacrum
7. Mucopolysaccharidosis (eg, Hurler, Hunter, Morquio); mucolipidosis
8. Myositis (fibrodyplasia) ossificans progressiva
9. Osteodysplasia (Melnick-Needles)
10. Osteopetrosis
11. Prader-Willi S.
12. Progeria
13. Pyknodysostosis

FRAGMENTED OR IRREGULAR FEMORAL HEAD

COMMON

1. Aseptic necrosis, all causes (see Gamut D-28)
2. Congenital dislocation of the hip
3. Legg-Perthes disease
4. Traumatic dislocation

UNCOMMON

1. Chondrodysplasia punctata (congenital stippled epiphyses, Conradi's disease)
2. Cretinism, hypothyroidism
3. Diastrophic dwarfism
4. Enchondromatosis (Ollier's disease)
5. Hemophilia
6. Hereditary arthro-ophthalmopathy (Stickler S.)
7. Infection
8. Leukemia
9. Mucopolysaccharidosis (eg, Hurler, Hunter, Morquio, Maroteaux-Lamy); pseudo-Hurler polydystrophy
10. Multiple epiphyseal dysplasia (Fairbank)
11. Osteochondritis dissecans
12. Osteochondromuscular dystrophy (Schwartz S.)
13. Renal osteodystrophy
14. Rhinotrichophalangeal S.
15. Rickets, all types
16. Slipped capital femoral epiphysis (late)

Reference:

 Greenfield GB: *Radiology of Bone Diseases.* Philadelphia, JB Lippincott Co, 1969, p 108.

SLIPPED CAPITAL FEMORAL EPIPHYSES

COMMON

1. Idiopathic
2. Renal osteodystrophy
3. Rickets
4. Trauma

UNCOMMON

1. Congenital coxa vara
2. Gaucher's disease
3. Gigantism (hyperpituitarism)
4. Hemophilia
5. Hyperparathyroidism, primary or secondary
6. Metaphyseal chondrodysplasia
7. Overweight
8. Pseudohypoparathyroidism
9. Scurvy
10. Steroid therapy
11. Syphilis

References:

1. Greenfield GB: *Radiology of Bone Diseases.* Philadelphia, JB Lippincott Co, 1969, p 224.

2. Steinbach HL, Young DA: The roentgen appearance of pseudohypoparathyroidism (PH) and pseudo-pseudohypoparathyroidism (PPH). *Am J Roentgenol* 97:49–66, 1966.

CONGENITAL SYNDROMES WITH AN ABNORMAL PELVIS
(See also Gamut D-110)

COMMON

1. Achondroplasia (small pelvis, short sacroiliac notch)
2. Down's S. (mongolism) (hypoplastic, flared iliac wings, decreased acetabular and iliac angles)
3. Mucopolysaccharidosis (eg, Hurler, Morquio) (flared iliac wings, shallow acetabula)

UNCOMMON

1. Achondrogenesis (sacral, pubic, ischial bones not ossified)
2. Asphyxiating thoracic dysplasia (flared ilia, trident pelvis)
3. Cleidocranial dysplasia (wide pubic symphysis)
4. Cockayne's S. (small square pelvis)
5. Diastrophic dwarfism (short thick iliac bones)
6. Ellis-Van Creveld S. (trident pelvis)
7. Kniest's disease (small pelvic bones)
8. Metaphyseal chondrodysplasias (abnormal acetabula)
9. Metatropic dwarfism (small iliac height and sacrosciatic notches)
10. Rubinstein-Taybi S. (flared ilia, small iliac index)
11. Spondyloepiphyseal dysplasia (squared ilia, delayed pubic and femoral head ossification)
12. Thanatophoric dwarfism (square ilia with small sacro-sciatic notches)
13. Trisomy 18 S. (vertical ilia, steep acetabular angles)

CONGENITAL SYNDROMES WITH DECREASED ACETABULAR ANGLE

COMMON

1. Achondroplasia
2. Down's S. (mongolism)

UNCOMMON

1. Absent abdominal musculature ("prune belly" S.)
2. Arthrogryposis
3. Asphyxiating thoracic dysplasia
4. Chondroectodermal dysplasia (Ellis-Van Creveld S.)
5. Cornelia de Lange S.
6. Exstrophy of the bladder
7. Hypophosphatasia
8. Osteogenesis imperfecta
9. Rubinstein-Taybi S.

PROTRUSIO ACETABULI (OTTO PELVIS), UNILATERAL OR BILATERAL

COMMON

1. Congenital
2. Degenerative joint disease
3. Idiopathic
4. Osteomalacia, rickets
5. Osteoporosis
6. Paget's disease
7. Rheumatoid arthritis
8. Trauma with medial dislocation of hip

UNCOMMON

1. Gout
2. Hydatid disease
3. Hyperparathyroidism
4. Hyperphosphatasia
5. Infectious arthritis (eg, pyogenic, tuberculous)
6. Mucopolysaccharidosis (esp. Morquio)
7. Neoplasm involving acetabulum, primary or metastatic, with medial dislocation of hip
8. Ochronosis
9. Osteogenesis imperfecta

References:

1. McEwen C, Poppel MH, Poker N, Jacobson HG: Protrusio acetabuli in rheumatoid arthritis. *Radiology* 66:33–40, 1956.

2. Murray RO, Jacobson HG: *The Radiology of Skeletal Disorders.* Baltimore, Williams & Wilkins Co, 1971.

BRIDGING OF THE PUBIC SYMPHYSIS

COMMON

1. Ankylosing spondylitis; rheumatoid arthritis
2. Degenerative changes
3. Idiopathic
4. Post-traumatic

UNCOMMON

1. Fluorosis
2. Infection (eg, osteitis pubis, tuberculosis, osteomyelitis)
3. Myositis ossificans (pseudomarsupial bones)
4. Ochronosis
5. Radiation therapy
6. Surgical fusion

Reference:

Schwarz G, Schwarz GS: Noninfectious symphysial bridging and pseudo-marsupial bones. *Am J Roentgenol* 97:687–692, 1966.

WIDENING OF THE PUBIC SYMPHYSIS

COMMON

1. Pregnancy
2. Traumatic dislocation

UNCOMMON

1. Cleidocranial dysplasia
2. Congenital anorectal malformations
3. Diastasis recti
4. Epispadias or hypospadias
5. Exstrophy of the bladder
6. Focal dermal hypoplasia (Goltz S.)
7. Hyperparathyroidism
8. Idiopathic
9. Infection (eg, tuberculosis, osteitis pubis)
10. Malignant tumor
11. Spondyloepiphyseal dysplasia congenita (delayed ossification)

Reference:

Muecke EC, Currarino G: Congenital widening of the pubic symphysis. *Am J Roentgenol* 103:179–185, 1968.

THINNED OR "RIBBON" RIBS

COMMON

1. Neurofibromatosis
2. Regenerated rib (postresection)

UNCOMMON

1. Angiomatosis (Gorham's disease)
2. Hyperparathyroidism
3. Idiopathic
4. Morquio S. (posterior portion)
5. Osteodysplasia (Melnick-Needles)
6. Osteogenesis imperfecta
7. Osteoporosis, severe
8. Paraplegia; poliomyelitis
9. Rheumatoid arthritis
10. Scleroderma
11. Trisomy 13 S.
12. Trisomy 18 S.

Reference:

   Murray RO, Jacobson HG: *The Radiology of Skeletal Disorders.* Balti-more, Williams & Wilkins Co, 1971, p. 31.

SHORT RIBS*

COMMON

1. Achondroplasia
2. [Rickets, all types]

UNCOMMON

1. Achondrogenesis
2. Asphyxiating thoracic dysplasia (Jeune's disease)
3. Campomelic dwarfism
4. Chondroectodermal dysplasia (Ellis-Van Creveld S.)
5. Enchondromatosis (Ollier's disease)
6. Mesomelic dwarfism variant
7. Morquio syndrome
8. Short-rib polysyndactyly syndrome
9. Spondylocostal dysostosis
10. Spondyloepiphyseal dysplasia congenita
11. Thanatophoric dwarfism

*Usually associated with small thorax

WIDE RIBS

COMMON

1. Achondroplasia
2. Anemia (esp. thalassemia)
3. Fibrous dysplasia
4. Mucopolysaccharidosis (eg, Hurler, Hunter, Sanfilippo, Morquio); mucolipidosis (eg, generalized gangliosidosis)
5. Normal variant
6. Paget's disease
7. Rickets (rosary)

UNCOMMON

1. Basal cell nevus syndrome (Gorlin)
2. Gaucher's disease; Niemann-Pick disease
3. Hyperphosphatasia
4. Hypochondroplasia
5. Infantile cortical hyperostosis (Caffey's disease)
6. Metaphyseal chondrodysplasia (Schmid)
7. Metaphyseal dysplasia (Pyle's disease)
8. Osteogenesis imperfecta congenita (thick bone type)
9. Osteomyelitis, healed; actinomycosis
10. Osteopetrosis
11. Polycythemia
12. Scurvy
13. Van Buchem's disease

References:

1. Dorst J: Personal communication.
2. Greenfield GB: *Radiology of Bone Diseases*. Philadelphia, JB Lippincott Co, 1969, p 224.

MULTIPLE SYMMETRICAL ANTERIOR RIB ENLARGEMENT

COMMON

1. Normal
2. Rickets

UNCOMMON

1. Asphyxiating thoracic dysplasia
2. Hypophosphatasia
3. Leukemia (chloromas)
4. Metaphyseal chondrodysplasia (Jansen, McKusick types)
5. Scurvy
6. Thalassemia
7. Thanatophoric dwarfism

Reference:

Austin JHM: Chloroma; report of a patient with unusual rib lesions. *Radiology* 93:671–672, 1969.

RESORPTION OR NOTCHING OF THE SUPERIOR RIB MARGINS

COMMON

1. Collagen disease (rheumatoid arthritis, lupus erythematosus, scleroderma)
2. Hyperparathyroidism

UNCOMMON

1. Coarctation of thoracic aorta (superior and inferior margins)
2. Idiopathic
3. Marfan's syndrome
4. Multiple cartilaginous exostoses
5. Neuroblastoma, thoracic
6. Neurofibromatosis
7. Osteodysplasia (Melnick-Needles)
8. Osteogenesis imperfecta
9. Poliomyelitis
10. Postoperative (erosion from rib retractors, chest tubes)
11. Progeria
12. Radiation therapy

References:

1. Greenfield GB: *Radiology of Bone Diseases.* Philadelphia, JB Lippincott Co, 1969, p 304.
2. Sargent EN, Turner AF, Jacobson G: Superior marginal rib defects. *Am J Roentgenol* 106:491–505, 1969.

CLASSIFICATION OF RIB NOTCHING

I. Arterial
  (a) high aortic obstruction
  (b) low aortic obstruction
  (c) subclavian obstruction

  (d) pulmonary oligemia

(1) coarctation of aorta

(2) aortic thrombosis

(3) Blalock-Taussig procedure (unilateral)

(4) pulseless disease (eg, Takayasu's)

(5) absent pulmonary artery (unilateral)

(6) Ebstein's anomaly

(7) emphysema

(8) pseudotruncus arteriosus

(9) pulmonary valvular stenosis or atresia

(10) tetralogy of Fallot

II. Venous

(11) superior vena cava obstruction

III. Arteriovenous

(12) A-V fistula of chest wall (intercostal artery-vein)

(13) pulmonary A-V fistula

IV. Neurogenic

(14) intercostal neurinoma

(15) neurofibromatosis

V. Osseous

(16) bulbar poliomyelitis

(17) hyperparathyroidism

(18) osteodysplasia (Melnick-Needles)

(19) thalassemia

(Continued)

VI. Idiopathic   (20) idiopathic
VII. Normal   (21) normal

Reference:

Felson B, Weinstein AW, Spitz HB: *Principles of Chest Roentgenology, A Programmed Text.* Philadelphia, WB Saunders Co, 1965, p. 197.

RIB LESION IN A CHILD

I. Congenital

   1. Achondroplasia

   2. Bifid rib, supernumerary rib, synostosis

   3. Cervical rib

   4. Coarctation of aorta

   5. Hypoplasia or absence

   6. Mucopolysaccharidosis (eg, Hurler, Morquio)

   7. Neurofibromatosis

   8. Osteopetrosis

   9. Other osteochondrodysplasias (see Gamut D-1)

  10. Thalassemia, sickle cell anemia

II. Inflammation

   1. Infantile cortical hyperostosis (Caffey's disease)

   2. Granulomatous disease of childhood

   3. Osteomyelitis (eg, bacterial, tuberculous, fungal)

III. Neoplasm

   1. Angioma

   2. Enchondroma

   3. Leukemia

   4. Mesenchymoma (hamartoma, chondroma)

   5. Metastasis (esp. neuroblastoma)

   6. Neurofibroma

   7. Osteochondroma

   8. Sarcoma (eg, Ewing's, osteosarcoma)

(Continued)

IV. Miscellaneous

    1. Fibrocystic lesion (cyst, nonossifying fibroma, fibrous dysplasia)

    2. Histiocytosis X

    3. Rib notching (see Gamut D-119)

    4. Rickets, all types

    5. Scurvy

    6. Trauma (eg, fracture, callus, regenerated rib)

SHORT LESION OF A RIB (LESS THAN 6 CM)
(See also Gamut D-122)

COMMON

1. Bone cyst
2. Brown tumor of hyperparathyroidism
3. Enchondroma
4. Eosinophilic granuloma (Histiocytosis X)
5. Fibrous dysplasia
6. Fracture, callus
7. Metastasis
8. Myeloma, plasmacytoma
9. Osteochondroma, exostosis
10. Osteomyelitis (eg, bacterial, tuberculous, fungal)

UNCOMMON

1. Angioma
2. Chondroblastoma
3. Chondromyxoid fibroma
4. Gaucher's disease
5. Giant cell tumor
6. Lipoma
7. Lymphoma (esp. Hodgkin's)
8. Mesenchymoma (hamartoma, chondroma)
9. Nonossifying fibroma
10. Osteoblastoma
11. Osteoid osteoma
12. Osteoma

LONG LESION OF A RIB (OVER 6 CM)
(See also Gamut D-121)

COMMON

1. Fibrous dysplasia
2. [Fused or bifid rib]
3. Metastasis
4. Myeloma, plasmacytoma
5. Osteomyelitis (eg, bacterial, tuberculous, fungal)
6. Sarcoma (eg, osteosarcoma, chondrosarcoma, Ewing's)
7. [Surgical removal; regeneration]

UNCOMMON

1. Aneurysmal bone cyst
2. Chondromyxoid fibroma
3. Hydatid cyst
4. Leterrer-Siewe or Hand-Schüller-Christian disease (Histio-cytosis X)
5. Paget's disease

MULTIPLE EXPANDING RIB LESIONS

COMMON

1. Anemia (eg, thalassemia, sickle cell)
2. Metastases
3. Multiple myeloma

UNCOMMON

1. Angiomatosis
2. Brown tumors of hyperparathyroidism
3. Engelmann's disease
4. Fibrous dysplasia
5. Gaucher's disease
6. Histiocytosis X
7. Hypophosphatasia
8. Infantile cortical hyperostosis (Caffey's disease)
9. Leukemia (chloromas)
10. Mucopolysaccharidosis (eg, Hurler, Morquio)
11. Multiple cartilaginous exostoses (diaphyseal aclasis)
12. Osteogenesis imperfecta
13. Pachydermoperiostosis
14. Paget's disease
15. Rickets (rosary)
16. Scurvy
17. Van Buchem's disease

CONGENITAL SYNDROMES WITH JOINT HYPERMOBILITY

COMMON

1. Down's S. (mongolism)
2. Marfan's S.
3. Morquio S.

UNCOMMON

1. Bird headed dwarfism (Seckel's S.)
2. Ehlers-Danlos S.
3. Focal dermal hypoplasia (Goltz S.)
4. Geroderma osteodysplastica
5. Hereditary arthro-ophthalmopathy (Stickler S.)
6. Metaphyseal chondrodysplasia (McKusick)
7. Oculocerebral-renal S.
8. Osteogenesis imperfecta
9. Pseudoachondroplastic dysplasia

Reference:

Smith DW: *Recognizable Patterns of Human Malformation.* Philadelphia, WB Saunders Co, 1970, p 287.

CONGENITAL SYNDROMES WITH LIMITED JOINT MOBILITY

COMMON

1. Achondroplasia (elbow)

2. Mucopolysaccharidosis (eg, Hurler, Hunter, Sanfilippo, Scheie, Maroteaux-Lamy); mucolipidosis (eg, Leroy's I cell, pseudo-Hurler polydystrophy, generalized gangliosidosis)

UNCOMMON

1. Arthrogryposis

2. Cerebrohepatorenal syndrome (third and fifth fingers)

3. Chondrodysplasia punctata (Conradi's disease)

4. Chondroectodermal dysplasia (Ellis-Van Creveld S.)

5. Cockayne's S.

6. Cornelia de Lange S. (elbow)

7. Diastrophic dwarfism

8. Dyschondrosteosis (elbow, wrist)

9. Dysplasia epiphysealis hemimelica (Trevor's disease) (unilateral knee and ankle)

10. Familial dwarfism with stiff joints

11. Hereditary arthro-ophthalmopathy (Stickler S.)

12. Kniest's disease

13. Leri's pleonosteosis

14. Metaphyseal chondrodysplasias

15. Metatropic dwarfism

16. Mietens-Weber S. (knee)

17. Multiple cartilaginous exostoses

18. Multiple epiphyseal dysplasia (hip)

(Continued)

19. Osteochondromuscular dystrophy (Schwartz S.)

20. Otopalatodigital S. (elbow)

21. Parastremmatic dwarfism

22. Popliteal pterygium S.

23. Progeria

24. Spondylometaphyseal dysplasia

25. Trisomy 13 S. (fingers)

26. Trisomy 18 S.

27. Weill-Marchesani S.

28. XXXXY S.

Reference:

Smith DW: *Recognizable Patterns of Human Malformation*. Philadelphia, WB Saunders Co, 1970, p 288.

CONGENITAL SYNDROMES WITH JOINT
DISLOCATION
(See also Gamut D-124)

1. Aminopterin-induced S. (hip)
2. Arthrogryposis (hip)
3. Bird-headed dwarfism (Seckel's S.) (hip)
4. Chondrodysplasia punctata (Conradi's disease)
5. Cornelia de Lange S. (elbow)
6. Dyschondrosteosis
7. Ehlers-Danlos S.
8. Fanconi S. (pancytopenia-dysmelia S.) (hip)
9. Geroderma osteodysplastica (hip)
10. Kniest's disease (hip)
11. Larsen's S. (elbow, knee, hip)
12. Mietens-Weber S. (hip)
13. Mucopolysaccharidosis (eg, Morquio) (hip, elbow, fingers)
14. Multiple cartilaginous exostoses
15. Neurofibromatosis
16. Oculodentodigital S.
17. Osteogenesis imperfecta
18. Otopalatodigital S. (elbow)
19. Popliteal pterygium S.
20. Pseudoachondroplastic dysplasia (hip)
21. Riley-Day S.
22. Russell-Silver S.
23. Whistling face S. (hip)

Reference:

Smith DW: *Recognizable Patterns of Human Malformation*. Philadelphia, WB Saunders Co, 1970, p 289.

POLYARTICULAR JOINT DISEASE

COMMON

1. Ankylosing spondylitis
2. Gout
3. Osteoarthritis
4. Rheumatoid arthritis

UNCOMMON

1. Acromegaly
2. Amyloidosis
3. Charcot joints
4. Familial Mediterranean fever
5. Hemochromatosis
6. Hemophilia
7. Jaccoud's arthritis
8. Lipoid dermatoarthritis
9. Lupus erythematosus
10. Ochronosis
11. Psoriatic arthritis
12. Reiter's syndrome
13. Scleroderma

RHEUMATOID-LIKE ARTHRITIS

COMMON

1. Ankylosing spondylitis
2. Gout
3. Lupus erythematosus
4. Psoriatic arthritis
5. Reiter's syndrome
6. Scleroderma

UNCOMMON

1. Erosive osteoarthritis, acute
2. Hemochromatosis
3. Lipoid dermatoarthritis (reticulohistiocytoma)
4. Sjögren's syndrome
5. Ulcerative colitis arthritis

DEGENERATIVE ARTHRITIS IN A YOUNG ADULT

COMMON

1. Aseptic necrosis (see Gamut D-28)
2. Erosive osteoarthritis
3. Hemophilia
4. Neuropathic joint
5. Postinfection (eg, pyogenic, tuberculous, smallpox)
6. Rheumatoid arthritis, juvenile
7. Scoliosis
8. Trauma, surgery, burn, frostbite

UNCOMMON

1. Acromegaly
2. Amyloidosis
3. Bone dysplasias
4. Ehlers-Danlos syndrome
5. Exostosis, intra-articular chondroma, Trevor's disease
6. Familial Mediterranean fever
7. Gout
8. Hemochromatosis
9. Macrodystrophia lipomatosa
10. Ochronosis
11. Scheuermann's disease
12. Wilson's disease (hepatolenticular degeneration)

ARTHRITIS WITH OSTEOPOROSIS

1. Hemophilia
2. Lupus erythematosus (late)
3. Pyogenic arthritis
4. Reiter's syndrome
5. Rheumatoid arthritis
6. Scleroderma
7. Tuberculous or fungal arthritis

ARTHRITIS WITHOUT SIGNIFICANT OSTEOPOROSIS

COMMON

1. Gout
2. Osteoarthritis (degenerative, traumatic, or erosive)
3. Psoriatic arthritis

UNCOMMON

1. Charcot joint
2. Jaccoud's arthritis (post-rheumatic fever)
3. Lupus erythematosus (early)
4. Sarcoidosis
5. Villonodular synovitis

ARTHRITIS WITH MULTIPLE SUBLUXATIONS
(USUALLY ULNAR DEVIATION)

COMMON

1. Rheumatoid arthritis

UNCOMMON

1. Charcot joint
2. Jaccoud's arthritis (post-rheumatic fever)
3. Lupus erythematosus
4. Other arthritis, advanced (eg, gouty, tuberculous, fungal, pyogenic)
5. Psoriatic arthritis

ARTHRITIS ASSOCIATED WITH PERIOSTITIS

COMMON

1. Psoriatic
2. Pyogenic
3. Reiter's syndrome
4. Rheumatoid (esp. juvenile)

UNCOMMON

1. Hemophilia
2. Tuberculous

FLUFFY CALCANEAL SPUR

COMMON

1. Psoriatic arthritis
2. Reiter's syndrome
3. Rheumatoid arthritis

UNCOMMON

1. Ankylosing spondylitis
2. Idiopathic; normal

Reference:

Sholkoff SD, Glickman MG, Steinbach HL: Roentgenology of Reiter's syndrome. *Radiology* 97:497–503, 1970.

CALCANEAL BONE RESORPTION
(PLANTAR OR POSTERIOR SURFACE)

COMMON

1. Psoriatic arthritis
2. Reiter's syndrome
3. Rheumatoid arthritis

UNCOMMON

1. Gout
2. Hyperparathyroidism
3. Lipoid dermatoarthritis (reticulohistiocytoma)
4. Osteomyelitis, decubitus ulcer

Reference:

Greenfield GB: *Radiology of Bone Diseases.* Philadelphia, JP Lippin-cott Co, 1969, p 304.

NEUROPATHIC (CHARCOT) JOINT

COMMON

1. Cushing's syndrome; systemic or local steroid therapy
2. Diabetic myelopathy or neuropathy
3. Spinal cord injury (eg, hemiplegia, paraplegia)
4. Tabes dorsalis

UNCOMMON

1. Congenital indifference to pain
2. Gangrene
3. Inflammatory disease of spinal cord (eg, arachnoiditis, acute myelitis, poliomyelitis)
4. Leprosy
5. Meningomyelocele; diastematomyelia; spina bifida vera
6. Multiple sclerosis
7. Neoplasm of spinal cord
8. Peripheral nerve injury
9. Pernicious anemia
10. Riley-Day syndrome
11. Scleroderma
12. Syringomyelia
13. Yaws

SOFT TISSUE MASS ABOUT A JOINT

COMMON

1. Aneurysm
2. [Fluid or blood in joint]
3. Infection
4. Neuropathic arthropathy (Charcot joint)
5. Synovial cyst (eg, Baker's cyst)
6. Synovial hypertrophy secondary to arthritis
7. Synovial osteochondromatosis

UNCOMMON

1. Amyloidosis
2. Chondroma, para-articular or intra-articular
3. Chondrosarcoma
4. Hemangioma of synovium
5. Localized nodular synovitis
6. Myositis ossificans
7. Parosteal sarcoma or other parosteal neoplasm (see Gamut D-50)
8. Pigmented villonodular synovitis
9. Synovioma

BENIGN SYNOVIAL LESION INVOLVING
A MAJOR JOINT

1. Amyloidosis
2. Hemangioma
3. Lipoma
4. Localized nodular synovitis
5. Pigmented villonodular synovitis
6. Synovial cyst (eg, Baker's cyst)
7. Synovial hypertrophy secondary to arthritis or infection
8. Synovial osteochondromatosis
9. Xanthoma

BONE LESIONS ON BOTH SIDES OF A JOINT

COMMON

*1. Degenerative arthritic cysts

*2. Gout

*3. Infection (esp. granulomatous)

 4. Metastases

 5. Multiple myeloma

UNCOMMON

*1. Amyloidosis

 2. Angiomas

 3. Enchondromas; Ollier's disease

*4. Hemophilia

*5. Jackhammer operator disease (driller's disease, post-vibration syndrome)

 6. Osteopoikilosis; osteopathia striata

*7. Pigmented villonodular synovitis

*8. Synovioma

*With joint involvement.

MULTIPLE FILLING DEFECTS IN KNEE JOINT ON ARTHROGRAPHY

COMMON

1. Cartilage fragments
2. Rheumatoid arthritis
3. Synovial, osteochondromatosis

UNCOMMON

1. Blood clots; hemophilic arthritis
2. Lipoma arborescens
3. Neoplasm
4. Pigmented villonodular synovitis
5. Synovial hemangioma
6. Tuberculosis

Reference:

Burgan DW: Lipoma arborescens of the knee: another cause of filling defects on a knee arthrogram. *Radiology* 101:583–584, 1971.

CALCIFIED LOOSE BODY IN A JOINT

COMMON

1. Degenerative joint disease with detached spur
2. Fracture with avulsed fragment in joint
3. Fragmentation of meniscus with calcification
4. Neuropathic (Charcot) joint
5. Osteochondritis dissecans (post-traumatic necrosis)
6. Synovial osteochondromatosis

UNCOMMON

1. [Dysplasia epiphysealis hemimelica (Trevor's disease) (unilateral epiphyseal osteochondroma involving knee or ankle)]
2. Sequestrum from osteomyelitis, tuberculosis, or pyogenic arthritis

CALCIFICATION OF ARTICULAR CARTILAGE

COMMON

1. Degenerative; post-traumatic
2. Idiopathic
3. Pseudogout (calcium pyrophosphate arthropathy)

UNCOMMON

1. Acromegaly
2. Gout
3. Hemochromatosis
4. Hyperparathyroidism
5. Hypophosphatasia
6. Ochronosis
7. Oxalosis
8. Wilson's disease

References:

1. Greenfield GB: *Radiology of Bone Diseases.* Philadelphia, JB Lippincott Co, 1969, p 420.
2. Moskowitz RW, Garcia F: Chondrocalcinosis articularis (pseudogout syndrome). *Arch Intern Med* 132:87–91, 1973.

PERIARTICULAR OR INTRA-ARTICULAR CALCIFICATION
(See also Gamuts D-141 and D-142)

COMMON

1. Charcot joint
2. Degenerative arthritis, loose body, "joint mouse"
3. Pseudogout (calcium pyrophosphate arthropathy)
4. Synovial osteochondromatosis
5. Synovitis, tendinitis (peritendinitis calcarea)

UNCOMMON

1. [Congenital stippled epiphyses (Conradi's disease)]
2. Dermatomyositis; calcinosis universalis
3. Diabetes mellitus
4. Dysplasia epiphysealis hemimelica (Trevor's disease); intracapsular chondroma
5. Gout
6. Hematoma, traumatic or spontaneous
7. Hemochromatosis
8. Hyperparathyroidism, primary or secondary
9. Hypervitaminosis D
10. Hypoparathyroidism
11. Lipocalcinogranulomatosis
12. Lupus erythematosus
13. Myositis ossificans
14. Ochronosis
15. Parosteal sarcoma
16. Rheumatoid arthritis

(Continued)

PERIARTICULAR OR INTRA-ARTICULAR CALCIFICATION
(Continued)

17. Scleroderma

18. Synovioma

19. Tuberculosis

20. Tumoral calcinosis

21. Werner's syndrome

Reference:

Greenfield GB: *Radiology of Bone Diseases.* Philadelphia, JB Lippincott Co, 1969, p 420.

CALCIFICATION IN THE MUSCLES AND SUBCUTANEOUS TISSUES
(See also Gamuts D-145, D-146 and D-148)

SYSTEMIC

COMMON

1. Dermatomyositis; calcinosis universalis
2. Gout; hyperuricemia
3. Hyperparathyroidism, primary and secondary
4. Scleroderma
5. Vascular (see Gamut D-150)

UNCOMMON

1. Basal cell nevus S. (Gorlin)
2. Bone destruction with hypercalcemia
3. Congenital fibromatosis
4. Ehlers-Danlos S.
5. Fat necrosis (pancreatitis; Weber-Christian disease)
6. Fluorosis
7. Homocystinuria
8. Hypervitaminosis A (ligaments)
9. Hypervitaminosis D
10. Hypoparathyroidism; pseudohypoparathyroidism, pseudopseudohypoparathyroidism
11. Idiopathic hypercalcemia (eg, William's S.)
12. Lupus erythematosus
13. Milk-alkali S.
14. Mucoviscidosis
15. Myositis (fibrodysplasia) ossificans progressiva
16. Neonatal subcutaneous fat necrosis (pseudosclerema)
17. Osteoporosis (immobilization)

(Continued)

CALCIFICATION IN THE MUSCLES AND SUBCUTANEOUS TISSUES
(Continued)

18. Paraplegia; poliomyelitis
19. Parasites (eg, cysticercosis, guinea worms, loa-loa)
20. Post-carbon monoxide poisoning
21. Progeria; Werner's S.
22. Pseudoxanthoma elasticum
23. Rheumatoid arthritis, ankylosing spondylitis (ligaments)
24. Tumoral calcinosis

NONSYSTEMIC

COMMON

1. Avulsed fracture fragment
2. Idiopathic
3. Inoculation (eg, calcified sterile abscess; antibiotic, bismuth, calcium gluconate, insulin, camphorated oil, or quinine injection; BCG vaccination)
4. Myositis ossificans, traumatic; hematoma
5. Peritendinitis calcarea

UNCOMMON

1. Burn, frostbite, electroshock
2. Epithelioma (pilo-matrixoma)
3. Foreign body granuloma
4. Healing infection or abscess (post-pyogenic myositis or fibrositis)

(Continued)

5. Leprosy (nerves)

6. Neoplasm, benign (eg, chondroma, fibromyxoma)

7. Neoplasm, malignant (eg, soft tissue osteosarcoma, chondrosarcoma, fibrosarcoma, liposarcoma, synovioma)

8. Scar

9. Volkman's contracture

References:

1. Edeiken J, Hodes PJ: *Roentgen Diagnosis of Diseases of Bone*, ed 2. Baltimore, Williams & Wilkins Co, 1973, pp 1139–1149.

2. Gayler BW, Brogdon BG: Soft tissue calcifications in the extremities in systemic disease. *Am J Med Sci* 590-605, 1965.

3. Greenfield GB: *Radiology of Bone Diseases.* Philadelphia, JB Lippincott Co, 1969, pp 411–426.

4. Kuhn JP, Rosenstein BJ, Oppenheimer EH: Metastatic calcification in cystic fibrosis. *Radiology* 97:59–64, 1970.

5. Teplick JG, Haskin ME: *Roentgenologic Diagnosis*, ed 2. Philadelphia, WB Saunders Co, 1971, vol 2, p. xxxvii.

WIDESPREAD CALCIFICATIONS IN THE SOFT TISSUES

COMMON

1. Dermatomyositis, calcinosis universalis
2. Hyperparathyroidism, primary or secondary
3. Scleroderma
4. Vascular (eg, atherosclerosis, varicosities, generalized arterial calcification of infancy)

UNCOMMON

1. Ehlers-Danlos S.
2. Gout; hyperuricemia
3. Homocystinuria
4. Hypervitaminosis D
5. Hypoparathyroidism; pseudohypoparathyroidism, pseudopseudohypoparathyroidism
6. Idiopathic hypercalcemia (eg, William's S.)
7. Immobilization osteoporosis
8. Intravascular coagulopathy
9. Lupus erythematosus
10. Milk-alkali S.
11. Mucoviscidosis
12. Myositis (fibrodysplasia) ossificans progressiva
13. Neuropathic calcification (eg, paraplegia)
14. Parasitic disease (eg, cysticercosis, guinea worms)
15. Progeria; Werner's S.
16. Pseudoxanthoma elasticum

(Continued)

17. Tumoral calcinosis

18. Widespread bone destruction

Reference:

Kuhn JB, Rosenstein BJ, Oppenheimer EH: Metastatic calcification in cystic fibrosis. *Radiology* 97:59–64, 1970.

SOLITARY LARGE CALCIFIED SOFT TISSUE MASS ADJACENT TO BONE
(See also Gamut D-144)

COMMON

1. Myositis ossificans
2. Osteochondroma

UNCOMMON

1. Aneurysm
2. Gouty tophus
3. Hyperparathyroidism, primary or secondary
4. Hypervitaminosis D
5. Paraplegia
6. Parosteal osteoma or chondroma
7. Parosteal sarcoma
8. Soft tissue osteosarcoma or chondrosarcoma
9. Synovioma
10. Tumoral calcinosis

CALCIFICATION ABOUT THE FINGER TIPS

COMMON

1. Scleroderma

UNCOMMON

1. Dermatomyositis; calcinosis universalis
2. Epidermolysis bullosa
3. Lupus erythematosus
4. Raynaud's disease
5. Rothmund's syndrome

Reference:

Greenfield GB: *Radiology of Bone Diseases.* Philadelphia, JB Lippin-cott Co, 1969, p 420.

CALCIFICATION IN A BURSA, TENDON OR LIGAMENT

BURSA

1. Bursal osteochondromatosis
2. Calcific bursitis
3. Gout
4. Hyperparathyroidism
5. Hypervitaminosis D
6. Pseudogout
7. Tumoral calcinosis

TENDON

1. Calcified ganglion
2. Calcinosis universalis
3. Diabetes mellitus
4. Gout
5. Ochronosis
6. Peritendinitis calcarea (usually post-traumatic or occupational)
7. Pseudogout

LIGAMENT

1. Ankylosing spondylitis; rheumatoid arthritis
2. Degenerative change
3. Fluorosis
4. Hypervitaminosis A
5. Idiopathic
6. Myositis (fibrodysplasia) ossificans progressiva
7. Pellegrini-Stieda disease (medial tibial collateral ligament)

Reference:

Greenfield GB: *Radiology of Bone Diseases.* Philadelphia, JB Lippincott Co, 1969, p 419.

CALCIFICATION IN LYMPH NODES

COMMON

1. Histoplasmosis
2. Tuberculosis

UNCOMMON

1. BCG vaccination
2. Coccidioidomycosis
3. Filariasis
4. Idiopathic
5. Lymphoma (postradiation therapy)
6. Metastasis from osteosarcoma or other calcifying neoplasm (eg, ovarian, thyroid, colon)

Reference:

Greenfield GB: *Radiology of Bone Diseases.* Philadelphia, JB Lippin-cott Co, 1969, p 419.

VASCULAR CALCIFICATION

COMMON

1. Aneurysm
2. Arteriosclerosis
3. Hemangioma; arteriovenous malformation
*4. Hyperparathyroidism, primary or secondary
5. Mönckeberg's sclerosis (medial sclerosis)
6. Phleboliths (eg, normal, varicose veins, hemangioma, Maffucci's syndrome, postradiation)
7. Premature atherosclerosis
   a. Familial hyperlipemia
   b. Generalized arterial calcification of infancy
   c. Progeria
   d. Secondary hyperlipemia
      (1) Cushing's syndrome
      (2) Diabetes mellitus
      (3) Glycogen storage disease
      (4) Hypothyroidism
      (5) Lipodystrophy
      (6) Nephrotic syndrome
      (7) Renal homotransplantation
   e. Werner's syndrome

UNCOMMON

1. Buerger's disease
2. Burn, frostbite
3. Calcified thrombus (eg, vena cava, portal vein, arterial)

(Continued)

   4. Gout, hyperuricemia
   5. Homocystinuria
   6. Hydramnios in infants
  *7. Hypervitaminosis D
   8. Hypoparathyroidism
  *9. Idiopathic hypercalcemia
 *10. Immobilization syndrome
 *11. Milk-alkali syndrome
  12. Mucoviscidosis
  13. Pseudoxanthoma elasticum
  14. Raynaud's disease
 *15. Sarcoidosis
  16. Takayasu's arteritis

*Hypercalcemia

Reference:

Teplick JG, Haskin ME: *Roentgenologic Diagnosis*, ed 2. Philadelphia, WB Saunders Co, 1971, vol 2, p xxii.

DISEASES AFFECTING MUSCLE TO FAT RATIO

I. DIMINUTION OF MUSCLE:CYLINDER RATIO (BELOW 0.64)

COMMON

1. Paralysis (eg, poliomyelitis, meningomyelocele)

UNCOMMON

1. Amyotonia congenita (Oppenheim)
2. Arthrogryposis multiplex congenita
3. Benign congenital hypotonia (Walton)
4. Cushingoid state with increased subcutaneous fat (steroid therapy, Cushing's syndrome)
5. Disseminated lipogranulomatosis
6. Prader-Willi S.
7. Spinal atrophy, progressive (Werdnig-Hoffmann)
8. Spondyloepiphyseal dysplasia congenita

II. INCREASE OF MUSCLE:CYLINDER RATIO (OVER 0.72)

A. DIMINUTION IN SUBCUTANEOUS FAT

COMMON

1. Malnutrition, debilitating disease (eg, anorexia nervosa)

(Continued)

UNCOMMON

1. Diencephalic syndrome
2. Hyperthyroidism
3. Progeria; Werner's syndrome
4. Renal tubular acidosis
5. Scleroderma, dermatomyositis
6. Total lipodystrophy

B. INCREASE IN MUSCLE MASS

UNCOMMON

1. Congenital muscular hypertrophy (de Lange)
2. Pseudohypertrophic stage of muscular dystrophy

References:

1. Greenfield GB: *Radiology of Bone Diseases.* Philadelphia, JB Lippincott Co, 1969, pp 440–441.
2. Litt RE, Altman DH: Significance of the muscle cylinder ratio in infancy. *Am J Roentgenol* 100:80–87, 1967.

THICKENING OF HEEL PAD
(GREATER THAN 22 MM)

COMMON

1. Acromegaly
2. Infection of soft tissues (eg, mycetoma)
3. Normal variant

UNCOMMON

1. Dilantin therapy
2. Generalized edema
3. Myxedema; thyroid acropachy
4. Obesity
5. Occupational
6. Trauma

Reference:

Greenfield GB: *Radiology of Bone Diseases.* Philadelphia, JB Lippincott Co, 1969, p 440.

SOFT TISSUE MASS WITH UNDERLYING BONE EROSION

COMMON

1. Carcinoma of skin or mouth
2. Decubitus ulcer
3. Giant cell tumor of tendon sheath
4. Gouty tophus
5. Rheumatoid arthritis

UNCOMMON

1. Amyloidosis
2. Angioma; Klippel-Trenaunay-Weber syndrome
3. Carcinoma developing in sinus tract of osteomyelitis or tropical ulcer
4. Epidermoid tumor
5. Fungus disease (eg, actinomycosis, blastomycosis)
6. Ganglion
7. Glomus tumor
8. Hemophilia
9. Hyperkeratosis plantaris
10. Kaposi sarcoma
11. Lipoid dermatoarthritis (reticulohistiocytoma)
12. Neurofibromatosis
13. Neuroma (eg, Morton's neuroma of toe)
14. Pigmented villonodular synovitis
15. Sarcoma of soft tissues
16. Sebaceous or other cyst
17. Surfer's knot
18. Synovioma

PRIMARY SOFT TISSUE TUMOR

I. Muscle
   1. Leiomyoma
   2. Leiomyosarcoma
   3. Rhabdomyosarcoma

II. Fat
   1. Hibernoma
   2. Lipoma; infiltrating angiolipoma; lipoma arborescens
   3. Liposarcoma

III. Connective Tissue
   1. Desmoid
   2. Fibromatoses
   3. Fibrosarcoma
   4. Fibrous histiocytoma
   5. Quasi-neoplastic benign proliferation of connective tissue (eg, nodular pseudosarcomatous fasciitis, juvenile xanthogranuloma, proliferative myositis)

IV. Nerve
   1. Malignant schwannoma
   2. Neurilemmoma
   3. Neurofibroma
   4. Neurofibrosarcoma
   5. Neuroma

V. Vessel
   1. Hemangioendothelioma
   2. Hemangioma
   3. Hemangiopericytoma
   4. Hemangiosarcoma
   5. Lymphangioma

(Continued)

VI. Synovium

    1. Ganglion

    2. Pigmented villonodular synovitis (giant cell tumor of tendon sheath)

    3. Synovioma

    4. Xanthoma

VII. Uncertain or Mixed Tissue Origin

    1. Alveolar soft part tumor

    2. Granular cell myoblastoma

    3. Mesenchymoma

VIII. Soft Tissue Osteosarcoma and Chondrosarcoma

IX. Other (Including Processes That May Mimic Tumor)

    1. Accessory muscle mass

    2. Aneurysm

    3. Arteriovenous malformation or fistula

    4. Bursal swelling, including iliopsoas bursa

    5. Dermatologic conditions

    6. Gardner's syndrome

    7. Hematoma

    8. Inflammatory mass

    9. Metastasis

    10. Secondary invasion from bone

    11. Wart, hyperkeratosis

Reference:

  Greenfield GB: *Radiology of Bone Diseases.* Philadelphia, JB Lippincott Co, 1969, p 431.

SWELLING OF THE INTERSTITIAL MARKINGS OF THE SOFT TISSUES ("RETICULATION" OF SOFT TISSUES)

COMMON

1. Infection of soft tissues (eg, cellulitis, tuberculosis, fungus disease, mycetoma)
2. Lymphatic obstruction
3. Neoplasm primary in soft tissues or secondary to bone neoplasm
4. Osteomyelitis
5. Thermal burn or electric shock
6. Trauma; spontaneous hemorrhage

UNCOMMON

1. [Acromegaly]
2. Infantile cortical hyperostosis (Caffey's disease)
3. Melorheostosis
4. Myositis (fibrodyplasia) ossificans progressiva (early)
5. Myxedema, thyroid acropachy
6. Neurofibromatosis
7. Sudeck's atrophy

Reference:

Greenfield GB: *Radiology of Bone Diseases.* Philadelphia, JB Lippincott Co, 1969, p 440.

LYMPHATIC OBSTRUCTION ON LYMPHANGIOGRAM (LYMPHEDEMA)

COMMON

1. [High pressure injection of contrast media]
2. Lymphoma (esp. Hodgkin's)
3. Metastases to lymph nodes
4. Postsurgical (esp. radical mastectomy); lymphocyst
5. Trauma

UNCOMMON

1. Filariasis
2. Inflammation, lymphadenitis
3. Lymphangiomatous malformation; lymphangioma of thoracic duct
4. [Primary lymphedema (Milroy's disease)]
5. Radiation therapy

Reference:

Escobar-Prieto A, Gonzalez G, Templeton A W, et al: Lymphatic channel obstruction: patterns of altered flow dyanmics. *Am J Roentgenol* 113:366–375, 1971.

SUBGAMUT D-156A
ROENTGEN SIGNS OF LYMPHATIC CHANNEL
OBSTRUCTION

1. Backflow
2. Collateral circulation
3. Dilatation of lymph vessels
4. Extravasation
5. Stasis of lymph flow

FILLING DEFECT IN LYMPH NODE ON LYMPHANGIOGRAM

COMMON

1. Granulomatous disease (eg, sarcoidosis, tuberculosis, fungus disease)
2. Lymphoma
3. Metastatic neoplasm (eg, carcinoma, melanoma, sarcoma)

UNCOMMON

1. Acute lymphadenitis (abscess)
2. Amyloidosis
3. Fatty replacement
4. Multiple myeloma
5. Normal anatomic hilum
6. Reactive hyperplasia of collagen disease (eg, rheumatoid arthritis)
7. Sjögren's syndrome

References:

1. Kuisk H: *Technique of Lymphography and Principles of Interpretation* St. Louis, Warren H Green Inc, 1971.
2. Wallace S, Jackson L, Dodd GD, Greening RR: Lymphangiographic interpretation. *Radiol Clin North Am* 3:467–485, 1965.

NOTES

NOTES

TABLE OF CONTENTS

E. CARDIOVASCULAR

CONGENITAL DISEASES OF THE HEART AND GREAT VESSELS

(Continued)

E

(Continued)

E

E

CARDIOVASCULAR ANOMALIES ASSOCIATED WITH VENTRICULAR SEPTAL DEFECT

A. Obstructive or Positional Anomalies of the Aorta
1. Corrected transposition of great vessels
2. Coarctation of aorta
3. Complete transposition of great vessels
4. Hypoplasia or interruption of aortic arch
5. Origin of both great vessels from right ventricle without pulmonary stenosis
6. Right aortic arch
7. Truncus arteriosus

B. Shunts
1. Aorticopulmonary window
2. Atrial septal defect
3. AV communis
4. Left ventricular-right atrial communication
5. Patent ductus arteriosus
6. Ruptured sinus of Valsalva aneurysm into right ventricle

C. Intracardiac Obstruction
1. Anomalous muscle bundle of right ventricle
2. Hypoplasia of right ventricle
3. Mitral stenosis
4. Pulmonary stenosis
5. Subaortic stenosis
6. Tetralogy of Fallot; pseudotruncus arteriosus

D. Valvular Incompetence, Any Valve

E

Reference:

Edwards JE: The pathology of ventricular septal defect. *Semin Roentgenol* 1:2-23, 1966.

CONGENITAL SYNDROMES
WITH CONGENITAL HEART DISEASE

COMMON

1. Asplenia or polysplenia S.
2. Down's S. (VSD, AV communis)
3. Hurler's S. (valvular or myocardial disease)
4. Marfan's S. (aortic or mitral insufficiency, cystic medial necrosis, dissecting aneurysm)
5. Rubella S. (PDA, VSD, pulmonary artery branch stenosis)
6. Scimitar (venolobar) S.
7. Turner's S. (coarctation of aorta, pulmonary stenosis)

UNCOMMON

1. Carpenter's S.
2. Cat-cry S.
3. Cerebrohepatorenal S. (PDA, septal defect)
4. Chondrodysplasia punctata
5. Cornelia De Lange S.
6. Ehlers-Danlos S. (medial necrosis of aorta, ASD, tetralogy)
7. Ellis-Van Creveld S. (septal defect, common atrium)
8. Fanconi's S.
9. Goltz's S.
10. Holt-Oram S. (ASD)
11. Larsen's S.
12. Laurence-Moon-Biedl S. (Tetralogy)
13. Myotonic dystrophy (arrhythmias)
14. No. 4 short arm deletion S.
15. No. 18 long arm deletion S.
16. Noonan's S.

(Continued)

E

17. Osteogenesis imperfecta (valvular incompetence)

18. Radial aplasia-thrombocytopenia S.

19. Rubinstein-Taybi S.

20. Trisomy 13 S. (VSD)

21. Trisomy 18 S. (VSD, PDA)

22. Ventriculoradial S. (VSD)

23. Weill-Marchesani S.

24. Williams' S. (supravalvular aortic stenosis, pulmonary artery branch stenosis)

25. XXXXX S. (PDA)

26. XXXXY S.

References:

1. Felson B, Editor: Dwarfs and Other Little People. *Semin Roentgenol* 8:260, 1973.
2. Meszaros WT: *Cardiac Roentgenology.*   Springfield, Charles C Thomas, 1969, p 330.
3. Rowe RD, Mehrizi A: *The Neonate With Congenital Heart Disease. Major Problems in Clinical Pediatrics.* Philadelphia, WB Saunders Co, 1968, vol 5.
4. Smith DW: *Recognizable Patterns of Human Malformation.* Philadelphia, WB Saunders Co, 1970, p 129.

LEFT TO RIGHT SHUNT IN CONGENITAL HEART DISEASE

COMMON

1. Atrial septal defect
2. Patent ductus arteriosus
3. Ventricular septal defect

UNCOMMON

1. AV communis, endocardial cushion defect
2. Anomalous origin of left coronary artery from pulmonary artery
3. Anomalous origin of right pulmonary artery from ascending aorta (hemitruncus)
4. Anomalous pulmonary venous return
5. Aorticopulmonary window
6. Coronary artery fistula to right heart or pulmonary artery
7. Left ventricular-right atrial shunt
8. Ruptured sinus of Valsalva aneurysm into right heart
9. Tetralogy of Fallot, acyanotic ("pink")

Reference:

Edwards JE, Carey LS, Neufeld HN, Lester RG: *Congenital Heart Disease.* Philadelphia, WB Saunders Co, 1965.

SUBGAMUT E-3A
ROENTGEN FINDINGS
IN THE COMMON LEFT TO RIGHT SHUNTS

	Pulm. Vasc.	Pulm. Art. Seg.	Aorta	SVC	LV	RV	LA	RA
1. ASD	↑	↑	↓	↓	N	↑	N	↑
2. PDA	↑	↑	↑	N	↑	N,↑	↑	N
3. VSD	↑	↑	N,↓	N	N,↑	↑	↑	N

RIGHT TO LEFT SHUNT OR ADMIXTURE LESION IN CONGENITAL HEART DISEASE

COMMON

1. Left to right shunt with reversal (Eisenmenger physiology)
2. Tetralogy of Fallot
3. Transposition of great vessels

UNCOMMON

1. Common atrium
2. Common ventricle
3. Cor biloculare
4. Ebstein's anomaly with ASD; Uhl's anomaly
5. Isolated hypoplasia of right ventricle with ASD
6. Origin of both great vessels from right ventricle without pulmonary stenosis
7. Pentalogy of Fallot
8. Pulmonary AV fistula
9. Pulmonary atresia with intact ventricular septum and ASD
10. Right pulmonary artery to left atrium fistula
11. Systemic venous connection to left atrium (eg, left SVC to LA)
12. Total anomalous pulmonary venous return
13. Tricuspid atresia
14. Trilogy of Fallot
15. Truncus arteriosus

References:

1. Edwards JE, Carey LS, Neufeld HN, Lester RG: *Congenital Heart Disease.* Philadelphia, WB Saunders Co, 1965.
2. Lester RG: Radiological concepts in the evaluation of heart disease. *Mod Concepts Cardiovasc Dis* 37:113-118, 1968.

SUBGAMUT E-4A
DIFFERENTIAL FEATURES OF MAJOR CYANOTIC
CONGENITAL HEART DISEASES*

	Cardiac Size	Pulm. Vasc.	Aortic Arch	EKG
1. Tetralogy of Fallot, including pseudotruncus (40%)	N, ↑	↓	R(25%)	RVH
2. Transposition of great vessels (15%)	↑	↑	L	RVH and/or LVH
3. Tricuspid atresia (10%)	N, ↑	↓	L	LVH
4. Trilogy of Fallot (5%)	↑	↓	L	RVH
5. Truncus arteriosus (10%)	↑	↑ or ↓	R(25%)	RVH and/or LVH

*80% of cyanotic congenital heart lesions are one of the five "T's."

SUBGAMUT E-4B
ONSET OF CYANOSIS IN CONGENITAL
HEART DISEASE

1. Marked cyanosis at birth or in first week:
   a. Asplenia syndrome
   b. Common ventricle with pulmonary stenosis and trans-position
   c. Ebstein's anomaly
   d. Hypoplastic left heart syndrome
   e. Origin of both great vessels from right ventricle with pulmonary stenosis
   f. Pulmonary atresia
   g. Tetralogy of Fallot, severe; pseudotruncus arteriosus
   h. Transposition of great vessels
   i. Tricuspid atresia

2. Mild or intermittent cyanosis at birth or appearance later in first month:
   a. AV communis
   b. Ebstein's anomaly
   c. Large left to right shunt with failure
   d. Tetralogy of Fallot
   e. Trilogy of Fallot
   f. Truncus arteriosus

3. Cyanosis during feeding or crying:
   a. Total anomalous pulmonary venous return below the diaphragm

Reference:

Rowe RD, Mehrizi A: *The Neonate With Congenital Heart Disease. Major Problems in Clinical Pediatrics.* Philadelphia, WB Saunders Co, 1968, vol 5.

RIGHT TO LEFT SHUNT AT ATRIAL LEVEL

COMMON

1. Atrial septal defect with pulmonary hypertension
2. Complete transposition of great vessels with interatrial communication
3. Total anomalous pulmonary venous return
4. Tricuspid atresia

UNCOMMON

1. Common atrium
2. Cor biloculare
3. Ebstein's anomaly with interatrial communication
4. Isolated hypoplasia of right ventricle
5. Normal newborn with patent foramen ovale
6. Pentalogy of Fallot
7. Primary pulmonary hypertension with interatrial communication
8. Pulmonary atresia with intact ventricular septum
9. Tricuspid stenosis with interatrial communication
10. Trilogy of Fallot (pulmonary stenosis with ASD)
11. Uhl's anomaly

Reference:

Meszaros WT: *Cardiac Roentgenology*. Springfield, Charles C Thomas, 1969, p 430.

RIGHT TO LEFT SHUNT AT VENTRICULAR LEVEL

COMMON

1. Complete transposition of great vessels with VSD
2. Eisenmenger's syndrome
3. Tetralogy of Fallot; pseudotruncus arteriosus

UNCOMMON

1. Common ventricle
2. Cor biloculare
3. Corrected transposition with VSD and predominant pulmonary stenosis
4. Origin of both great vessels from right ventricle
5. Truncus arteriosus

Reference:

Meszaros WT: *Cardiac Roentgenology.* Springfield, Charles C Thomas, 1969, p 443.

RIGHT TO LEFT SHUNT AT DUCTUS LEVEL

COMMON

1. Coarctation of aorta, preductal
2. Patent ductus arteriosus with pulmonary hypertension

UNCOMMON

1. Aortic atresia
2. Interruption of aortic arch
3. Mitral atresia; congenital mitral stenosis
4. Pulmonary vein atresia
5. Total anomalous pulmonary venous return

Reference:

Meszaros WT: *Cardiac Roentgenology.* Springfield, Charles C Thomas, 1969, p 414.

CONGENITAL HEART DISEASE ASSOCIATED WITH ANTERIOR RIGHT AORTIC ARCH (MIRROR-IMAGE BRANCHING)

1. Pseudotruncus arteriosus (40%)*

2. Tetralogy of Fallot (25%)

3. Transposition of great vessels with pulmonary stenosis (usually)

4. Tricuspid atresia (5%)

5. Truncus arteriosus (25%)

*(%) refers to percentage of all cases of that entity

VASCULAR RINGS AND OTHER ANOMALIES OF THE AORTIC ARCH AND BRACHIOCEPHALIC ARTERIES

COMMON

1. Aberrant right subclavian artery

*2. Double aortic arch

3. Right aortic arch, right descending aorta, and aberrant left subclavian artery

4. Right aortic arch, right descending aorta, and mirror image branching

UNCOMMON

1. Anomalous left common carotid artery

2. Anomalous innominate artery

3. Cervical aorta (high, usually right-sided aortic arch)

*4. Left aortic arch, left descending aorta, and right ductus arteriosus

5. Left aortic arch, right descending aorta, and right ductus arteriosus

*6. Pulmonary sling (aberrant left pulmonary artery)

7. Right aortic arch, left descending aorta, and encircling ductus

8. Right aortic arch, right descending aorta, and isolated left subclavian artery (congenital subclavian steal)

9. Right aortic arch, right descending aorta, and left ductus arteriosus

*Usually symptomatic

Reference:

Swischuk LE: *Radiology of the Newborn and Young Infant.* Baltimore, Williams & Wilkins Co, 1973.

ANOMALOUS ARTERIAL COMMUNICATION IN THE CHEST

A. Direct Communication of Aorta and Pulmonary Artery

    1. Aorticopulmonary window

    2. Patent ductus arteriosus

    3. Pseudotruncus arteriosus

    4. Truncus arteriosus

B. Aortic or Systemic Artery Anomaly

    1. Fistula

        a. Aortico-left ventricular tunnel

        b. Brachiocephalic artery to systemic vein (eg, transverse cervical artery to internal jugular vein fistula)

        c. Coronary artery fistula

        d. Postoperative aortic-cardiac fistula

        e. Ruptured sinus of Valsalva aneurysm into heart

        f. Systemic-pulmonary AV fistula (bronchial, brachiocephalic, or chest wall artery to pulmonary artery or vein)

    2. Anomalous origin of systemic artery

        a. Origin of left coronary artery from pulmonary artery

        b. Origin of subclavian artery from pulmonary artery

C. Pulmonary Artery Anomaly

    1. Fistula

        a. Pulmonary AV fistula

        b. Right pulmonary artery to left atrium fistula

    2. Anomalous origin of pulmonary artery

        a. Left pulmonary artery from right pulmonary artery (pulmonary artery sling)

(Continued)

b. Left or right pulmonary artery from descending aorta

c. Right pulmonary artery from ascending aorta (hemi-truncus)

3. Anomalous artery arising from aorta to supply a lung segment

a. Pulmonary sequestration

b. Scimitar (venolobar) syndrome

Reference:

Franken EA, Hurwitz RA: 1973 Radiological Society of North America Scientific Exhibit.

FLAT OR CONCAVE PULMONARY ARTERY SEGMENT IN CONGENITAL HEART DISEASE

COMMON

1. Tetralogy of Fallot; pseudotruncus arteriosus
2. Transposition of great vessels, complete

UNCOMMON

1. Asplenia syndrome
2. Common ventricle with pulmonary stenosis
3. Corrected transposition (pulmonary artery medially positioned)
4. Ebstein's anomaly; Uhl's anomaly
5. Origin of both great vessels from right ventricle with pulmonary stenosis
6. Pentalogy of Fallot
7. Pulmonary atresia with intact ventricular septum
8. Tricuspid atresia or stenosis
9. Truncus arteriosus

PULMONARY ARTERIAL VASCULARITY IN COMMON CONGENITAL HEART DISEASES
(See also Gamuts E-13, E-14, and E-40)

	Incidence of all congenital heart disease†
1. Increased Vascularity with Prominent Pulmonary Artery Segment	
a. AV communis	4%
b. Anomalous pulmonary venous return	
c. Atrial septal defect	11%
d. Patent ductus arteriosus	12%
e. Ventricular septal defect	22%
2. Increased Vascularity with Flat or Concave Pulmonary Artery Segment	
*a. Transposition of great vessels	6%
*b. Truncus arteriosus	3%
3. Normal Vascularity	
a. Aortic stenosis	3%
b. Coarctation of aorta	7%
c. Endocardial fibroelastosis	2%
d. Pulmonary valvular stenosis	4%
e. Small left to right shunt	
4. Decreased Vascularity	
*a. Ebstein's anomaly	
*b. Pulmonary atresia or severe stenosis	
*c. Tetralogy of Fallot	12%
*d. Tricuspid atresia	3%
*e. Trilogy of Fallot	

*Cyanotic lesions

†Note: Incidence based on analysis of 2200 cases of CHD.
     12 lesions account for 89% of all CHD.
     3 shunt lesions (ASD, VSD, PDA) account for 45% of all CHD.

CONGENITAL HEART DISEASE WITH DIMINISHED PULMONARY ARTERIAL VASCULARITY
(See also Gamut E-12)

COMMON

1. Tetralogy of Fallot; pseudotruncus arteriosus

UNCOMMON

1. Asplenia syndrome (Ivemark)
2. Common ventricle with pulmonary atresia or stenosis
3. Ebstein's anomaly with ASD
4. Origin of both great vessels from right ventricle with pulmonary stenosis
5. Pentalogy of Fallot (pulmonary stenosis with ASD and VSD)
6. Pulmonary atresia with intact ventricular septum and ASD
7. Pulmonary insufficiency; absent pulmonary valve
8. Pulmonary stenosis, severe
   a. Supravalvular (coarctations of pulmonary artery)
   b. Valvular
   c. Subvalvular (infundibular stenosis; anomalous muscle bundle of right ventricle)
9. Right ventricular hypoplasia with tricuspid insufficiency and infundibular pulmonary stenosis
10. Transposition of great vessels, complete or corrected, with pulmonary atresia or stenosis
11. Tricuspid atresia or stenosis with pulmonary atresia or stenosis
12. Tricuspid insufficiency
13. Trilogy of Fallot (pulmonary stenosis with ASD)
14. Truncus arteriosus, type IV (occasionally types II or III)
15. Tumor of right atrium (eg, myxoma) obstructing tricuspid valve

(Continued)

16. Uhl's anomaly (parchment right ventricle)

References:

1. Edwards JE, Carey LS, Neufeld HN, and Lester RG: *Congenital Heart Disease.* Philadelphia, WB Saunders Co, 1965.
2. Lester RG: Radiological concepts in the evaluation of heart disease. *Mod Concepts Cardiovasc Dis* 37:113-118, 1968.
3. Schiebler GL, Miller RH, Gessner IH: The triad of cyanosis, decreased pulmonary vascularity and cardiomegaly. *Radiol Clin North Am* 6:361-365, 1968.
4. Swischuk LE: *Radiology of the Newborn and Young Infant.* Baltimore, WIlliams & Wilkins Co, 1973.
5. Wesenberg RL: *The Newborn Chest.* New York, Harper & Row, 1973.

CYANOTIC CONGENITAL HEART DISEASE
WITH INCREASED PULMONARY VASCULARITY
(See also Gamut E-12)

COMMON

1. Total anomalous pulmonary venous return
2. Transposition of great vessels, complete

UNCOMMON

1. Common atrium
2. Common ventricle without pulmonary stenosis
3. Cor biloculare
4. Left to right shunt with reversal — Eisenmenger physiology (esp. PDA and VSD)
5. Origin of both great vessels from right ventricle without pulmonary stenosis (including Taussig-Bing syndrome)
6. Tricuspid atresia without pulmonary stenosis
7. Truncus arteriosus, types I, II, and III

INTRINSIC PULSATION OF PULMONARY ARTERY ("HILAR DANCE") IN CONGENITAL HEART DISEASE

COMMON

1. Atrial septal defect
2. Ventricular septal defect

UNCOMMON

1. Anomalous left coronary artery arising from pulmonary artery
2. Anomalous pulmonary venous return
3. Aorticopulmonary window
4. Coronary artery fistula
5. Corrected transposition of great vessels with VSD
6. Intracardiac rupture of congenital sinus of Valsalva aneurysm
7. [Pulmonary AV fistula]
8. Pulmonary insufficiency; absent pulmonary valve
9. Transposition of great vessels
10. Truncus arteriosus

CONGESTIVE HEART FAILURE IN A NEONATE
(0–4 WEEKS)
(See also Gamuts E-17 and E-30)

COMMON

1. Coarctation of aorta, severe
2. Hypoplastic left heart syndrome
3. Left to right shunt, large (VSD, PDA, AV communis)
4. Tetralogy of Fallot, severe; pseudotruncus arteriosus
5. Transposition of great vessels

UNCOMMON

1. Anemia, severe (eg, erythroblastosis)
2. Arrhythmia, tachycardia, complete heart block
3. Arteriovenous fistula or hemangioma (peripheral, pulmonary, hepatic, or cerebral)
4. Asplenia or polysplenia syndrome
5. Cardiac tumor (see Gamut E-33)
6. Common ventricle; double inlet left ventricle
7. Cor triatriatum
8. Hemitruncus
9. Iatrogenic (eg, fluid overload, sodium chloride poisoning)
10. Intracranial disease with increased intracranial pressure
11. Maternal diabetes
12. Myocardiopathy (see Gamut E-32)
    a. Anomalous left coronary artery arising from pulmonary artery
    b. Endocardial fibroelastosis
    c. Glycogen storage disease (Pompe's)

(Continued)

d. Myocardial ischemia (eg, from neonatal hypoxia, infantile coronary arteriosclerosis)

e. Myocarditis (esp. toxoplasma, Coxsackie B, rubella)

13. Neonatal hypoglycemia; hyperthyroidism

14. Origin of both great vessels from right ventricle

15. Polycythemia (eg, maternal-fetal hemorrhage; placental or twin-to-twin transfusion)

16. Premature (prenatal) closure of foramen ovale

17. Pulmonary atresia

18. [Pulmonary lymphangiectasia]

19. Pulmonary vein atresia

20. [Total anomalous pulmonary venous return with obstruction]

21. Tricuspid atresia

22. Truncus arteriosus, severe

References:

1. Wesenberg RL: *The Newborn Chest.* New York, Harper & Row, 1973.

2. Swischuk LE: *Radiology of the Newborn and Young Infant.* Baltimore, Williams & Wilkins Co, 1973.

CARDIOMEGALY IN A NEONATE (0–4 WEEKS)
(See also Gamuts E-16 and E-29)

COMMON

1. Coarctation of aorta, severe
2. Hypoplastic left heart syndrome
3. Left to right shunt in failure (VSD, PDA, AV communis)
4. Tetralogy of Fallot, severe; pseudotruncus arteriosus
5. Transposition of great vessels

UNCOMMON

1. Anemia, severe (eg, erythroblastosis)
2. Arteriovenous fistula, peripheral
3. Asplenia or polysplenia syndrome
4. Common ventricle
5. Myocardiopathy (eg, endocardial fibroelastosis, glycogen storage disease, anomalous left coronary artery, myocarditis)
6. Origin of both great vessels from right ventricle
7. Pulmonary atresia
8. Tricuspid atresia
9. Truncus arteriosus, severe

ABNORMAL CARDIAC POSITION
OR DISPLACEMENT

CONGENITAL

1. Absence of a pulmonary artery
2. Agenesis or hypoplasia of a lobe or lung; venolobar syndrome
3. Asplenia or polysplenia syndrome
4. Congenital absence of left pericardium
5. Dextrocardia, "mirror-image" type with situs inversus
6. Dextroversion (dextrorotation) with situs solitus or situs indeterminate
7. Levoversion (levocardia with situs inversus)
8. Mesoversion (mesocardia)
9. Pectus excavatum

ACQUIRED

1. Atelectasis or fibrosis, unilateral
2. Diaphragmatic hernia or elevation
3. Emphysema, unilateral
4. Mass lesion (eg, neoplasm, aneurysm)
5. Pleural fluid or thickening; pneumothorax
6. Pneumonectomy
7. Scoliosis (heart shifted to concave side)
8. Technical (rotation of patient)

RIGHT ATRIAL ENLARGEMENT

COMMON

1. Left to right shunt into right atrium (eg, ASD, AV communis, anomalous pulmonary venous return, left ventricular-right atrial shunt, ruptured sinus of Valsalva aneurysm into right atrium)
2. Pulmonary atresia or stenosis
3. Right heart failure, any cause
4. Right ventricle enlargement producing right atrial enlargement (see Gamut E-20)
5. Tricuspid insufficiency

UNCOMMON

1. Aneurysm of right atrium
2. Aortic atresia
3. Congenital or idiopathic right atriomegaly
4. Ebstein's anomaly; Uhl's anomaly
5. Endocardial fibroelastosis
6. Hypoplastic left heart syndrome
7. Tetralogy of Fallot
8. Transposition of great vessels with interatrial communication
9. Tricuspid atresia or stenosis, including carcinoid syndrome
10. Trilogy of Fallot
11. Tumor of right atrium or ventricle (eg, myxoma)

Reference:

Meszaros WT: *Cardiac Roentgenology.* Springfield, Charles C Thomas, 1969, pp 68, 327.

RIGHT VENTRICULAR ENLARGEMENT

COMMON

1. Chronic left heart failure (eg, myocardiopathy, mitral insufficiency)
2. Cor pulmonale: right heart failure; pulmonary hypertension, primary or secondary (eg, emphysema, fibrosis) (see Gamut E-41)
3. Left to right shunt (see Gamut E-3)
4. Mitral stenosis
5. Pulmonary stenosis
6. Tetralogy of Fallot

UNCOMMON

1. Ebstein's anomaly; Uhl's anomaly
2. Hypoplastic left heart syndrome
3. Myxoma of left atrium
4. Origin of both great vessels from right ventricle
5. Pulmonary atresia (with tricuspid insufficiency)
6. Pulmonary insufficiency; absent pulmonary valve
7. Pulmonary venous obstruction (eg, cor triatriatum)
8. Transposition of great vessels
9. Tricuspid insufficiency
10. Trilogy of Fallot
11. Truncus arteriosus

Reference:

Meszaros WT: *Cardiac Roentgenology.* Springfield, Charles C Thomas, 1969, pp 65–66.

FILLING DEFECT IN RIGHT VENTRICLE
ON ANGIOCARDIOGRAPHY

COMMON

1. Jet of unopacified blood (eg, VSD with left to right shunt)
2. Thrombus

UNCOMMON

1. Aneurysm or diverticulum of ventricular septum
2. Anomalous muscle bundle
3. Bernheim's syndrome (?) (left ventricular hypertrophy with encroachment on right ventricle)
4. Endocardial fibroelastosis (bulging of ventricular septum)
5. Foreign body (eg, catheter)
6. Idiopathic myocardial hypertrophy (eg, idiopathic hypertrophic subaortic stenosis)
7. Metastatic neoplasm
8. Primary neoplasm (eg, myxoma)
9. Prolapsed valve

LEFT ATRIAL ENLARGEMENT

COMMON

1. Mitral stenosis or insufficiency (congenital or acquired)
2. Patent ductus arteriosus; aorticopulmonary window
3. Relative mitral insufficiency (eg, congestive heart failure, acute rheumatic fever, aortic stenosis or insufficiency, idiopathic hypertrophy of left ventricle, coarctation of aorta)
4. Ventricular septal defect

UNCOMMON

1. Atrial septal defect with late reversal of shunt (esp. ostium primum type)
2. Congenital or idiopathic left atriomegaly
3. Coronary artery fistula
4. Endocardial fibroelastosis
5. Mitral annulus syndrome
6. Myocardiopathy (see Gamut E-32)
7. Origin of both great vessels from right ventricle
8. Parachute mitral valve complex
9. Ruptured papillary muscle
10. Thrombus in left atrium (esp. ball-valve)
11. Transposition of great vessels
12. Tricuspid atresia
13. Trilogy of Fallot
14. Truncus arteriosus
15. Tumor of left atrium (eg, myxoma)

LEFT VENTRICULAR ENLARGEMENT

COMMON

1. Aortic insufficiency
2. Aortic stenosis
3. Arteriosclerotic heart disease
4. Coarctation of aorta
5. Congestive heart failure
6. High output heart disease (see Gamut E-31)
7. Hypertension
8. Mitral insufficiency
9. Myocardial infarction with failure; left ventricular aneurysm
10. Myocardiopathy (see Gamut E-32)
11. Patent ductus arteriosus; aorticopulmonary window
12. Ventricular septal defect

UNCOMMON

1. AV communis
2. Idiopathic hypertrophic subaortic stenosis (IHSS)
3. Origin of both great vessels from right ventricle
4. Pulmonary atresia with intact ventricular septum
5. Transposition of great vessels
6. Tricuspid atresia or stenosis
7. Truncus arteriosus
8. Tumor of left ventricle

EXTRA BUMP ALONG THE UPPER LEFT HEART BORDER (THE THIRD MOGUL)

COMMON

1. Aneurysm of left ventricle
2. Left atrial appendage enlargement in rheumatic or congenital heart disease
3. [Thymus gland; mediastinal mass]

UNCOMMON

1. Absence of the pericardium
2. Common ventricle with outlet chamber and left-sided ascending aorta
3. Coronary artery aneurysm or AV fistula
4. Corrected transposition with left-sided ascending aorta
5. Ebstein's anomaly
6. Levoposition of right atrial appendage
7. Myocardiopathy with left ventricular hypertrophy (eg, idiopathic, familial, African)
8. Sinus of Valsalva aneurysm (left)
9. Tetralogy of Fallot
10. Tumor or cyst of heart or pericardium

Reference:

Daves M: Skiagraphing the mediastinal moguls. *New Physician.* Jan 1970, p 49.

MITRAL INSUFFICIENCY

COMMON

1. Functional (eg, hypertension, aortic insufficiency, myocardiopathy)
2. Rheumatic heart disease

UNCOMMON

1. Bacterial endocarditis
2. Congenital
3. Corrected transposition (with anomalous left AV valve)
4. Idiopathic hypertrophic subaortic stenosis
5. Marfan's syndrome
6. Ostium primum defect with cleft mitral valve leaflet
7. Papillary muscle injury (eg, myocardial infarction, trauma)

Reference:

Meszaros WT: *Cardiac Roentgenology*. Springfield, Charles C Thomas, 1969, p 235.

AORTIC INSUFFICIENCY

COMMON

1. Aortitis (syphilitic, Takayasu's)
2. Rheumatic heart disease

UNCOMMON

1. Aortico-left ventricular tunnel
2. Bacterial endocarditis
3. Congenital bicuspid aortic valve
4. Cystic medial necrosis of aorta (eg, Marfan's syndrome)
5. Sinus of Valsalva aneurysm
6. Subvalvular aneurysm of left ventricle
7. Trauma to aortic cusp
8. Ventricular septal defect with prolapsed aortic cusp

Reference:

Meszaros WT: *Cardiac Roentgenology.* Springfield, Charles C Thomas, 1969, p 249.

SMALL HEART

COMMON

1. Asthenia
2. [Emphysema]
3. Normal
4. Senile atrophy
5. Wasting diseases (eg, malnutrition, tuberculosis, cancer, lymphoma, ulcerative colitis, scleroderma, anorexia nervosa)

UNCOMMON

1. Adrenal insufficiency
2. Constrictive pericarditis (see Subgamut E-27A)
3. Dehydration (eg, dysentery)

SUBGAMUT E-27A
CONSTRICTIVE PERICARDITIS

1. Histoplasmosis

2. Idiopathic

3. Pyogenic infection (esp. staphylococcal or pneumococcal)

4. Radiation therapy

5. Traumatic pericarditis; hemopericardium

6. Tuberculosis

7. Uremia

8. Viral pericarditis

Reference:

Harrison TR: *Principles of Internal Medicine*, ed 7. New York, McGraw-Hill Inc, 1974, p 1215–1217.

HYPERTENSIVE CARDIOVASCULAR DISEASE

1. Essential hypertension

2. Adrenal disease
   a. Adrenocortical adenoma
   b. Adrenogenital syndrome
   c. Carcinoma
   d. Cushing's syndrome
   e. Pheochromocytoma
   f. Primary aldosteronism

3. Central nervous system disorder
   a. Familial dysautonomia (Riley-Day syndrome)
   b. Pituitary disease (eg, Cushing's syndrome)

4. Coarctation of aorta

5. Collagen disease
   a. Lupus erythematosus
   b. Polyarteritis nodosa

6. Hyperthyroidism

7. Renal disease
   a. Agenesis or hypoplasia
   b. Chronic pyelonephritis
   c. Glomerulonephritis
   d. Polycystic kidneys

8. Renovascular disease
   a. Fibromuscular hyperplasia
   b. Perirenal hematoma
   c. Renal artery stenosis

Reference:

LoPresti JM: Personal communication

LARGE HEART WITHOUT MURMUR
IN AN INFANT OR CHILD
(See also Gamut E-17)

COMMON

1. Anemia
2. Coarctation of aorta
3. Endocardial fibroelastosis
4. Myocarditis, various types
5. [Pericardial effusion (see Gamut E-35)]

UNCOMMON

1. Cardiac tumor, primary (eg, rhabdomyosarcoma, myxoma) or secondary to metastasis or local invasion
2. Coronary insufficiency, myocardial infarction (eg, anomalous origin of left coronary artery from pulmonary artery, medial calcification of coronaries in the infant, progeria)
3. Glycogen storage disease (Pompe's)
4. Hurler's syndrome
5. Nutritional deficiency (eg, beriberi)
6. Patent ductus arteriosus in failure
7. [Pectus excavatum]
8. Pulmonary atresia

CONGESTIVE HEART FAILURE
IN AN OLDER CHILD
(See also Gamut E-16)

COMMON

1. Acute glomerulonephritis; uremia
2. Anemia, severe
3. Congenital heart disease
4. Myocardiopathy (see Gamut E-32)
5. Rheumatic heart disease

UNCOMMON

1. Arrhythmia
2. Arteriovenous fistula (peripheral, pulmonary, hepatic, or cerebral)
3. Cardiac tumor (see Gamut E-33)
4. Fluid overload
5. Sodium chloride poisoning

HIGH OUTPUT HEART DISEASE

1. Anemia (eg, sickle cell anemia)
2. Arteriovenous fistula, peripheral
3. Beriberi
4. Hypervolemia (overtransfusion, fluid overload)
5. Paget's disease
6. Pickwickian obesity
7. Polycythemia vera
8. Pregnancy
9. Pyrexia
10. Thyrotoxicosis

Reference:

Teplick JG, Haskin ME: *Roentgenologic Diagnosis,* ed 2. Philadelphia, WB Saunders Co, 1971, vol 2, p xx.

MYOCARDIOPATHY

COMMON

1. Amyloidosis
2. Collagen disease (lupus erythematosus, polyarteritis nodosa, scleroderma, rheumatoid disease)
*3. Endocardial fibroelastosis
*4. Infectious myocarditis (rheumatic, septic, diphtheritic, Chagas' disease, toxoplasmic, Coxsackie and other viral)
5. Ischemia
6. Nutritional deficiency (eg, beriberi, alcoholism, cirrhosis)
7. Thyrotoxicosis

UNCOMMON

1. Acromegaly
2. Anemia
3. Annular subvalvular left ventricular aneurysm (African)
*4. Anomalous origin of left coronary artery from pulmonary artery
5. Beer drinker's heart (cobalt toxicity)
6. Endomyocardial fibrosis (African myocardiopathy)
7. Familial
*8. Glycogen storage disease (Pompe's)
9. Hemochromatosis
*10. Hurler's syndrome
11. Idiopathic
*12. Idiopathic myocardial hypertrophy, symmetric or asymmetric (idiopathic hypertrophic subaortic stenosis)

(Continued)

13. Leukemia

*14. Medial calcification of coronary arteries in infants

15. Myxedema

*16. Neoplasm, metastatic or primary (eg, rhabdomyoma)

17. Neuromuscular dystrophy (eg, Friedreich's ataxia, progressive muscular dystrophy)

18. Postpartum heart disease

19. Potassium and magnesium depletion

*20. Progeria (coronary atherosclerosis)

21. Sarcoidosis

22. Toxic (drugs, chemicals)

23. Uremia

*Seen in infants

References:

1. Harrison TR: *Principles of Internal Medicine*, ed 7. New York, McGraw-Hill Inc, 1974, p 1217–1220.
2. Meszaros WT: *Cardiac Roentgenology.* Springfield, Charles C Thomas, 1969.
3. Rowe RD, Mehrizi A: *The Neonate With Congenital Heart Disease. Major Problems in Clinical Pediatrics.* Philadelphia, WB Saunders Co, 1968, vol. 5.

CARDIAC AND/OR PERICARDIAL TUMOR OR CYST

COMMON

1. Invasive pulmonary or mediastinal tumor (eg, lymphoma, thymoma)
2. Metastasis (esp. from lung, breast, or melanoma)
3. Myxoma
4. Pericardial cyst

UNCOMMON

1. Angioma
2. Fibroma, fibrous hamartoma, fibrolipoma
3. Hydatid cyst
4. Lipoma
5. Lymphoma
6. Mesothelioma
7. Rhabdomyoma
8. Sarcoma (eg, angiosarcoma, rhabdomyosarcoma)
9. Teratoma

Reference:

Davis GD, Kincaid OW, Hallermann FJ: Roentgen aspects of cardiac tumors. *Semin Roentgenol* 4:384–394, 1969.

CALCIFICATION IN THE HEART
OR GREAT VESSELS

COMMON

1. Aneurysm of aorta, including dissecting aneurysm
2. Aortitis (eg, syphilis, Takayasu's)
3. Arteriosclerosis of aorta
4. Coronary artery arteriosclerosis; Mönckeberg's medial sclerosis
5. Mitral annulus (atherosclerosis)
6. Myocardial infarction, myocardial aneurysm
7. [Pericardial calcification (eg, atrioventricular groove; tuberculous, traumatic, or viral pericarditis; constrictive pericarditis; asbestosis)]
8. Valvular (esp. aortic or mitral stenosis)

UNCOMMON

1. Annular subvalvular left ventricular aneurysm
2. Cardiac tumor (esp. myxoma)
3. Coronary artery aneurysm
4. Ductus arteriosus
5. Endocardial (eg, jet from ASD or VSD)
6. Endocardial fibroelastosis
7. Hydatid cyst
8. Left atrial wall (rheumatic endocarditis, mitral disease)
9. Pulmonary artery thrombus
10. Pulmonary hypertension
11. Sinus of Valsalva aneurysm or arteriosclerosis
12. Thrombus in heart chamber or great vessel (eg, aorta, inferior vena cava)
13. Trauma, surgery (eg, incision, graft, coronary by-pass)

References:

1. Meszaros WT: *Cardiac Roentgenology.* Springfield, Charles C Thomas, 1969, p 8.
2. Shapiro JH, Jacobson HG, Rubinstein BM, Poppel MH, Schwedel JB: *Calcifications Of The Heart.* Springfield, Charles C Thomas, 1963.
3. Teplick JG, Haskin ME: *Roentgenologic Diagnosis,* ed 2. Philadelphia, WB Saunders Co, 1971.

PERICARDIAL EFFUSION

COMMON

1. Collagen disease (rheumatoid disease, lupus erythematosus, scleroderma, polyarteritis nodosa)
2. Congestive heart failure
3. Pericarditis (viral, Coxsackie, bacterial, amebic, toxoplasmic, tuberculous, histoplasmic, rheumatic)
4. Postcardiac surgery (incl. coronary artery bypass)
5. Postmyocardial infarction (Dressler syndrome)
6. Trauma, including iatrogenic
7. Tumor of pericardium or heart (primary or secondary) (see Gamut E-33)
8. Uremia; nephrosis

UNCOMMON

1. Amyloidosis
2. Anticoagulant therapy, excessive
3. Beriberi; hypoproteinemia
4. Blood dyscrasia (eg, severe anemia, erythroblastosis fetalis, bleeding diathesis)
5. Dissecting aneurysm with leakage
6. Endomyocardial fibrosis (African)
7. Gout
8. Idiopathic
9. Myxedema
10. Pancreatitis
11. Radiation therapy

(Continued)

12. Sarcoidosis

References:

1. Harrison TR: *Principles of Internal Medicine*, ed 7. New York, McGraw-Hill Inc, 1974, pp 1211–1215.
2. Teplick JG, Haskin ME: *Roentgenologic Diagnosis,* ed 2. Philadelphia, WB Saunders Co, 1971, vol 2, pxxi.

PNEUMOPERICARDIUM

COMMON

1. Iatrogenic (eg, surgery, pericardiocentesis, resuscitation, diagnostic)

UNCOMMON

1. Congenital absence of the pericardium with pneumothorax
2. Idiopathic
3. [Intracardiac gas (eg, sepsis, abortion)]
4. Perforation from adjacent abscess or neoplasm of lung, mediastinum, esophagus, stomach, or liver
5. Pericarditis due to gas-forming organism
6. Pneumomediastinum or interstitial pulmonary air trapping with extension into pericardium
7. Trauma

PULMONARY VENOUS OBSTRUCTION OR HYPERTENSION (INCREASED PULMONARY VENOUS VASCULARITY)

COMMON

1. Left ventricular failure, any cause
2. Mitral stenosis or insufficiency

UNCOMMON

1. Aortic stenosis or insufficiency
2. Coarctation of aorta (severe)
3. Hypoplastic left heart syndrome (aortic and/or mitral atresia, hypoplasia or interruption of aortic arch, hypoplasia of left ventricle)
4. Left atrial myxoma or ball-valve thrombus
5. Myocardiopathy (see Gamut E-32)
6. Obstruction or stenosis of pulmonary veins

   a. Congenital
      (1) Atresia or stenosis
      (2) Cor triatriatum
      (3) Total anomalous pulmonary venous return below or above the diaphragm with stenosis of venous trunk

   b. Acquired
      (1) Constrictive pericarditis (see Subgamut E-27A)
      (2) Mediastinal tumor
      (3) Mediastinitis or mediastinal fibrosis
      (4) Thrombosis of pulmonary veins

7. Parachute mitral valve complex

References:

1. Lester RG: Radiological concepts in the evaluation of heart disease. *Mod Concepts Cardiovasc Dis* 37:113-118, 1968.
2. McLoughlin MJ: Cor triatriatum sinister. *Clin Radiol* 21:287-296, 1970.
3. Meszaros WT: *Cardiac Roentgenology.* Springfield, Charles C Thomas, 1969, p 97.
4. Robinson AE, Capp MP, Chen JT, Lester RG: Left-sided obstructive diseases of the heart and great vessels. *Semin Roentgenol* 3:410-419, 1968.

DILATATION OF THE MAIN PULMONARY ARTERY SEGMENT

COMMON

1. Congestive heart failure, high output heart disease (see Gamut E-31)

2. Cor pulmonale: right heart failure, pulmonary hypertension, primary or secondary (eg, emphysema, fibrosis) (see Gamut E-41)

3. Idiopathic

4. Left to right shunt (eg, ASD, VSD, PDA, Eisenmenger physiology) (see Gamut E-3)

5. [Mediastinal or left hilar mass]

6. Mitral stenosis or insufficiency, acquired or congenital

7. Normal, under age 30

8. Pregnancy

9. Pulmonary thrombosis or embolism

10. Pulmonary valvular stenosis (poststenotic dilatation)

11. [Technical or positional factors (eg, lordotic view, patient rotation, asthenia, dextroscoliosis, pectus excavatum)]

UNCOMMON

1. Absent pulmonary valve

2. Aneurysm of pulmonary artery

3. Aorta-pulmonary artery fistula (traumatic, eg, ruptured aneurysm)

4. Aortopulmonary surgical shunt (eg, Pott's procedure)

5. Coarctation of pulmonary artery or its branches

6. [Congenital absence of the pericardium]

7. Hypoplastic left heart syndrome

8. Marfan's syndrome

(Continued)

9. Metastatic tumor embolism

10. Origin of both great vessels from right ventricle

11. Parachute mitral valve complex

12. Tricuspid atresia without pulmonary stenosis

13. Trilogy of Fallot

14. Truncus arteriosus, type I

PULMONARY ARTERY ANEURYSM

COMMON

1. Congenital heart disease (eg, patent ductus arteriosus, valvular pulmonary stenosis)

UNCOMMON

1. Arteriovenous fistula

2. Atherosclerosis

3. Cystic medial necrosis (eg, Marfan's syndrome)

4. Idiopathic; congenital (?)

5. Infection (mycotic aneurysm)

6. Syphilis

7. Trauma, including surgical (false aneurysm)

References:

1. Reid JM, Stevenson JG: Aneurysm of the pulmonary artery. *Dis Chest* 36:104–107, 1959.
2. Viamonte M Jr, Le Page JR: Pitfalls in the radiologic evaluation of mediastinal abnormalities. *Radiol Clin North Am* 6:451–465, 1968.

INCREASED PULMONARY ARTERIAL VASCULARITY
(See also Gamuts E-12, E-14, and E-37)

COMMON

1. High output heart disease (eg, pregnancy, hyperthyroidism, Pickwickian obesity, polycythemia vera) (see Gamut E-31)
2. Left to right shunts (see Gamut E-3)

UNCOMMON

1. Aorta-pulmonary artery fistula (eg, traumatic, ruptured aneurysm)
2. Common atrium
3. Common ventricle without pulmonary stenosis
4. Cor biloculare
5. Origin of both great vessels from right ventricle without pulmonary stenosis (incl. Taussig-Bing syndrome)
6. Total anomalous pulmonary venous return
7. Transposition of great vessels
8. Tricuspid atresia without pulmonary stenosis
9. Truncus arteriosus, types I, II, and III

References:

1. Teplick JG, Haskin ME: *Roentgenologic Diagnosis,* ed 2. Philadelphia, WB Saunders Co, 1971, p xx.
2. Meszaros WT: *Cardiac Roentgenology.* Springfield, Charles C Thomas, 1969, pp 324–325.

PULMONARY ARTERIAL HYPERTENSION
(COR PULMONALE)

A. Chronic hypoxia

  1. Chest deformity (eg, kyphoscoliosis, thoracoplasty)
  2. Chronic airway obstruction (eg, enlarged tonsils and adenoids)
  3. High altitude dwelling
  4. Neuromuscular disease (eg, poliomyelitis, amyotrophic lateral sclerosis, myasthenia gravis)
  5. Pickwickian obesity
  6. Pleural thickening, massive

B. Diffuse lung disease

  1. Bronchiectasis
  2. Chronic bronchitis
  3. Emphysema
  4. Interstitial fibrosis (see Gamut F-13)
  5. Lymphangitic metastases
  6. Mucoviscidosis
  7. Tuberculosis, extensive

C. Diffuse pulmonary arterial or heart disease

  1. Arteritis (eg, polyarteritis nodosa, Wegener's syndrome)
  2. Hypoplastic left heart syndrome
  3. Left to right shunt (Eisenmenger physiology)
  4. Left ventricular failure, chronic (eg, aortic valvular disease)
  5. Mitral stenosis or insufficiency (long-standing)
  6. Primary pulmonary hypertension, idiopathic; pulmonary arteriolar sclerosis
  7. Pulmonary artery stenosis
  8. Schistosomiasis

(Continued)

D. Pulmonary thromboembolism (eg, recurrent pulmonary emboli, sickle cell anemia, polycythemia vera)

E. Ventriculoatrial shunt for hydrocephalus

References:

1. Meszaros WT: *Cardiac Roentgenology.*   Springfield, Charles C Thomas, 1969, p 78.
2. Teplick JG, Haskin ME: *Roentgenologic Diagnosis*, ed 2. Philadelphia, WB Saunders Co, 1971, vol 1, p xx.

SMALL ASCENDING AORTA AND/OR AORTIC ARCH

COMMON

1. Atrial septal defect
2. Coarctation of aorta (long infantile type)
3. Decreased cardiac output (eg, endocardial fibroelastosis or other myocardiopathy; constrictive pericarditis)
4. Mitral stenosis and/or insufficiency
5. [Technical (eg, rotated chest, dextroscoliosis, pectus excavatum)]
6. Ventricular septal defect

UNCOMMON

1. AV communis
2. Hypoplastic left heart syndrome
3. Supravalvular aortic stenosis
4. Transposition of great vessels, complete
5. Tricuspid atresia with transposition

Reference:

Meszaros WT: *Cardiac Roentgenology*. Springfield, Charles C Thomas, 1969, pp 148–149.

PROMINENT ASCENDING AORTA
AND/OR AORTIC ARCH

COMMON

1. Aneurysm of aorta (eg, syphilitic, mycotic, atherosclerotic, traumatic, idiopathic, and dissecting) (see Subgamut E-43A)

2. Aortic insufficiency

3. Aortic valvular stenosis (eg, congenital, rheumatic, atherosclerotic)

4. Aortitis (eg, syphilitic, rheumatoid, Takayasu's)

5. Atherosclerosis; senile aorta with tortuosity and unfolding

6. Coarctation of aorta

7. Hypertensive heart disease

8. [Mediastinal lesion simulating large aorta]

9. Patent ductus arteriosus

10. Tetralogy of Fallot; pseudotruncus arteriosus

UNCOMMON

1. Aneurysm of sinus of Valsalva or coronary artery

2. Aortic-left ventricular tunnel

3. Asplenia syndrome (aorta usually transposed)

4. Corrected transposition (left-sided ascending aorta)

5. Ehlers-Danlos syndrome

6. Marfan's syndrome

7. Osteogenesis imperfecta

8. Pseudocoarctation of aorta

9. Pseudoxanthoma elasticum

10. Pulmonary atresia with intact ventricular septum

11. Subvalvular aortic stenosis

(Continued)

PROMINENT ASCENDING AORTA
AND/OR AORTIC ARCH
(CONTINUED)

12. Tricuspid atresia without transposition
13. Truncus arteriosus
14. Ventrical septal defect with reversal of shunt

Reference:

Teplick JG, Haskin ME: *Roentgenologic Diagnosis*, ed 2. Philadelphia, WB Saunders Co, 1971, vol 1 p xxi.

SUBGAMUT E-43A
PREDISPOSING CAUSES OF DISSECTING
ANEURYSM

1. Aortic stenosis

2. Atherosclerosis

3. Coarctation of aorta

4. Cystic medial necrosis of aorta (eg, Marfan's syndrome)

5. Ehlers-Danlos syndrome

6. Hypertension

7. Intramural injection of contrast medium

8. Pregnancy

9. Trauma

Reference:

Meszaros WT: *Cardiac Roentgenology.* Springfield, Charles C Thomas, 1969, p 160.

ENLARGED AZYGOS VEIN*

COMMON

1. Absence or obstruction of the inferior vena cava (eg, azygos continuation, often with polysplenia)
2. Congestive heart failure
3. [Enlarged azygos node; mediastinal tumor]
4. Obstruction of the superior vena cava
5. Portal hypertension; splenic vein thrombosis

UNCOMMON

1. Arteriovenous fistula
2. Constrictive pericarditis (see Subgamut E-27A)
3. Idiopathic
4. Pericardial effusion (see Gamut E-35)
5. Pregnancy
6. Total anomalous pulmonary venous return to the azygos vein
7. Traumatic azygos aneurysm
8. Tricuspid insufficiency

*Note: The azygos vein decreases in size with inspiration, upright position, and Valsalva maneuver.

INFERIOR VENA CAVA OBSTRUCTION

COMMON

1. Direct tumor invasion (eg, renal cell carcinoma, Wilms' tumor, hepatoma)
2. Lymphadenopathy
3. Retroperitoneal tumor
4. Surgical plication
5. Thromboembolism
6. Transient compression (eg, ascites, pregnancy, acute gastric dilatation)

UNCOMMON

1. Adhesions
2. Aortic aneurysm
3. Compression by liver mass or enlarged liver
4. [Congenital absence of inferior vena cava]
5. Retroperitoneal fibrosis
6. Sarcoma of inferior vena cava (eg, leiomyosarcoma, angiosarcoma)
7. Web at junction of inferior vena cava and right atrium

NOTES

NOTES

TABLE OF CONTENTS

F. CHEST

ALVEOLAR LESIONS

INTERSTITIAL LESIONS

F

PULMONARY NODULAR OR MASS LESIONS

PULMONARY CYSTIC OR DESTRUCTIVE LESIONS

MISCELLANEOUS PULMONARY LESIONS

(Continued)

F

MEDIASTINAL LESIONS

F

PLEURAL AND EXTRAPLEURAL LESIONS

MISCELLANEOUS THORACIC LESIONS

F

F

LOCALIZED ALVEOLAR SHADOWS, SOLITARY OR MULTIPLE

COMMON

1. Infarction
2. Pneumonia, acute or organizing
3. Pulmonary contusion
4. Tuberculosis

UNCOMMON

1. Alveolar cell carcinoma
2. Fungus disease
3. Löffler's syndrome
4. Lymphoma
5. Parasitic disease
6. Pseudolymphoma
7. Pulmonary collapse
8. Pulmonary edema, localized
9. Pulmonary infiltration with eosinophilia (PIE)
10. Radiation pneumonitis

LOBAR ENLARGEMENT

COMMON

1. Klebsiella pneumonia
2. Pneumococcal pneumonia

UNCOMMON

1. Carcinoma of the lung (drowned lung)
2. [Interlobar fluid]
3. Lung abscess
4. Tuberculosis

SUBGAMUT F-2A
PNEUMONIA INVOLVING AN ENTIRE LOBE

COMMON

1. Pneumococcal

UNCOMMON

1. E. coli
2. Klebsiella
3. Staphylococcal
4. Streptococcal
5. Tuberculous
6. Viral

LOBAR OR SEGMENTAL COLLAPSE

COMMON

1. Bronchial adenoma, papilloma
2. Bronchogenic carcinoma
3. Foreign body (eg, peanut)
4. Mucous plug (postoperative, postanesthesia, inflammatory)

UNCOMMON

1. Aortic aneurysm
2. Asthma
3. Bronchiectasis
4. Broncholithiasis
5. Bronchomalacia
6. Cardiac enlargement (esp. dilated left atrium)
7. Endotracheal tube positioned too low
8. Inflammatory stricture of bronchus (eg, tuberculosis)
9. Lymphadenopathy, "middle lobe syndrome"
10. Mediastinal neoplasm
11. Mucoid impaction (eg, asthma, aspergillus sensitivity)
12. Mucoviscidosis
13. Organized pneumonia; pulmonary fibrosis
14. Pertussis
15. Pneumonia
16. Poliomyelitis, bulbar
17. Radiation therapy

Reference:

Teplick JG, Haskin ME: *Roentgenologic Diagnosis*, ed 2. Philadelphia, WB Saunders Co, 1971, vol 2, p xxv.

RECURRENT PNEUMONIA
(See also Gamut F-5)

COMMON

1. Alcoholism with aspiration
2. Asthma
3. Bronchial tumor (adenoma, carcinoma)
4. Bronchiectasis
5. Chronic sinusitis, including Kartagener's syndrome
6. Eosinophilic pneumonia
7. Esophageal disease with aspiration
8. Foreign body
9. Mucoviscidosis
10. Neuromuscular disorders with aspiration (brain damage, myasthenia gravis, pseudobulbar palsy, etc.)
11. Opportunistic infection
12. Parasitic diseases (ascariasis, strongyloidiasis, hookworm disease, paragonimiasis, dirofilariasis, schistosomiasis)

UNCOMMON

1. Choanal atresia
2. Extrinsic compression of tracheobronchial tree (eg, vascular ring)
3. Immunologic disorders
4. Inhalation diseases (farmer's lung, silo filler's disease, byssinosis, etc.)
5. Laryngeal disease
6. Lupus erythematosus; scleroderma
7. Pulmonary sequestration
8. Rheumatoid or ankylosing spondylitis
9. Riley-Day syndrome
10. Sickle cell disease
11. Tracheoesophageal fistula
12. Tracheostomy

CHRONIC ASPIRATION PNEUMONIA IN A CHILD
(See also Gamuts F-4 and F-39)

COMMON

1. Brain damage, neuromuscular disorders (muscular dystrophy, etc.)
2. Esophageal disease (atresia, stenosis, achalasia, chalasia, etc.)
3. Idiopathic
4. Tracheoesophageal fistula

UNCOMMON

1. Choanal atresia
2. Cleft palate
3. Hiatus hernia
4. Laryngeal wall deficiency, congenital
5. Micrognathia (eg, Riley-Day syndrome)
6. Vascular ring

Reference:

Gatewood OMB, Vanhoutte JJ: The role of the barium swallow examination in evaluation of pediatric pneumonias. *Am J Roentgenol* 97:203-210, 1966.

DISSEMINATED ALVEOLAR DISEASE, ACUTE OR CHRONIC

I. ACUTE

COMMON

1. Hyaline membrane disease; aspiration syndrome; transient tachypnea of the newborn
2. Pneumonia, including opportunistic or other unusual etiology (chickenpox, cytomegalic inclusion disease, *E. coli*, influenza, leptospirosis, Löffler's, measles giant cell, mycoplasma, pneumocystis, psittacosis)
3. Pulmonary edema

UNCOMMON

1. Pulmonary hemorrhage (anticoagulants, aspirated blood, Goodpasture's syndrome, idiopathic, idiopathic hemosiderosis, hemophilia, leukemia, trauma)

II. CHRONIC

COMMON

1. Alveolar cell carcinoma
2. Alveolar proteinosis
3. Lymphoma
4. Sarcoidosis

UNCOMMON

1. Alveolar microlithiasis
2. Desquamative interstitial pneumonitis (DIP), lymphocytic interstitial pneumonitis (LIP)
3. Hair spray pneumonia
4. Mineral oil aspiration, lipoid pneumonia
5. Tuberculosis, fungus disease

SUBGAMUT F-6A
ROENTGEN SIGNS OF ALVEOLAR DISEASE

1. Air bronchogram or alveologram
2. Alveolar nodules (acinar or peribronchiolar)
3. Butterfly shadow
4. Coalescence (early)
5. Early appearance after onset of symptoms
6. Fluffy margins
7. Segmental or lobar distribution

PULMONARY EDEMA
(See also Gamuts F-8 and F-15)

COMMON

1. Agonal
2. Aspiration (eg, Mendelsohn's syndrome)
3. Cerebral (stroke, head trauma, epilepsy)
4. Drug hypersensitivity, allergy (eg, penicillin, hexamethonium, nitrofuradantin), and poisoning
5. Fluid overload, overtransfusion
6. Glomerulonephritis, acute
7. Heart disease (left heart failure, mitral stenosis, hypoplastic left heart syndromes)
8. Narcotics (heroin, etc.)
9. Oxygen toxicity (shock lung)
10. Pulmonary embolism or infarct
11. Uremia

UNCOMMON

1. Cardiopulmonary bypass
2. Hanging, suffocation
3. High altitude
4. Hypoproteinemia
5. Inhalation of noxious gas
6. Intravascular coagulation defect
7. Liver disease
8. [Lymphangiectasia]
9. Malaria

(Continued)

10. Mediastinal tumor with venous or lymphatic obstruction
11. Near drowning
12. Neoplasm of heart (esp. left atrial myxoma)
13. Pneumothorax post-thoracentesis (unilateral)
14. Pregnancy
15. Pulmonary veno-occlusive disease
16. Radiation therapy
17. Retained fetal lung fluid (transient tachypnea)
18. Shock (eg, insulin reaction, shock therapy)
19. Thoracic trauma
20. Transfusion reaction

PULMONARY EDEMA IN AN INFANT
(See also Gamuts F-7 and F-15)

COMMON

1. Agonal
2. Fluid overload
3. [Hyaline membrane disease]
4. Hypoplastic left heart syndromes (mitral or aortic stenosis or atresia, cor triatriatum, hypoplastic aorta)
5. Oxygen toxicity (shock lung), early
6. Retained fetal lung fluid (transient tachypnea)

UNCOMMON

1. Anomalous pulmonary venous return, total
2. Drug hypersensitivity
3. [Lymphangiectasia]
4. Myocardiopathy
5. Obstructive tumor or thrombus in left atrium
6. Stenosis of pulmonary veins

ALVEOLAR PATTERN IN PATIENTS WITH LYMPHOMA

COMMON

1. Bacterial pneumonia
2. Cytomegalic inclusion virus pneumonia
3. Fungus disease (moniliasis, aspergillosis, histoplasmosis, torulosis)
4. Pneumocystis carinii pneumonia

UNCOMMON

1. Drug reaction (eg, methotrexate)
2. Lymphomatous or leukemic infiltrate
3. Mycoplasma pneumonia
4. Pulmonary edema (congestive failure)
5. Pulmonary hemorrhage

PULMONARY HEMORRHAGE

COMMON

1. Contusion
2. Goodpasture's syndrome

UNCOMMON

1. Anticoagulant therapy
2. Aspiration from a bleeding pulmonary lesion
3. Hemophilia, leukemia, and other bleeding states
4. Idiopathic
5. Idiopathic hemosiderosis
6. Mitral stenosis

ALVEOLAR PATTERNS THAT CHANGE TO INTERSTITIAL

1. Alveolar sarcoidosis
2. Desquamative, lymphocytic, and giant cell interstitial pneumonitis (DIP, LIP, GCIP)
3. Hemosiderosis
4. Idiopathic
5. Oxygen toxicity (shock lung)
6. Sensitivity pneumonitis (eg, farmer's lung, bagassosis)
7. Viral pneumonia

DIFFUSE MILIARY NODULES IN THE LUNGS (LESS THAN 5 MM DIAMETER)

COMMON

*1. Fungus disease (eg, histoplasmosis, coccidioidomycosis, blastomycosis, torulosis)

2. Histiocytosis X

3. Interstitial fibrosis (subliminal honeycombing)

4. Metastatic malignancy (eg, thyroid; lymphangitic carcinomatosis)

5. Pneumoconiosis

6. Sarcoidosis

*7. Tuberculosis, miliary

UNCOMMON

1. Alveolar cell carcinoma

2. Alveolar microlithiasis

3. Amyloidosis

*4. Bronchiolitis fibrosa obliterans

*5. Embolism from oily contrast medium (lymphangiography, hysterosalpingography)

6. Hemosiderosis (mitral stenosis)

7. Lymphoma

*8. Melioidosis (septicemic form)

9. Parasitic disease (schistosomiasis, filariasis)

*10. Pneumonia of unusual etiology (eg, chickenpox, measles)

11. Rheumatoid lung

12. Tuberous sclerosis

*Acute

SUBGAMUT F-12A
DIFFUSE MILIARY NODULES IN THE LUNGS
OF A NEWBORN

*1. Acute bronchiolitis

*2. Hyaline membrane disease

 3. Lymphangiectasia

 4. Total anomalous pulmonary venous return below the diaphragm

*Acute

HONEYCOMB LUNG (INTERSTITIAL FIBROSIS)

COMMON

1. [Bronchiectasis]
2. Histiocytosis X
3. Idiopathic interstitial fibrosis (Hamman-Rich)
4. Pneumoconiosis
5. Sarcoidosis

UNCOMMON

1. [Adenomatoid malformation of newborn (unilateral)]
2. Amyloidosis
3. Chemical inhalation (late stage)
4. Desquamative, lymphocytic, and giant cell interstitial pneumonitis (DIP, LIP, GCIP)
5. Drug therapy (eg, nitrofurantoin, hexamethonium, busulfan)
6. Gaucher's disease
7. Idiopathic pulmonary hemosiderosis (late)
8. Lipoid pneumonia
9. [Lymphangiomyomatosis]
10. [Mikity-Wilson syndrome, respirator or shock lung]
11. [Mucoviscidosis]
12. Muscular cirrhosis (leiomyomatosis) ?
13. Neurofibromatosis
14. Niemann-Pick disease
15. Rheumatoid lung
16. Scleroderma; dermatomyositis
17. Sensitivity pneumonitis, recurrent (eg, farmer's lung, bagassosis)
18. Tuberous sclerosis

Reference:

Felson B: Disseminated interstitial diseases of the lung. *Ann Radiol* 9:325–345, 1966.

SUBGAMUT 13A
ROENTGEN SIGNS OF INTERSTITIAL DISEASE

1. Discrete miliary nodules

2. Honeycombing

3. Kerley's lines

4. Late appearance after onset of symptoms

5. Late coalescence

6. Small irregular shadows, reticular stranding

Reference:

Felson B: The roentgen diagnosis of disseminated pulmonary alveo-lar diseases. *Semin Roentgenol* 2:3–21, 1967.

DISSEMINATED SMALL IRREGULAR SHADOWS (RETICULAR, RETICULONODULAR, LINEAR, "ILL-DEFINED")

COMMON

1. Idiopathic
2. Lymphangitic metastases
3. Organic dust inhalation (see Gamut F-44)
4. Pneumoconiosis (see Gamut F-43)

UNCOMMON

1. Acute bronchiolitis; bronchiolitis fibrosa obliterans (eg, chemical inhalation)
2. Amyloidosis
3. Drug hypersensitivity (eg, nitrofurantoin)
4. Embolism from oily contrast media; fat embolism
5. Fungus disease
6. Honeycomb lung[1]
7. Interstitial fibrosis (see Gamut F-13)
8. Interstitial nodules[1] (see Gamut F-12)
9. Interstitial pulmonary edema[1]
10. Lymphoma
11. Mucoviscidosis
12. Oxygen toxicity; Mikity-Wilson syndrome
13. Parasitic disease (eg, schistosomiasis, filariasis, paragonimiasis)
14. Pulmonary fibrosis
15. Riley-Day syndrome; other aspiration pneumonia
16. Sarcoidosis

[1]Interstitial disease in which the pattern of miliary nodules, honeycombing, or Kerley's lines cannot be recognized, though present pathologically.

(Continued)

17. Scleroderma; dermatomyositis

18. Sjögren's syndrome

19. "Small airways disease"

20. Tuberculosis

21. Viral pneumonia (eg, measles, chickenpox)

References:

1. Fraser RG, Paré JAP: *Diagnosis of Diseases of the Chest.* Philadel-phia, WB Saunders Co, 1970.

2. Teplick JG, Haskin ME: *Roentgenologic Diagnosis*, ed 2. Philadelphia, WB Saunders Co, 1971, vol 2, p XXIII.

INTERSTITIAL EDEMA PATTERN, ACUTE KERLEY'S LINES — A, B, AND C
(See also Gamuts F-7, F-8, and F-16)

COMMON

1. Pneumonia, esp. interstitial
2. Pulmonary edema, interstitial
3. Retained fetal lung fluid (transient tachypnea)

UNCOMMON

1. Glomerulonephritis, acute
2. Hypoproteinemic state (eg, cirrhosis, burns, nephrosis, allergic conditions, exudative skin disorders)
3. Pulmonary hemorrhage (see Gamut F-10)

KERLEY'S LINES, CHRONIC — A, B, AND C
(See also Gamut F-15)

COMMON

1. Bronchogenic carcinoma, hilar
2. Idiopathic (esp. in elderly)
3. Lymphangitic metastases
4. Pneumoconiosis
5. Rheumatic mitral stenosis

UNCOMMON

1. Alveolar cell carcinoma
2. Alveolar lymphoma
3. Alveolar proteinosis
4. Desquamative interstitial pneumonitis (DIP)
5. Idiopathic pulmonary hemosiderosis (late)
6. Interstitial fibrosis, any cause (see Gamut F-13)
7. Left atrial tumor
8. Lymphangiectasia, diffuse
9. Mediastinal tumor with lymphatic obstruction
10. Mineral oil aspiration, lipoid pneumonia
11. Newborn cardiovascular syndromes (total anomalous venous return below the diaphragm; hypoplastic left heart syndromes)
12. Pulmonary vein stenosis or thrombosis
13. Radiation fibrosis
14. Sarcoidosis
15. Thoracic duct ligation, obstruction, or injury

SOLITARY PULMONARY NODULE
(UNDER 4 CM DIAMETER)

COMMON

1. Bronchial adenoma
2. Bronchogenic carcinoma; alveolar cell carcinoma
3. [Chest wall lesion (skin tumor, nipple shadow, rib lesion); artefact]
4. Granuloma (eg, tuberculosis, histoplasmosis, coccidio-domycosis, torulosis, idiopathic, talc)
5. Hamartoma
6. Metastasis (eg, from sarcoma, colon, ovary, testis, Wilms')

UNCOMMON

1. Abscess
2. Amyloid tumor
3. Arteriovenous malformation
4. Bulla, infected
5. Cyst, fluid filled (bronchogenic, bronchiectatic, hydatid)
6. [Encapsulated fluid in pleural fissure; fibrin ball]
7. Extramedullary hematopoiesis
8. Fungus ball
9. Gumma
10. Hematoma
11. Inflammatory pseudotumor; organized pneumonia (see Gamut F-18)
12. Lipoid granuloma (paraffinoma)
13. Lymph node, intrapulmonary
14. Lymphoma

(Continued)

15. Mast cell disease

16. [Mediastinal mass]

17. [Mesothelioma of pleura]

18. Mucoid impaction (eg, aspergillus sensitivity)

19. Neoplasm, benign (chemodectoma, chondroma, endometrioma, fibroma, granular cell myoblastoma, hemangioma, hemangiopericytoma, leiomyoma, lipoma, neurofibroma)

20. Parasite granuloma (eg, heart worm, ascaris)

21. Plasmacytoma

22. Pneumoconiosis, conglomerate mass

23. Pulmonary infarct

24. Pulmonary sequestration

25. Pulmonary varix; anomalous pulmonary vein

26. Rheumatoid nodule

27. Sarcoma of lung

28. Splenosis

References:

1. Felson B: *Chest Roentgenology*. Philadelphia, WB Saunders Co, 1973, p 315.
2. Reeder MM, Hochholzer L, Evans RG: RPC of the Month from the AFIP: Amyloid tumor of the lung. *Radiology* 93:1369–1375, 1969.

LARGE SOLITARY PULMONARY MASS
(GREATER THAN 4 CM DIAMETER)

COMMON

*1. Abscess
 2. Bronchogenic carcinoma; alveolar cell carcinoma
*3. Metastasis (eg, from sarcoma, testis, Wilms', hepatoma)

UNCOMMON

 *1. Arteriovenous malformation
  2. Bronchial adenoma
 *3. Cyst, fluid filled (bronchogenic, bronchiectatic, hydatid)
 *4. Granuloma (tuberculosis or fungus disease, esp. torulosis)
 *5. Hamartoma
 *6. Hematoma
 *7. Inflammatory pseudotumor; organized nodular pneumonia (types — fibroxanthoma, fibroma, plasma cell granuloma, sclerosing hemangioma of Liebow, pseudolymphoma)
 *8. Lipoid pneumonia
 *9. [Loculated interlobar or pleural fluid]
*10. Lymphoma
*11. [Mediastinal mass]
 12. [Mesothelioma of pleura]
 13. Pneumoconiosis, conglomerate mass
*14. Pulmonary sequestration
*15. Sarcoma of lung, primary
 16. Wegener's granuloma

*Seen in children

Reference:
Reeder MM: RPC of the Month from the AFIP: Hydatid cyst of the lung. *Radiology* 95:429–437, 1970.

SUPERIOR SULCUS (APICAL) MASS

COMMON

1. Bronchogenic carcinoma (Pancoast tumor)
2. Innominate artery aneurysm or buckling
3. Neurogenic tumor
4. Thyroid, retrosternal

UNCOMMON

1. Bronchogenic or tracheal cyst
2. Cystic hygroma (lymphangioma)
3. Lymphoma
4. Mediastinal tumor, other
5. Mesothelioma or other pleural tumor
6. Rib lesion

MASS-LIKE PULMONARY INFILTRATE RADIATING FROM THE HILUM

COMMON

1. Bronchogenic carcinoma
2. Lymphoma (esp. Hodgkin's)
3. Organizing pneumonia

UNCOMMON

1. Actinomycosis
2. Blastomycosis
3. Pneumoconiosis (conglomerate mass)
4. Pseudolymphoma

SHAGGY PULMONARY NODULE, SOLITARY OR MULTIPLE (FUZZY, ILL DEFINED BORDERS)

COMMON

1. Bronchogenic carcinoma; alveolar cell carcinoma
2. Fungus disease
3. Infarct, bland or septic
4. Pneumoconiosis
5. Tuberculosis

UNCOMMON

1. Eosinophilic granuloma
2. Inflammatory pseudotumor (esp. pseudolymphoma)
3. Lipid pneumonia (paraffinoma)
4. Lymphoma
5. Metastasis (esp. choriocarcinoma)
6. Parasitic disease
7. Rheumatoid nodule
8. Sarcoidosis, alveolar type
9. Wegener's granuloma

MULTIPLE DISCRETE PULMONARY NODULES OR MASSES (NONMILIARY) WITH WELL DEFINED MARGINS (OVER 5 MM IN DIAMETER)

COMMON

1. [Chest wall lesions (neurofibromatosis, nipple shadows, rib lesions); foreign bodies; artefacts]
2. Granulomas (eg, histoplasmosis, tuberculosis, torulosis, blastomycosis, coccidioidomycosis, idiopathic)
3. Metastases

UNCOMMON

1. Alveolar cell carcinoma; rarely multiple primary bronchogenic carcinomas
2. Amyloid tumors
3. Arteriovenous malformations
4. Bronchial adenomas, multiple
5. Bronchiectatic cysts, fluid filled
6. [Encapsulated pleural effusions]
7. Eosinophilic granuloma
8. Gaucher's disease; Niemann-Pick disease
9. Hamartomas
10. Heart worms (Dirofilariasis)
11. Hemosiderosis with bone formation in rheumatic mitral disease
12. Hydatid cysts
13. Leiomyomatosis (benign metastasizing leiomyoma)
14. Lymphoma
15. Mucoid impactions
16. Papillomatosis of the lung

(Continued)

17. Paraffinomas

18. Paragonimiasis

19. Pneumoconiosis, conglomerate masses

20. Polyarteritis nodosa

21. Pulmonary infarcts

22. Rheumatoid nodules

23. Sarcoidosis

24. Septic embolism with abscesses

25. Wegener's granulomatosis

Reference:

Fraser RG, Paré JAP: *Diagnosis of Diseases of the Chest.* Philadelphia, WB Saunders Co, 1970, p 275.

SHARPLY DEFINED CAVITARY LESIONS OF THE LUNGS (SINGLE (S) OR MULTIPLE (M), THIN OR THICK WALLED)

COMMON

	Type of Lesion	Thin Walled	Thick Walled
1. Abscess, bacterial or amebic	SM		x
2. Bronchogenic carcinoma	S	x	x
3. Granuloma due to tuberculosis (typical or atypical mycobacteria); fungus disease; idiopathic	SM	x	x
4. Metastatic neoplasm	SM	x	x

UNCOMMON

	Type of Lesion	Thin Walled	Thick Walled
1. Bleb or bulla, non-infected or infected	SM	x	x
2. Cystic bronchiectasis	M	x	
3. Hamartoma	S		x
4. Hematoma, laceration of lung	S	x	x
5. Hernia of bowel through diaphragm	SM	x	x
6. Histiocytosis X	M	x	
7. [Honeycomb lung, oxygen toxicity, Mikity-Wilson]	M	x	
8. Hydatid cyst	SM	x	x
9. Hydropneumothorax, encapsulated	SM	x	
10. Infarct	SM	x	x
11. Interlobar bronchopleural fistula	S	x	

(Continued)

	Type of Lesion	Thin Walled	Thick Walled
12. Lung cysts (eg, bronchogenic, congenital, traumatic)	S	x	
13. Lymphoma, Hodgkin's disease	SM		x
14. Melioidosis	SM	x	x
15. Organized pneumonia, inflammatory pseudotumor (eg, pseudolymphoma)	SM		x
16. Paragonimiasis	SM	x	x
17. Polyarteritis nodosa	M	x	
18. Pneumatocele	SM	x	
19. Pneumoconiosis, conglomerate mass	S		x
20. Rheumatoid granuloma, ankylosing spondylitis granuloma	M	x	x
21. Sarcoidosis, cystic	M	x	
22. Sequestration	S	x	x
23. Wegener's granuloma	SM	x	x

Reference:

Felson B: *Chest Roentgenology*. Philadelphia, WB Saunders Co, 1973, p 321.

MOBILE MASS IN A PULMONARY CAVITY
(MENISCUS SIGN)

COMMON

1. Aspergillus fungus ball

UNCOMMON

1. Abscess with inspissated pus
2. Blood clot in tuberculous cavity, infarct, or pulmonary laceration
3. Bronchogenic carcinoma, bronchial adenoma, sarcoma
4. Gangrene of lung
5. Granuloma (tuberculous, fungus, or idiopathic)
6. Hydatid cyst
7. Torulosis
8. Tuberculous cavernolith

CYST-LIKE PULMONARY LESIONS IN A CHILD, SOLITARY OR MULTIPLE

COMMON

1. [Diaphragmatic hernia with bowel in chest]
2. Pneumatocele
3. Sequestration

UNCOMMON

1. Adenomatoid malformation
2. Bronchiectasis
3. Bulla
4. Coccidioidomycosis; rarely other fungus disease
5. Histiocytosis X
6. Hydatid cyst
7. Laceration
8. Lung abscess
9. Paragonimiasis
10. Tuberculosis

MULTIPLE CAVITARY LESIONS IN THE LUNGS

COMMON

1. Bullae
2. Cystic bronchiectasis
3. Fungus disease
4. Honeycomb lung (see Gamut F-13)
5. Metastases
6. Pneumatoceles
7. Septic emboli (abscesses); narcotic addiction
8. Tuberculosis

UNCOMMON

1. Carcinoma of lung, multiple primaries
2. [Hernia of bowel through diaphragm]
3. Hydatid cysts
4. Hydropneumothorax, encapsulated (post-thoracentesis or bronchopleural fistula)
5. Lymphoma, Hodgkin's disease
6. Melioidosis
7. Paragonimiasis
8. Pseudolymphoma (lymphoid pseudotumors)
9. Pulmonary infarcts
10. Rheumatoid granulomas
11. Sarcoidosis, cystic
12. Wegener's granulomatosis; polyarteritis nodosa

Reference:

Reeder MM, Hochholzer L: RPC of the Month from the AFIP: Rheumatoid nodules of the lungs. *Radiology* 92:1106–1111, 1969.

HYPERINFLATION OF BOTH LUNGS
(BILATERAL OVEREXPANDED RADIOLUCENT
LUNGS)
(See also Gamut F-28)

COMMON

1. Asthma
2. Bronchiolitis, acute diffuse of infants
3. Bronchopneumonia, diffuse infantile
4. Congenital heart disease (usually cyanotic)
5. Emphysema, diffuse bullous
6. Tracheal or laryngeal obstruction or compression (foreign body, vascular ring, tumor, tracheomalacia, etc.)

UNCOMMON

1. Bronchiolitis fibrosa obliterans
2. Hyperventilation (metabolic disturbances, acidosis, gastro-enteritis, etc.)
3. Mucoviscidosis (early)
4. Oxygen toxicity (shock lung)
5. Tracheoesophageal fistula

UNILATERAL HYPERLUCENT LUNG;
UNILATERAL SEGMENTAL, LOBAR, OR PULMONARY OLIGEMIA
(See also Gamut F-34)

COMMON

1. [Absent pectoral muscles, surgical or congenital; mastectomy]
2. Bullous emphysema; cystic bronchiectasis
3. Contralateral increased density caused by pleural, chest wall, or pulmonary disease
4. Lateral decubitus film, normal variant
5. Lobar collapse with compensatory overdistension of remaining lobes
6. Obstructive hyperaeration (foreign body, neoplasm, inflammation)
7. [Pneumothorax]
8. [Rotation (scoliosis, poor positioning)]

UNCOMMON

1. Absent or hypoplastic pulmonary artery; pulmonary branch stenosis
2. Bronchogenic cyst; sequestration; congenital segmental bronchial atresia
3. Congenital lobar emphysema
4. Pneumatocele
5. Postlobectomy
6. Pulmonary artery embolism, thrombosis, or obstruction by carcinoma
7. Swyer-James (Macleod) syndrome
8. Venolobar syndrome

INFANTILE LOBAR EMPHYSEMA

COMMON

1. Cartilage ring anomaly (absence, hypoplasia, or malacia)
2. Idiopathic

UNCOMMON

1. Bronchial atresia, segmental
2. Bronchial kinking
3. Foreign body
4. Mucosal flap or enlarged fold of bronchus
5. Neoplasm
6. Patent ductus arteriosus
7. Pulmonary artery sling

BRONCHIAL LESION

COMMON

1. Absent bronchus (congenital, surgical)
2. Bronchial adenoma
3. Bronchogenic carcinoma
4. Extrinsic pressure (eg, lymph nodes, mediastinal tumor, enlarged left atrium)
5. Foreign body
6. Metastatic endobronchial malignancy (hypernephroma, melanoma, breast)
7. Mucous plug, mucoid impaction (see Subgamut F-30A)
8. Stricture, inflammatory (tuberculosis, fungus, other)

UNCOMMON

1. Amyloidosis
2. Broncholith
3. Fracture or laceration of bronchus
4. Granular cell myoblastoma
5. Hamartoma
6. Lymphoma
7. Mesenchymal tumor (benign or malignant spindle cell tumor, lipoma, chondroma, angioma)
8. Parasites (Ascaris, Paragonimus)
9. Polyp, papilloma
10. Rhinoscleroma
11. Silicotic conglomerate mass
12. Wegener's granuloma

SUBGAMUT F-30A
MUCOID IMPACTION OF A BRONCHUS

1. Aspergillus sensitivity
2. Asthma, other allergic states
3. Atresia of bronchus, congenital
4. Bronchial adenoma
5. Bronchogenic carcinoma
6. Bronchogenic cyst
7. Idiopathic

BRONCHIECTASIS

COMMON

1. Chronic bronchitis
2. Foreign body
3. Idiopathic
4. Mucoviscidosis
5. Postinfection
6. Tuberculosis

UNCOMMON

1. Bronchial compression
2. Fungus disease
3. Immunologic disorder (eg, dysgammaglobulinemia, Wiscott-Aldrich syndrome)
4. Kartagener's triad
5. Mucoid impaction
6. Riley-Day syndrome (familial autonomic dysfunction)
7. Other bronchial lesion (see Gamut F-30)

SUBGAMUT F-31A
TYPES OF BRONCHIECTASIS

1. Ampullary, varicose
2. Bronchiolectasis
3. Cylindrical, fusiform
4. Cystic
5. Reversible, pseudobronchiectasis
6. Saccular

UNILATERAL OR BILATERAL DISPLACEMENT OF A HILUM

COMMON

1. Bronchogenic carcinoma
2. Emphysema
3. Inflammatory process (tuberculosis, fungus)
4. Lobar collapse
5. Lobectomy
6. Mediastinal mass
7. Pneumoconiosis
8. Pneumothorax

UNCOMMON

1. Absent pulmonary artery
2. Lobar agenesis
3. Sarcoidosis, fibrotic
4. Swyer-James (Macleod) syndrome

UNILATERAL HILAR ENLARGEMENT
(See also Gamut F-54)

COMMON

1. Inflammatory lymphadenopathy (eg, primary tuberculosis, fungus disease, esp. histoplasmosis, coccidioidomycosis)
2. Intrabronchial neoplasm (eg, bronchogenic carcinoma, adenoma)
3. Lymphoma
4. Metastatic neoplasm
5. Valvular pulmonic stenosis (poststenotic dilatation of left pulmonary artery)

UNCOMMON

1. Aneurysm of a pulmonary artery
2. Arteriovenous fistula
3. Blocked contralateral pulmonary artery (eg, carcinoma, Swyer-James syndrome, congenital absence of pulmonary artery)
4. [Mediastinal mass superimposed on hilus (eg, thymoma)]
5. [Pneumonia, juxtahilar (silhouette sign)]
6. Pulmonary artery coarctation (poststenotic dilatation)
7. Pulmonary embolism
8. Sarcoidosis

UNILATERAL SMALL HILAR SHADOW
(See also Gamut F-28)

COMMON

1. Hyperaeration of one lung (emphysema)
2. Lobar collapse with hilum displaced behind the heart
3. Normal variant
4. Obstructive overdistension of one lung
5. Rotation (scoliosis, poor positioning)
6. Surgical resection of one lobe

UNCOMMON

1. Congenital absence, hypoplasia, or coarctation of a pulmonary artery
2. Pulmonary artery embolism
3. Swyer-James (Macleod) syndrome (idiopathic unilateral hyperlucent lung)
4. Tumor (primary or metastatic) or inflammatory process blocking a pulmonary artery

GENERALIZED PULMONARY OLIGEMIA
(See also Gamut F-27)

COMMON

1. Bullous emphysema
2. Chronic obstructive emphysema
3. Congenital heart disease with right to left shunt

UNCOMMON

1. Compression of main pulmonary artery (eg, by neoplasm or lymphadenopathy)
2. Mitral stenosis (chronic postcapillary hypertension)
3. Primary pulmonary hypertension
4. Pulmonary artery stenosis or coarctation
5. Secondary pulmonary hypertension, other causes (eg, schistosomiasis, etc.)
6. Widespread embolic disease to small arteries

Reference:

Fraser RG, Paré JAP: *Diagnosis of Diseases of the Chest*. Philadelphia, WB Saunders Co, 1970, p 499.

INCREASED PULMONARY ARTERIAL CIRCULATION TO ONE LUNG

COMMON

1. Obstruction of pulmonary artery flow on contralateral side (eg, embolism, neoplasm, pulmonary artery sling) (see Gamut F-34)

2. Pulmonary A-V fistula (congenital or acquired)

UNCOMMON

1. Left to right shunt with increased flow to one lung (eg, patent ductus arteriosus)

2. [Scimitar syndrome; hypogenetic lung; pulmonary artery atresia, stenosis, or coarctation (opposite lung)]

3. Surgical procedure for cyanotic congenital heart disease (Waterson, Blalock, Potts)

4. Unilateral origin of a pulmonary artery from the aorta; truncus arteriosus with single pulmonary artery

Reference:

Chen JTT, Capp MP, Johnsrude IS, et al: Roentgen appearance of pulmonary vascularity in the diagnosis of heart disease. *Am J Roentgenol* 112:559–570, 1971.

PULMONARY DISEASE WITH EOSINOPHILIA

COMMON

1. Aspergillus sensitivity
2. Asthma
3. Drug sensitivity (eg, furadantin, penicillin, isoniazid, sulfa)
4. Eosinophilic leukemia
5. Idiopathic, acute (Löffler's syndrome)
6. Idiopathic, chronic (PIE)
7. Parasitic diseases, including tropical eosinophilia (see Gamut F-4)

UNCOMMON

1. Brucellosis
2. Carcinoma (eg, lung)
3. Coccidioidomycosis
4. Desquamative interstitial pneumonitis (DIP)
5. Polyarteritis nodosa
6. Wegener's granuloma

Reference:

Carrington CB, Addington WW, Goff AM, et al: Chronic eosinophilic pneumonia. *N Engl J Med* 280:787–798, 1969.

LOCALIZED NONRESOLVING PULMONARY INFILTRATE

COMMON

1. Bronchial obstruction (eg, adenoma, carcinoma, foreign body, mucous plug)
2. Bronchiectasis
3. Chronic aspiration pneumonia (Zenker's diverticulum, achalasia, chalasia, hiatus hernia, esophageal atresia, stenosis or web, scleroderma, neuromuscular disorders)
4. Organized pneumonia
5. Pneumonia, untreated or antibiotic resistant (eg, mycoplasma, tuberculosis, actinomycosis, blastomycosis, Friedländer's)

UNCOMMON

1. Foreign body in pulmonary tissue (eg, splinter, Lycoperdon)
2. Idiopathic
3. Immunologic disorders
4. Lung abscess
5. Mineral oil pneumonitis; lipoid pneumonia
6. Pulmonary sequestration
7. Radiation pneumonitis
8. Steroid or immunosuppressant therapy

Reference:

Kreel L: *Outline of Radiology.* New York, Appleton-Century-Crofts, 1971, pp 10–11.

CHRONIC PULMONARY INFILTRATE
IN A CHILD
(See also Gamuts F-4 and F-5)

COMMON

1. Aspiration
2. Asthma, aspergillus sensitivity (mucoid impaction)
3. Bronchiectasis
4. Foreign body
5. Mucoviscidosis
6. Parasitic disease (see Gamut F-4)
7. Pulmonary sequestration
8. Tuberculosis

UNCOMMON

1. Adenomatoid malformation
2. Bronchial obstruction (stricture, tumor, etc.)
3. Fungus disease
4. Histiocytosis X
5. Idiopathic pulmonary fibrosis
6. Idiopathic pulmonary hemosiderosis
7. Immunologic disorders
8. Lipoid pneumonia
9. Pneumonia, organized
10. Sarcoidosis

BILATERAL BASILAR INFILTRATE

COMMON

1. Asbestosis
2. Aspiration pneumonia
3. Bronchiectasis
4. Idiopathic interstitial fibrosis (Hamman-Rich)
5. Scleroderma; dermatomyositis

UNCOMMON

1. Alveolar proteinosis
2. Desquamative interstitial pneumonitis (DIP)
3. Lipoid pneumonia
4. Lupus erythematosus
5. Mucoviscidosis
6. Rheumatoid lung

PLEURAL-BASED LESION ARISING FROM LUNG OR PLEURA

COMMON

1. Mesothelioma, benign or malignant
2. Metastasis
3. Pleural fluid, loculated or interlobar
4. Pulmonary infarct
5. Rib or chest wall lesion

UNCOMMON

1. Fibrin ball
2. Fungus infection (actinomycosis, torulosis, blastomycosis)
3. Granuloma of lung
4. Lipoma
5. Mesenchymal tumor
6. Neurilemmoma of intercostal nerve
7. Rheumatoid nodule

COMBINED SKIN AND WIDESPREAD LUNG DISORDER

COMMON

1. Lupus erythematosus
2. Sarcoidosis
3. Scleroderma; dermatomyositis

UNCOMMON

1. Acanthosis nigricans
2. Allergy, drug sensitivity, parasitic infestation
3. Amyloidosis
4. Bleeding disorder (see Gamut F-10)
5. Burns
6. Chickenpox
7. Erythema nodosum
8. Fungus disease
9. Histiocytosis X
10. Juvenile xanthogranuloma
11. Lymphoma, mycosis fungoides
12. Malignant neoplasm of the skin with metastases (eg, melanoma, Kaposi's sarcoma)
13. Measles
14. Neurofibromatosis
15. Osler's familial telangiectasia
16. Rheumatoid arthritis
17. Tuberous sclerosis
18. Wegener's granuloma

Reference:

Rubin EH, Siegelman SS: *The Lungs in Systemic Diseases.* Springfield, Charles C Thomas, 1969.

PULMONARY DISORDER CAUSED BY INHALATION OF DUST (PNEUMOCONIOSIS)
(See also Gamut F-44)

COMMON

1. Anthracosis and anthracosilicosis
2. Asbestosis
3. Silicosis

UNCOMMON

1. Aluminum inhalation
2. Antimony inhalation
3. Bagassosis (sugar cane)
4. Barium pneumoconiosis
5. Berylliosis
6. Byssinosis (cotton)
7. Cadmium inhalation
8. Carcinogenic dust (arsenic, chromate, uranium, asbestos, thorium)
9. Cerium pneumoconiosis (arc lamp)
10. Diatomaceous earth pneumoconiosis
11. Farmer's lung (moldy hay, wheat dust), tabacosis
12. Fog-fever and the heaves
13. Graphite pneumoconiosis
14. Hemp dust inhalation disease
15. Kaolinosis (clay and china clay)
16. Lipid pneumonitis
17. Lycoperdonosis (puff ball fungus)
18. Malt worker's pneumonia

(Continued)

19. Manganese pneumoconiosis
20. Maple bark stripper's disease
21. Mica pneumoconiosis
22. Mushroom picker's pneumonia
23. Osmium pneumoconiosis
24. Paprika splitter's lung
25. Pigeon breeder's lung, bird fancier's lung, ostrich feather lung
26. Pituitary snuff user's lung
27. Platinum pneumoconiosis
28. Radioactive ore disease (radon)
29. Sequoiosis
30. Siderosis
31. Silver pneumoconiosis; argyrosiderosis (ferric oxide + silver)
32. Smallpox handler's disease
33. Stannosis
34. Suberosis (cork)
35. Talc pneumoconiosis
36. Thatched roof dust disease
37. Thesaurosis (hair spray) ?
38. Vanadium pneumoconiosis
39. Wheat weevil disease

PULMONARY DISORDER CAUSED BY INHALATION OF NOXIOUS VAPORS
(See also Gamut F-43)

A. Halogens
   1. Bromine
   2. Chlorine

B. Halogenated hydrocarbons
   1. Carbon tetrachloride
   2. Chloropicrin
   3. Methyl bromide
   4. Methyl chloride
   5. Trichloroethylene

C. Oxides of nitrogen
   1. Nitric oxide (electric arc welding)
   2. Nitrogen dioxide (silo filler's disease)

D. Irritant gases
   1. Ammonia
   2. Hydrogen fluoride
   3. Hydrogen sulfide
   4. Lewisite
   5. Mustard gas
   6. Nickel carbonyl
   7. Phosgene
   8. Sulfur dioxide

E. Others
   1. Acetone
   2. Acrolein
   3. Hair spray
   4. Insecticides
   5. Isoamyl acetate
   6. Oxygen (high concentration)
   7. Smoke

UPPER AIRWAY OBSTRUCTION IN A CHILD

COMMON

1. Croup
2. Foreign body
3. Mass, extrinsic (neoplasm, cystic hygroma, thyroglossal cyst, etc.)
4. Mass, intrinsic (papillomas, hemangioma, duplication cyst, etc.)
5. Tracheal stricture (traumatic, postoperative, or congenital)
6. Vascular ring

UNCOMMON

1. Allergy (spasm, edema)
2. Choanal atresia
3. Diphtheria
4. Epiglottitis
5. Esophageal atresia, tracheoesophageal fistula
6. Laryngeal web
7. Laryngomalacia; tracheomalacia
8. Laryngospasm (eg, tetany)
9. Macroglossia
10. Micrognathia with glossoptosis (eg, Pierre-Robin syndrome; Möbius syndrome; isolated micrognathia)
11. Peritonsillar abscess
12. Tonsils and adenoids, enlarged

References:

1. Dunbar JS: Upper respiratory tract obstruction in infants and children. *Am J Roentgenol* 109:227–246, 1970.
2. Schapiro RL, Evans ET: Surgical disorders causing neonatal respiratory distress. *Am J Roentgenol* 114:305–321, 1972.

INTRATRACHEAL MASS

COMMON

1. Adenoma (carcinoid, cylindroma)
2. Carcinoma, primary or secondary invasive (from thyroid, esophagus, or lung)
3. Foreign body; tube
4. Intubation stricture

UNCOMMON

1. Amyloidosis; tracheopathia osteoplastica
2. Granuloma
3. Hamartoma
4. Inspissated secretions
5. Mesenchymal tumor (eg, hemangioma, fibroma, xanthoma, leiomyoma)
6. Metastasis (esp. kidney, melanoma)
7. Papilloma or polyp
8. Polychondritis
9. Rhinoscleroma
10. Thyroid tumor, benign
11. Trauma (eg, laceration, hematoma)
12. Wegener's granuloma

Reference:

Fleming RJ, Medina J, Seaman WB: Roentgenographic aspects of tracheal tumors. *Radiology* 79:628–636, 1962.

SUPERIOR VENA CAVAL OBSTRUCTION

COMMON

1. Aneurysm of aorta or great arteries
2. Lymphadenopathy
3. Mediastinal fibrosis (histoplasmosis, irradiation, idiopathic)
4. Tumor of lung, esophagus, or mediastinum

UNCOMMON

1. Mediastinal emphysema, severe
2. Pericarditis, constrictive
3. Thrombosis of superior vena cava

Reference:

Mikkelsen WJ: Varices of the upper esophagus in superior vena caval obstruction. *Radiology* 81:945–948, 1963.

SMALL OR ABSENT THYMUS IN AN INFANT

COMMON

1. Agammaglobulinemia, dysgammaglobulinemia
2. Stress from serious illness (eg, burn, birth trauma)

UNCOMMON

1. Agenesis (DiGeorge syndrome)
2. Congenital heart disease (eg, complete transposition of the great vessels)
3. Drugs (eg, nitrogen mustard, cytoxan, prednisone)
4. Radiation therapy
5. Steroid therapy

"ANTERIOR" MEDIASTINAL LESION
(See also Gamuts F-50 and F-51)

Anterior to a curved vertical line extending along the posterior border of the heart and anterior margin of the trachea

COMMON

*1. Aneurysm of ascending aorta or sinus of Valsalva; buckled innominate artery

2. Lymphoma (esp. nodular sclerosing Hodgkin's)

3. Morgagni hernia; hepatic herniation

4. Pericardial cyst

*5. Retrosternal thyroid

6. Teratoid lesion (benign or malignant teratoma, dermoid cyst, seminoma, choriocarcinoma, embryonal cell carcinoma)

7. Thymic lesion (benign or malignant thymoma, thymic cyst*, thymolipoma, lymphoma arising in thymus, thymic hyperplasia)

UNCOMMON

1. Anomalous left superior vena cava

2. Bronchogenic cyst

*3. Cardiac tumor or aneurysm

4. Chemodectoma

5. Cystic hygroma, lymphangioma

*6. Hematoma

7. Lymphoid hyperplasia, benign

*8. Mediastinitis; mediastinal abscess or fibrosis

*9. Mesenchymal tumor

*Can calcify

(Continued)

"ANTERIOR" MEDIASTINAL LESION
(Continued)

10. Neurofibroma

11. Pericardial tumor

12. Superior vena caval dilatation

References:

1. Felson B: *Chest Roentgenology.* Philadelphia, WB Saunders Co, 1973, p 419.
2. Leigh TF, Weens HS: *The Mediastinum.* Springfield, Charles C Thomas, 1959.

"MIDDLE" MEDIASTINAL LESION
(See also Gamuts F-49 and F-51)
Between anterior and posterior mediastinum

COMMON

*1. Aneurysm of aorta or major arteries; right aortic arch

2. Azygos vein enlargement

*3. Bronchogenic cyst

4. Esophageal lesion (eg, achalasia, leiomyoma*, carcinoma)

5. Hiatal hernia

*6. Lymph node enlargement (see Gamut F-53)

*7. Thyroid tumor

8. Varices, mediastinal or esophageal

UNCOMMON

1. Chemodectoma

2. Enteric cyst

*3. Hematoma

*4. Mediastinitis; mediastinal abscess or fibrosis

5. Mesenchymal tumor

6. Pancreatic pseudocyst

7. Parathyroid tumor

8. Tracheal tumor or cyst

9. Vagus or phrenic neurinoma

*Can calcify

References:

1. Felson B: *Chest Roentgenology*. Philadelphia, WB Saunders Co, 1973, p 419.
2. Leigh TF, Weens HS: *The Mediastinum*. Springfield, Charles C Thomas, 1959.

"POSTERIOR" MEDIASTINAL LESION
(See also Gamuts F-49 and F-50)
In posterior thoracic gutter

COMMON

*1. Aneurysm of descending aorta

*2. Neurogenic tumor

*3. Spine disease, paraspinal lesion

UNCOMMON

1. Bochdalek hernia

*2. Bronchogenic cyst

3. Chemodectoma

4. Enteric cyst

5. Extramedullary hematopoiesis

6. Glomus tumor

*7. Hematoma

8. Lymphoid hyperplasia

9. Lymphoma

*10. Mediastinitis; mediastinal abscess or fibrosis

11. Meningocele, lateral

12. Mesenchymal tumor

13. Neurenteric cyst

*14. Pheochromocytoma

*15. [Pleural fluid, loculated]

16. Pseudocyst of pancreas

17. Sequestration, extrapulmonary

18. Thoracic kidney

*19. Thyroid tumor

*Can calcify

(Continued)

References:

1. Felson B: *Chest Roentgenology*. Philadelphia, WB Saunders Co, 1973, p 419.
2. Leigh TF, Weens HS: *The Mediastinum*. Springfield, Charles C Tomas, 1959.

RIGHT ANTERIOR CARDIOPHRENIC
ANGLE MASS

COMMON

1. Epicardial fat pad, "lipoma"
2. Morgagni hernia
3. [Localized paralysis of right hemidiaphragm, partial eventration of diaphragm]
4. Pericardial cyst
5. Pleural effusion, encapsulated; pleural adhesions
6. Right middle lobe disease

UNCOMMON

1. Cardiac tumor or aneurysm
2. Diaphragmatic mass
3. Fat pad necrosis
4. Herniation of liver, traumatic or congenital (ectopic)
5. Mediastinal mass, anterior (eg, thymic lesion, teratoid tumor or cyst, lymphoma)
6. Pericardial effusion, encapsulated
7. Pulmonary neoplasm
8. [Right atrial dilatation]

MEDIASTINAL LYMPH NODE ENLARGEMENT

COMMON

1. Bronchogenic carcinoma
2. [Expiration film]
3. Histoplasmosis or other fungus disease
4. Lymphoma
5. Metastatic malignancy, other
6. Pneumoconiosis
7. Sarcoidosis
8. Tuberculosis

UNCOMMON

1. Erythema nodosum, other than sarcoidosis
2. Idiopathic
3. [Mediastinal tumor, aortic aneurysm, prominent superior vena cava]
4. Tularemia
5. Viral disease (eg, psittacosis, infectious mononucleosis)
6. Wegener's granulomatosis

References:

1. Fraser RG, Paré JAP: *Diagnosis of Diseases of the Chest.* Philadelphia, WB Saunders Co, 1970.
2. Teplick JG, Haskin ME: *Roentgenologic Diagnosis*, ed 2. Philadelphia, WB Saunders Co, 1971, vol 2, p xxvi.

UNILATERAL OR BILATERAL HILAR LYMPH NODE ENLARGEMENT

COMMON

1. Bronchogenic carcinoma
2. [Embolism]
3. [Expiratory film]
4. [Heart disease (shunts, failure, cor pulmonale, valvular pulmonic stenosis, etc.)]
5. Histoplasmosis or other fungus disease
6. Lymphoma
7. Metastatic malignancy
8. Pneumoconiosis (eg, silicosis, berylliosis)
9. Sarcoidosis
10. Tuberculosis

UNCOMMON

1. Allergic reaction
2. Brucellosis
3. Erythema nodosum
4. Idiopathic (eg, inflammatory lymphadenitis)
5. [Mediastinal tumor]
6. [Polycythemia vera]
7. Tularemia
8. Viral disease (eg, psittacosis, infectious mononucleosis)

References:

1. Paul LW, Juhl JH: *The Essentials of Roentgen Interpretation*, ed 3. New York, Harper & Row, 1972.
2. Shanks SC, Kerley P: *A Textbook of X-Ray Diagnosis*. Philadelphia, WB Saunders Co, 1970.
3. Rabin CB, Editor: *Roentgenology of the Chest*. Springfield, Charles C Thomas, 1958.

SUBGAMUT F-54A
MARKED HILAR LYMPHADENOPATHY

1. Inflammatory lymphadenitis, including tuberculosis
2. Lymphoma
3. Metastasis (esp. undifferentiated or oat cell bronchogenic carcinoma)
4. Sarcoidosis

PNEUMOMEDIASTINUM

COMMON

1. Asthma

2. Birth trauma

3. Bronchial or tracheal injury

4. [Esophageal air (e.g., dilated esophagus, diverticulum, belch)]

5. [Hiatal hernia]

6. Hyaline membrane disease

7. Iatrogenic (surgical procedure or endoscopy of esophagus, trachea, bronchi, or neck; retroperitoneal gas insufflation; anterior pneumomediastinography; overinflation during anesthesia)

8. "Spontaneous"

UNCOMMON

1. [Abscess, mediastinal]

2. [Communicating enterogenous or bronchogenic cyst (duplication)]

3. Drilling teeth

4. Esophageal perforation

5. Retroperitoneal rupture of duodenum or colon

6. Rib fracture with pulmonary laceration

7. Resuscitation attempt

References:

1. Felson B: The mediastinum. *Semin Roentgenol* 4:41–58, 1969.
2. Gray JM, Hanson GC: Mediastinal emphysema: aetiology, diagnosis, and treatment. *Thorax* 21:325–332, 1966.
3. Kreel L: *Outline of Radiology.* New York, Appleton-Century-Crofts, 1971.

PNEUMOTHORAX

COMMON

1. [Giant bulla]
2. Iatrogenic (eg, post-thoracotomy, diagnostic, therapeutic, resuscitation, thoracentesis, tracheotomy)
3. Mediastinal emphysema
4. "Spontaneous"; ruptured bulla
5. Trauma

UNCOMMON

1. Bronchopleural fistula from lung abscess, tuberculosis, fungus or other granulomatous disease
2. Chemical pneumonitis
3. Esophageal rupture
4. Honeycomb lung (esp. eosinophilic granuloma)
5. Hyaline membrane disease
6. Mucoviscidosis
7. Oxygen toxicity, Mikity-Wilson syndrome, shock lung
8. Pneumatocele, ruptured
9. Pneumoconiosis
10. Pneumonia
11. Pneumoperitoneum with passage of air through diaphragm
12. Pulmonary infarction
13. Pulmonary neoplasm, primary or metastatic (esp. osteosarcoma)

PLEURAL FLUID WITH OTHERWISE NORMAL APPEARING CHEST
(See also Gamut F-58)

COMMON

1. Cirrhosis with ascites (permeation of diaphragm)
2. Idiopathic
3. Infection (tuberculosis, fungus, bacteria, virus)
4. Lupus erythematosus
5. Lymphoma
6. Malignant neoplasm, metastatic or primary (eg, meso-thelioma)
7. Pancreatitis, pancreatic pseudocyst or carcinoma
8. Pregnancy
9. Pulmonary infarction
10. Subphrenic or liver abscess (eg, amebic, pyogenic)
11. Trauma (blood, chyle)

UNCOMMON

1. Asbestosis
2. Chylothorax, spontaneous
3. Constrictive pericarditis
4. Esophageal rupture
5. Hemorrhage, spontaneous (eg, anticoagulants, coagula-tion defect, hemophilia)
6. Hypoproteinemia
7. Iatrogenic (ventriculopleural shunt or other surgery, improperly inserted intravenous catheter, peritoneal dialy-sis, instillation of drugs)
8. Lymphatic or thoracic duct obstruction (eg, filariasis, malignant tumor)

(Continued)

9. Mediterranean fever

10. Myxedema

11. Niemann-Pick disease

12. Ovarian neoplasm (Meig's syndrome) and other abdominal malignancy with ascites (permeation of diaphragm)

13. Polyserositis, familial

14. Postmyocardial infarction syndrome

15. Renal disease (nephrotic syndrome, acute glomerulonephritis, hydronephrosis)

16. Rheumatoid disease

17. Waldenström's macroglobulinemia

18. Whipple's disease

References:

1. Fraser RG, Paré JAP: Diagnosis of Diseases of the Chest. Philadelphia, WB Saunders Co, 1970.

2. Rabin CB, Editor: *Roentgenology of the Chest.* Springfield, Charles C Thomas, 1958.

3. Teplick JG, Haskin ME: *Roentgenologic Diagnosis*, ed 2. Philadelphia, WB Saunders Co, 1971, vol 2, p xxvi.

4. Rabin CB, Blackman NS: Bilateral pleural effusion: its significance in association with a heart of normal size. *J Mt Sinai Hosp* 24:45–53, 1957.

PLEURAL FLUID ASSOCIATED WITH OTHER RADIOGRAPHIC EVIDENCE OF CHEST DISEASE
(See also Gamut F-57)

COMMON

*1. Bronchogenic carcinoma

*2. Congestive heart failure

 3. Inflammatory lung disease (bacterial, fungal, viral)

*4. Lymphoma

*5. Metastatic carcinoma

*6. Postoperative (eg, postpneumonectomy)

*7. Pulmonary infarction

*8. Subphrenic abscess

*9. Trauma to chest (blood, chyle)

UNCOMMON

 *1. Aneurysm of aorta with rupture

  2. Asbestosis

  3. Dermoid cyst, ruptured

 *4. Esophageal rupture

  5. Hydrocarbon pneumonitis

  6. Löffler's syndrome

  7. Lupus erythematosus

 *8. Mesothelioma (malignant)

  9. Myxedema

 10. Niemann-Pick disease

 11. Neoplasm of chest wall or rib cage with invasion of pleura (eg, myeloma, metastasis, bone sarcoma)

(Continued)

*12. Parasitic disease (eg, amebiasis, paragonimiasis, hydatid disease)

13. Pericarditis (esp. constrictive)

14. Postmyocardial infarction syndrome

15. Radiation therapy

16. Rheumatoid disease

17. Sarcoidosis

18. Superior vena cava or azygos vein obstruction

19. Wegener's granulomatosis

*Can be massive

Reference:

Fraser RG, Paré JAP: *Diagnosis of Diseases of the Chest.* Philadelphia, WB Saunders Co, 1970.

CHYLOTHORAX

COMMON

1. Iatrogenic (surgical injury to thoracic duct)
2. Idiopathic
3. Trauma to thoracic duct (eg, fractured rib or vertebra)
4. Tumor involving thoracic duct or mediastinum (esp. lymphoma)

UNCOMMON

1. Aneurysm of thoracic duct with rupture
2. Anomaly of thoracic duct (eg, atresia)
3. Cirrhosis of liver
4. Filariasis
5. Lymphangioma, lymphangiomyomatosis
6. Lymphadenopathy (eg, tuberculous)
7. Thrombosis of left subclavian vein

Reference:

Bower GC: Chylothorax: observations in 20 cases. *Chest* 46:464–468, 1964.

PLEURAL CALCIFICATION

COMMON

1. Empyema, organized
2. Hemothorax, organized
3. Idiopathic
4. Pleural effusion, organized
5. Pneumoconiosis (asbestosis, silicates)
6. Tuberculosis

UNCOMMON

1. Armillifer (tongue worm) infestation
2. Histoplasmosis
3. Mineral oil aspiration
4. Oleothorax
5. Pneumoconiosis from tin or barium

EXTRAPLEURAL LESION

COMMON

1. Mediastinal mass (see Gamuts F-49 to F-51)
2. Rib fracture; chest wall hematoma
3. Rib neoplasm, primary or metastatic
4. Spinal, paraspinal, sternal, or subphrenic lesion

UNCOMMON

1. Inflammation of chest wall
2. Lipoma, extrapleural
3. Lobar agenesis with extrapleural adipose tissue
4. Neurofibroma and other soft tissue tumors
5. Rib lesion, other (see Gamut F-62)
6. Sympathectomy and other operations

EXTRAPLEURAL SOFT TISSUE MASS ASSOCIATED WITH RIB DESTRUCTION

COMMON

1. Bone sarcoma (eg, Ewing's, osteosarcoma, chondrosarcoma, fibrosarcoma)
2. Fracture with hematoma or callus
3. Metastasis
4. Myeloma
5. Osteomyelitis of rib with soft tissue abscess, including tuberculosis, actinomycosis, and other fungus disease

UNCOMMON

1. Aneurysmal bone cyst
2. Brown tumor; osteitis fibrosa cystica
3. Giant cell tumor
4. Histiocytosis X
5. Lymphoma
6. Myelofibrosis with extramedullary hematopoiesis (eg, thalassemia)
7. Neurogenic tumor
8. Pleural based lesion eroding rib (see Gamut F-41)

CONGENITAL SYNDROMES WITH PECTUS EXCAVATUM OR CARINATUM

COMMON

1. Homocystinuria
2. Marfan's S.
3. Morquio S.
4. Osteogenesis imperfecta
5. Turner's S.

UNCOMMON

1. Down's S. (mongolism)
2. Hallerman-Streiff S.
3. Klinefelter's S.
4. Metaphyseal chondrodysplasia (McKusick)
5. Mietens-Weber S.
6. Mohr S.
7. Noonan's S.
8. Oculocerebral-renal S.
9. Osteochondromuscular dystrophy (Schwartz-Jampel)
10. Otopalatodigital S.
11. Whistling face S.

Reference:

Smith DW: *Recognizable Patterns of Human Malformation.* Philadelphia, WB Saunders Co, 1970, p 285.

CONGENITAL SYNDROMES WITH
SMALL THORACIC CAGE

COMMON

1. Asphyxiating thoracic dysplasia
2. Ellis-van Creveld S.
3. Metaphyseal dysostosis, Jansen-type
4. Metatropic dwarfism

UNCOMMON

1. Achondrogenesis; achondroplasia
2. Diastrophic dwarfism
3. Osteogenesis imperfecta
4. Pseudoachondroplastic form of spondyloepiphyseal dysplasia

References:

1. Felson B, Editor: Dwarfs and Other Little People. *Semin Roentgenol* 8:133–263, 1973.
2. Smith DW: *Recognizable Patterns of Human Malformation.* Philadelphia, WB Saunders Co, 1970, p 285.

BILATERAL ELEVATED DIAPHRAGM

COMMON

1. Abdominal tumor or cyst (eg, ovarian cyst, carcinoma)
2. Ascites
3. Liver and spleen enlargement
4. Obesity, severe
5. Pneumoperitoneum
6. Pregnancy
7. [Subpulmonary effusion, bilateral]

UNCOMMON

1. [Diaphragmatic hernia, bilateral or large]
2. Lobar collapse, bilateral
3. Lupus erythematosus
4. Pleural disease, bilateral
5. Pulmonary infarction, bilateral
6. Subphrenic abscess, bilateral
7. Trauma, bilateral

UNILATERAL HIGH DIAPHRAGM

COMMON

1. Distended stomach or splenic flexure (left)
2. Eventration
3. Fractured rib (guarding)
4. Normal; idiopathic
5. Phrenic nerve paralysis or injury (See Gamut F-67)
6. Pleural disease (eg, fibrosis, acute pleurisy, pneumonia, pulmonary infarct)
7. Postoperative
8. Pulmonary collapse
9. Ruptured spleen or liver with subphrenic hematoma
10. Scoliosis (on side of concavity)
11. Subphrenic inflammatory disease (eg, subphrenic, perinephric, hepatic, or splenic abscess, pancreatitis, cholecystitis, perforated ulcer)
12. Subphrenic mass (enlarged liver, carcinoma of stomach)
13. [Subpulmonary effusion]

UNCOMMON

1. High retroperitoneal mass (eg, thoracic kidney, retroperitoneal neoplasm)
2. [Traumatic diaphragmatic hernia]
3. Tumor or cyst of diaphragm

PARALYZED OR FIXED HEMIDIAPHRAGM

COMMON

1. [Diaphragmatic hernia, esp. traumatic]
2. Eventration
3. Phrenic nerve paralysis (eg, neoplasm, inflammation, or aneurysm of thoracic or cervical region)
4. Subphrenic inflammatory disease (eg, hepatic, splenic, perinephric, or subphrenic abscess; pancreatitis; cholecystitis)

UNCOMMON

1. Herpes
2. Idiopathic
3. Muscle disease (eg, myotonia congenita)
4. Neoplastic involvement of diaphragm, primary or secondary
5. Neurologic disease (eg, poliomyelitis, peripheral neuritis, Erb's palsy, hemiplegia)
6. Pneumonia
7. Postoperative (phrenic nerve section)
8. Pulmonary infarct
9. Radiation therapy
10. Trauma (eg, phrenic nerve or brachial plexus injury)

LONG LINEAR SHADOWS IN THE THORAX, SOLITARY OR MULTIPLE

COMMON

1. Bulla, pneumatocele, or thin-walled cavity (curvilinear)
2. Kerley's lines
3. Normal pleural fissure
4. Normal pulmonary arteries and veins
5. Plate-like atelectasis
6. Pneumothorax (edge of lung)
7. Pulmonary scar
8. Skin fold; artefact

UNCOMMON

1. Anomalous pulmonary vein (eg, scimitar syndrome, other forms of anomalous pulmonary venous return)
2. Bronchial arteries in cyanotic congenital heart disease
3. Bronchial wall thickening (eg, bronchiectasis, chronic bronchitis)
4. Bronchiectatic bronchus filled with secretion
5. Dilated vessels associated with arteriovenous malformation
6. Mucoid impaction of bronchus
7. Pleural band or scar

FAT SHADOW IN THE THORAX

COMMON

1. Fat pad, pericardial or chest wall
2. Lipoma
3. Teratoma (dermoid)

UNCOMMON

1. Excessive fat from steroids
2. Hibernoma
3. Omental hernia
4. Thymolipoma

EGGSHELL CALCIFICATIONS

COMMON

1. Idiopathic
2. Silicosis; coal worker's pneumoconiosis

UNCOMMON

1. Aneurysm of great vessels
2. Blastomycosis
3. Pulmonary artery calcification in chronic pulmonary hypertension (atrial septal defect, cor pulmonale)
4. Sarcoidosis

Reference:

Felson B: *Chest Roentgenology.* Philadelphia, WB Saunders Co, 1973, p. 465.

SOLITARY THORACIC CALCIFICATION

COMMON

1. Cardiovascular
2. Chest wall (rib callus, costal cartilage calcification, myositis ossificans, parasites, benign or malignant tumor of rib, breast, or chest wall)
3. Granuloma, nonspecific
4. Histoplasmoma
5. Mediastinal mass (eg, teratoma, thymoma, neurogenic tumor, substernal thyroid, bronchogenic cyst)
6. Pericardial
7. Pleural (eg, asbestosis, tuberculosis, hemothorax, empyema)
8. Tuberculosis, inactive

UNCOMMON

1. Amyloid tumor
2. Bronchial adenoma (carcinoid)
3. Bronchogenic carcinoma engulfing preexisting granuloma
4. Broncholith
5. Bulla
6. [Foreign body]
7. Fungus ball
8. Hamartoma
9. Hematoma
10. Lymphoma, treated
11. Metastasis (eg, osteosarcoma, chondrosarcoma, colloid carcinoma, psammomatous carcinoma, cystosarcoma phylloides)

(Continued)

12. Parasite (see Gamut F-72)
13. Pulmonary artery atherosclerosis
14. Pulmonary thromboembolism

MULTIPLE OR WIDESPREAD THORACIC CALCIFICATIONS

COMMON

1. Histoplasmosis, coccidioidomycosis
2. [Postlymphangiography, postbronchography]
3. Silicosis, coal workers' pneumoconiosis
4. Tracheobronchial cartilage (physiologic)
5. Tuberculosis (not miliary)

UNCOMMON

1. Alveolar microlithiasis
2. Amyloidosis; tracheopathia osteoplastica
3. Broncholiths
4. Chickenpox pneumonia
5. [Foreign bodies]
6. Fungus balls
7. Lymphoma after radiation therapy
8. Metabolic (primary or secondary hyperparathyroidism, hypervitaminosis D, milk-alkali syndrome, intravenous calcium administration)
9. Metastases (eg, osteosarcoma, chondrosarcoma, colloid carcinoma, psammomatous carcinoma, cystosarcoma phylloides)
10. Parasites (Paragonimus, Armillifer, Cysticercus, or guinea worm in lung, thoracic muscles, or subcutaneous tissues)
11. Pulmonary artery atherosclerosis
12. Pulmonary hemosiderosis (mitral stenosis)
13. Pulmonary osteopathia (bony metaplasia of lung)

(Continued)

14. Sarcoidosis

15. [Tin or barium pneumoconiosis]

References:

1. Felson B: Thoracic calcifications. *Chest* 56:330–343, 1969.
2. Salzman E: *Lung Calcifications in X-Ray Diagnosis.* Springfield, Charles C Thomas, 1968.

RETROCARDIAC LESION IN A CHILD

1. Collapse of left lower lobe
2. Diaphragmatic or hiatal hernia
3. Lymphadenopathy
4. Mediastinal lesion (see Gamuts F-50 and F-51)
5. Pleural effusion
6. Pneumonia
7. Pulmonary neoplasm or cyst
8. Pulmonary sequestration
9. Spine disease, paraspinal abscess

BLURRING OF THE HEART BORDER ON PA CHEST FILM

COMMON

1. Idiopathic
2. Infiltrate in lingula, right middle lobe, or anterior segment of an upper lobe
3. Mediastinal lesion
4. Normal blood vessel
5. Pericardial fat pad
6. Pleural fluid
7. Pleuropericardial adhesion; postinfarction myocardial scar

UNCOMMON

1. Congenital venolobar syndrome
2. Funnel breast
3. Pericarditis, constrictive

COMPLETE OPACIFICATION OF
ONE HEMITHORAX

COMMON

1. Collapse of lung
2. Consolidation of lung
3. Pleural effusion, massive (see Subgamut F-75A); empyema; hemothorax; chylothorax
4. Postpneumonectomy (fibrothorax)

UNCOMMON

1. Adenomatoid malformation of lung (airless)
2. Agenesis of a lung
3. Cardiomegaly, massive
4. Diaphragmatic hernia
5. Eventration of diaphragm
6. Fibrosis of lung or pleura
7. Hematoma of chest wall
8. Mediastinal or pulmonary mass, unilateral
9. Mesothelioma of pleura

SUBGAMUT F-75A
MASSIVE PLEURAL FLUID

COMMON

1. Congestive heart failure
2. Empyema
3. Metastasis
4. Nephrosis
5. Postpneumonectomy
6. Trauma, hemothorax
7. Tuberculosis

UNCOMMON

1. Chylothorax
2. Idiopathic
3. Lymphoma
4. Mesothelioma, malignant
5. Pulmonary infarction

NOTES

NOTES

TABLE OF CONTENTS

G. GASTROINTESTINAL AND ABDOMEN

ESOPHAGUS

STOMACH

(Continued)

G

G

SMALL AND LARGE BOWEL

COLON AND RECTUM

G

GALLBLADDER, BILIARY TRACT, AND LIVER

SPLEEN AND PANCREAS

(Continued)

G

GAMUT   G-86   Mass in Region of the Pancreas

G-87   Pancreatic Angiographic Abnormality
(Via celiac, superior mesenteric, or subselective arteriography)

G-88   Pancreatic Calcification

MISCELLANEOUS, INCLUSIVE

G-89   Abdominal Calculi that Layer in Upright Position

G-90   Nonvisceral Abdominal Calcification

G-91   Abdominal Calcification in an Infant or Young Child
(See also Gamuts G-79 and G-90)

G-92   Abdominal Disease Associated With Pleural Effusion

G-93   Spontaneous Pneumoperitoneum Without Peritonitis

G-94   Abnormal Gas in the Right Upper Quadrant
(Outside the gut)

G-95   Abnormal Gas in the Left Upper Quadrant
(Outside the gut)

G-96   Large Abdominal Gas Pocket

G-97   Perforated Hollow Viscus in a Newborn

G-98   Gasless Abdomen in a Newborn

G-99   Gasless Abdomen in an Adult

G-100 Large Abdominal Mass in an Infant or Child

G-101 Peritoneal Fluid in an Infant

G-102 Obstruction of Abdominal Lymphatics, Cisterna Chyli, or Thoracic Duct on Lymphangiography (Chylous ascites)

G-103 Celiac Artery Abnormality

G

VALLECULAR SIGN: RETENTION OF BARIUM IN THE HYPOPHARYNX (ROENTGEN COUNTERPART OF DYSPHAGIA)

COMMON

1. Bulbar palsy; pseudobulbar palsy
2. Foreign body
3. Neoplasm, malignant
4. Scleroderma; dermatomyositis
5. Thyroid tumor

UNCOMMON

1. Cricopharyngeal achalasia (muscular incoordination)
2. Hematoma of the neck
3. Myasthenia gravis; other primary muscular disorder
4. Stricture (eg, lye)

ESOPHAGEAL MOTILITY DISORDER

COMMON

1. Cardiospasm (achalasia)
2. Diffuse esophageal spasm
3. Presbyesophagus
4. Neurologic disease (pseudobulbar palsy, multiple sclerosis, cerebral disease, bulbar poliomyelitis, Riley-Day syndrome)
5. Obstructive lesion, extrinsic or intrinsic (Schatzki ring, stricture, tumor, foreign body, web)
6. Scleroderma; dermatomyositis; rheumatoid arthritis

UNCOMMON

1. Amyloidosis
2. Chagas' disease
3. Diabetes
4. Drugs (atropine, Probanthine, curare)
5. Esophagitis (moniliasis, radiation, caustic, peptic, reflux)
6. Muscle disease (myotonic dystrophy, muscular dystrophy, myasthenia gravis)
7. Thyrotoxicosis; myxedema

References:

1. Teplick JG, Haskin ME: *Roentgenologic Diagnosis*, ed 2. Philadelphia, WB Saunders Co, 1971, vol 2, p xxvii.
2. Zboralske FF, Dodds WJ: Roentgenographic diagnosis of primary disorders of esophageal motility. *Radiol Clin North Am* 7:147–162, 1969.

SEGMENTAL (TERTIARY) CONTRACTIONS
OF THE ESOPHAGUS

COMMON

1. Gastroesophageal reflux
2. Neuromuscular disorder
3. Normal; idiopathic
4. Obstruction
5. Presbyesophagus

UNCOMMON

1. Achalasia
2. Chagas' disease
3. Spasm, diffuse idiopathic

Reference:

Bennett JR, Hendrix TR: Diffuse esophageal spasm: a disorder with more than one cause. *Gastroenterology* 59:273–279, 1970.

EXTRINSIC DEFECT ON
THE CERVICAL ESOPHAGUS

COMMON

1. Cricopharyngeal muscle
2. Lymph node enlargement
3. Soft tissue abscess or hematoma
4. Spinal spur
5. Thyroid mass

UNCOMMON

1. Aneurysm or buckling of carotid or innominate artery
2. [Leiomyoma or lipoma of esophagus]
3. Parathyroid tumor
4. [Pharyngeal venous plexus]
5. Spinal neoplasm or inflammation
6. Tracheal or laryngeal cyst or neoplasm
7. [Web, sideropenic (Plummer-Vinson syndrome)]

EXTRINSIC DEFECT ON
THE THORACIC ESOPHAGUS

COMMON

1. Anomalous artery or vein, pulmonary or systemic (see Gamut G-6)
2. Aorta (aneurysm, coarctation, right, left, or double arch, tortuosity)
3. Bronchogenic or enteric cyst (duplication)
4. Cardiac enlargement (esp. left atrium)
5. Hernia, paraesophageal
6. Lymph node enlargement
7. Mediastinal mass
8. Normal (left main stem bronchus, aortic knob)
9. Pericardial effusion, tumor, or cyst
10. Pulmonary mass

UNCOMMON

1. Azygos or hemiazygos vein dilatation
2. Spinal abnormality (eg, kyphosis, scoliosis)
3. Tracheal tumor
4. Vagus nerve tumor

EXTRINSIC VASCULAR DEFECT ON THE ESOPHAGUS OR TRACHEA

COMMON

1. Aberrant right subclavian artery
2. Right aortic arch (with or without aberrant left subclavian artery)

UNCOMMON

1. Anomalous innominate artery
2. Aortic diverticulum
3. Corrected transposition (medially placed pulmonary artery)
4. Double aortic arch
5. Enlarged bronchial artery
6. Pulmonary artery sling (anomalous origin of left pulmonary artery)
7. Pulmonary vein draining into back of left atrium

SOLITARY INTRAMURAL DEFECT OF THE ESOPHAGUS

COMMON

1. Extrinsic lesion invading the wall (carcinoma of the lung, granulomatous lymph nodes)
2. Gastric neoplasm with upward extension
3. Mucosal lesion invading the wall (eg, carcinoma)
4. Neoplasm, benign (spindle cell tumor, lipoma, angioma)

UNCOMMON

1. Abscess
2. Cyst, bronchogenic or enteric (duplication)
3. [Foreign body]
4. Lymphoma
5. Melanoma
6. Metastatic neoplasm
7. Sarcoma
8. Varix

CONSTRICTION OF THE DISTAL ESOPHAGUS

COMMON

1. Benign cyst or neoplasm (eg, duplication cyst, leiomyoma)
2. Carcinoma or sarcoma of esophagus or gastric cardia
3. Cardiospasm (achalasia)
4. Extrinsic pressure (from heart, aorta, mediastinal mass or lymphadenopathy)
5. Physiologic (muscular ring, inferior esophageal sphincter, normal sling fibers of diaphragm)
6. Stricture (eg, peptic or reflux esophagitis, corrosives, instrumentation)
7. Schatzki ring (mucosal ring)

UNCOMMON

1. Cartilage ring
2. Hiatal hernia
3. Peptic esophageal ulcer
4. Spasm, local or diffuse, idiopathic

Reference:

Teplick JG, Haskin ME: *Roentgenologic Diagnosis*, ed 2. Philadelphia, WB Saunders Co, 1971, vol 2, p xxvii.

ESOPHAGEAL LESION IN A CHILD

COMMON

1. Atresia
2. Chalasia
3. Esophagitis
4. Foreign body
5. Hiatal hernia, including short esophagus
6. Vascular compression, extrinsic (aberrant right subclavian artery, anomalous left pulmonary artery, aortic diverticulum, double aortic arch, ligamentum arteriosum, right aortic arch)

UNCOMMON

1. Achalasia
2. Diverticulum
3. Duplication cyst (enteric, neurenteric, bronchogenic)
4. Intraluminal diaphragm
5. Neoplasm
6. Stenosis, congenital or traumatic
7. Ulcer
8. Varices

Reference:

LoPresti JM: Personal communication.

DIVERTICULUM OF THE ESOPHAGUS

I. Upper third

    1. Lateral pharyngeal pouch

    *2. Zenker's (pulsion type, posterior wall)

II. Middle third

    *1. Traction (retracted by adherent lymph node)

III. Lower third

    1. Congenital epiphrenic

    2. [Mucosal tear, spontaneous (Mallory-Weiss) or post-instrumentation]

    3. [Penetrating peptic ulcer]

    4. Postoperative (eg, muscle splitting operation for achalasia)

*Common

Reference:

Kreel L: *Outline of Radiology.* New York, Appleton-Century-Crofts, 1971, pp 110–112.

ESOPHAGEAL VARICES

COMMON

1. Portal hypertension
*2. Superior vena cava obstruction from bronchogenic carcinoma, other neoplasms, chronic fibrosing mediastinitis (downhill varices)

UNCOMMON

*1. Arteriovenous fistula
2. Idiopathic
3. Mediastinal tumor without vena cava obstruction
*4. Operation (resection of retrosternal tumor)

*Varices may be confined to upper esophagus

ESOPHAGOBRONCHIAL FISTULA

COMMON

1. Carcinoma of esophagus or lung
2. Congenital, with or without esophageal atresia

UNCOMMON

1. Abscess
2. Actinomycosis
3. Caustic esophagitis (eg, lye)
4. Diverticulum of esophagus with perforation
5. Esophageal lung (sequestration)
6. Granulomatous lymph node, with or without broncholith (histoplasmosis, tuberculosis)
7. Lymphoma
8. Rupture of esophagus, spontaneous
9. Trauma (operative, instrumentation, foreign body)

ABNORMAL POSITION OF THE STOMACH (ROTATION OR DISPLACEMENT)

COMMON

1. Cascade stomach
2. Displacement by enlargement of adjacent organ (liver, spleen, kidney, pancreas, aorta) or by adjacent mass
3. Eventration or paralysis of diaphragm
4. Hernia (hiatal, Morgagni, Bochdalek, traumatic, pericardial)

UNCOMMON

1. Absent diaphragm
2. Volvulus

Reference:

Kreel L: *Outline of Radiology*. New York, Appleton-Century-Crofts, 1971, pp 133–134.

FILLING DEFECTS IN THE STOMACH, SOLITARY OR MULTIPLE (INTRALUMINAL, MUCOSAL, OR INTRAMURAL)

COMMON

1. Benign tumor (eg, carcinoid, glomus tumor, hamartoma, spindle cell tumor, angioma, lipoma, villous adenoma)

2. Bezoar

*3. Blood clot

4. Carcinoma

5. Ectopic pancreas

*6. Foreign body

*7. Giant rugal fold

*8. Lymphoma

*9. Metastatic neoplasm (esp. melanoma, lymphoma, and Kaposi's sarcoma)

*10. Peptic ulcer

*11. Polyp, adenomatous or hamartomatous (eg, Peutz-Jeghers)

12. Postoperative defect

*13. Varix

UNCOMMON

1. Duplication cyst

2. Granuloma with eosinophils (inflammatory fibroid polyp)

3. Jejunogastric intussusception

4. Prolapse of esophageal mucosa

5. Sarcoma

*May be solitary or multiple

Reference:

Teplick JG, Haskin ME: *Roentgenologic Diagnosis*, ed 2. Philadelphia, WB Saunders Co, 1971, vol 2, p xxviii.

LARGE GASTRIC FOLDS, LOCAL OR WIDESPREAD
(See also Gamut G-16)

COMMON

1. Carcinoma
2. Hypertrophic gastritis
3. Lymphoma
4. Normal variant
5. Pancreatitis, acute
6. Peptic ulcer
7. Postoperative stomach
8. Varices

UNCOMMON

1. Amyloidosis
2. Corrosive gastritis
3. Crohn's disease
4. Eosinophilic gastritis
5. Menetrier's disease
6. Metastatic neoplasm; extension from carcinoma of pancreas
7. Multiple polyps
8. Phlegmonous gastritis
9. Postfreezing gastritis
10. Postradiation gastritis
11. Pseudolymphoma
12. Zollinger-Ellison syndrome

LINITUS PLASTICA OF THE STOMACH
(See also Gamuts G-15 and G-17)

COMMON

1. Carcinoma

UNCOMMON

1. Amyloidosis
2. Corrosive gastritis
3. Crohn's disease
4. Eosinophilic gastritis
5. Idiopathic gastritis
6. Lymphoma; pseudolymphoma
7. Metastatic neoplasm; extension from carcinoma of pancreas
8. Phlegmonous gastritis
9. Postfreezing gastritis
10. Postradiation gastritis
11. Sarcoidosis
12. Syphilis
13. Tuberculosis

NARROWING AND/OR DEFORMITY OF ANTRUM OF STOMACH
(See also Gamut G-16)

COMMON

1. Antral gastritis
2. Carcinoma of stomach
3. Hypertrophic pyloric stenosis (infantile, adult)
4. Pancreatitis; carcinoma of the pancreas
5. Peptic ulcer scarring
6. Prolapse of gastric mucosa

UNCOMMON

1. Adhesions
2. Amyloidosis
3. Congenital perigastric bands
4. Corrosive gastritis
5. Crohn's disease
6. Eosinophilic gastritis
7. Gastroenterostomy
8. Lymphoma; pseudolymphoma
9. Metastatic neoplasm
10. Peptic ulcer perforation, walled off
11. Postfreezing gastritis
12. Postradiation therapy
13. Sarcoidosis
14. Strongyloidiasis; schistosomiasis
15. Syphilis
16. Tuberculosis
17. Web (diaphragm), prepyloric

Reference:

Teplick JG, Haskin ME: *Roentgenologic Diagnosis*, ed 2. Philadelphia, WB Saunders Co, 1971, vol 2, p xxviii.

GASTRIC DILATATION, RETENTION, OR OBSTRUCTION

COMMON

1. Aerophagia
2. Diabetic gastropathy
3. Drugs (eg, Probanthine, atropine, morphine)
4. Hypertrophic pyloric stenosis (infantile, adult)
5. Iatrogenic (intubation)
6. Idiopathic
7. "Paralytic ileus," nonobstructive distension (eg, post-operative, trauma, acute pancreatitis)
8. Pylorospasm
9. Obstructive pyloroduodenal lesion (ulcer, fibrosis, or neoplasm)
10. Vagotomy

UNCOMMON

1. Bezoar
2. Body cast
3. Gastritis, acute
4. High small bowel obstruction
5. Hypokalemia
6. Lead poisoning
7. Porphyria
8. Tracheoesophageal fistula with esophageal atresia
9. Uremia
10. Volvulus, with or without hiatal hernia

Reference:

Teplick JG, Haskin ME: *Roentgenologic Diagnosis*, ed 2. Philadelphia, WB Saunders Co, 1971, vol 2, p xxviii.

INTERSTITIAL EMPHYSEMA OF THE STOMACH

UNCOMMON

1. Corrosive gastritis
2. Gastric distension
3. Gastroscopy
4. Ischemia
5. Necrotizing gastroenterocolitis
6. Peptic ulcer with intramural perforation
7. Phlegmonous gastritis
8. Pneumatosis cystoides
9. Postfreezing gastritis

GASTROCOLIC OR
GASTRODUODENOCOLIC FISTULA

COMMON

1. Carcinoma of the colon, stomach, or pancreas

UNCOMMON

1. Actinomycosis
2. Crohn's disease
3. Foreign body
4. Marginal ulcer
5. Pancreatitis
6. Perforated diverticulum
7. Perforated peptic ulcer
8. Tuberculosis

INCREASED RETROGASTRIC AND/OR RETRODUODENAL SPACE

COMMON

1. Obesity
2. Pancreatic mass (carcinoma, cystadenoma, pseudocyst, pancreatitis)
3. Retroperitoneal hematoma
4. Retroperitoneal lymph node enlargement (eg, lymphoma, tuberculosis)
5. Retroperitoneal neoplasm (eg, sarcoma, renal or adrenal tumor)

UNCOMMON

1. Aortic aneurysm
2. Ascites
3. Choledochal cyst
4. Hepatomegaly, esp. caudate lobe
5. Leiomyoma or leiomyosarcoma of posterior wall of stomach
6. Postoperative
7. Retroperitoneal abscess
8. Retroperitoneal edema

DUODENAL OBSTRUCTION IN AN INFANT (DOUBLE BUBBLE SIGN)

COMMON

1. Annular pancreas
2. Duodenal atresia or stenosis

UNCOMMON

1. Choledochal cyst
2. Congenital peritoneal bands (Ladd's bands)
3. Diaphragm or web
4. Duplication of duodenum, intraluminal diverticulum
5. Midgut volvulus
6. Preduodenal portal vein
7. Retroperitoneal tumor

Reference:

Kassner EG, Sutton AL, DeGroot TJ: Bile duct anomalies associated with duodenal atresia; paradoxical presence of small bowel gas. *Am J Roentgenol* 116:577–583, 1972.

DILATATION OF THE DUODENUM

COMMON

1. Congenital atresia, stenosis, or diaphragm
2. Drugs (Probanthine, atropine, morphine)
3. Idiopathic
4. Ileus, localized (eg, acute pancreatitis, cholecystitis)
5. Obstruction from extrinsic mass (eg, lymphadenopathy, metastatic or invasive neoplasm from pancreas or kidney, aortic aneurysm, choledochal cyst)
6. Scleroderma; dermatomyositis
7. Superior mesenteric artery syndrome
8. Vagotomy

UNCOMMON

1. Annular pancreas
2. Chagas' disease
3. Cholecystoduodenocolic bands
4. Gallstone impaction
5. Hematoma of duodenum
6. Inflammatory disease causing obstruction (eg, Crohn's disease, strongyloidiasis)
7. Intraluminal diverticulum
8. Midgut volvulus
9. Postbulbar duodenal ulcer
10. Preduodenal portal vein
11. Primary neoplasm of duodenum
12. Sprue
13. Zollinger-Ellison syndrome

Reference:

Eaton SB Jr, Ferrucci JT Jr: Personal communication.

SUPERIOR MESENTERIC ARTERY SYNDROME (CONSTRICTION OF TRANSVERSE DUODENUM)

COMMON

1. Normal variant
2. Scleroderma
3. Weight loss; severe burns; body cast

UNCOMMON

1. [Aortic aneurysm]
2. [Band, congenital or acquired]
3. Congenital small vascular angle
4. [Internal hernia]
5. [Lymphadenopathy]
6. [Retroperitoneal inflammatory or neoplastic disease]
7. Thickening of root of mesentery (eg, Crohn's disease, pancreatitis, tuberculosis)

Reference:

Wallace RG, Howard WB: Acute superior mesenteric artery syndrome in the severely burned patient. *Radiology* 94:307–310, 1970.

WIDENING OF THE DUODENAL LOOP

COMMON

1. Normal variant
2. Pancreatic mass

UNCOMMON

1. Aortic aneurysm
2. Choledochal cyst
3. Duodenal hematoma
4. Duodenal spindle cell tumor, benign or malignant
5. Gastric tumor
6. Retroperitoneal lymph node enlargement (eg, lymphoma)
7. Retroperitoneal neoplasm, primary or metastatic

THICKENED FOLDS IN THE DUODENUM

COMMON

1. Edema (eg, cirrhosis, cardiac failure)
2. Hypertrophy of Brünner's glands
3. Intramural hemorrhage
4. Normal variant
5. Pancreatitis, acute or chronic
6. Parasitic diseases (giardiasis, strongyloidiasis, hookworm disease)
7. Peptic duodenitis

UNCOMMON

1. Amyloidosis
2. Corrosive duodenitis
3. Crohn's disease
4. Eosinophilic enteritis
5. Intestinal lymphangiectasia (Gordon's protein losing enteropathy)
6. Lymphoma
7. Mastocytosis
8. Mucoviscidosis
9. Postoperative
10. Sprue; celiac disease
11. Varices
12. Whipple's disease
13. Zollinger-Ellison syndrome

POSTBULBAR DUODENAL ULCERATION

COMMON

1. Carcinomatous invasion from pancreas, colon, right kidney, or gallbladder
2. Peptic ulcer

UNCOMMON

1. Aorticoduodenal fistula
2. Carcinoma, primary
3. Ectopic pancreas
4. Lymphoma
5. Metastasis (eg, melanoma, Kaposi's sarcoma)
6. Spindle cell tumor, benign or malignant
7. Zollinger-Ellison syndrome

Reference:

Eaton SB Jr, Ferrucci JT Jr: Personal communication.

SOLITARY INTRINSIC DUODENAL MASS

COMMON

1. Brünner's gland adenoma or hypertrophy
2. Ectopic pancreas
3. Peptic ulcer with edema or deformity
4. Polyp, adenomatous or hamartomatous
5. Prolapse of gastric mucosa

UNCOMMON

1. Benign tumor (angioma, carcinoid, lipoma, myxoma, papilloma, spindle cell tumor, villous adenoma, and their malignant counterparts)
2. Blood clot
3. Carcinoma
4. Duplication cyst
5. Foreign body
6. Gallstone impaction at papilla
7. Intraluminal diverticulum
8. Lymphoma
9. Metastasis
10. Papilla of Vater enlargement
11. Varix

EXTRINSIC INDENTATION ON THE DUODENUM

COMMON

1. Duodenocolic apposition
2. Enlarged gallbladder or common bile duct
3. Enlarged right kidney
4. [Hematoma, intramural]
5. Hepatic tumor, cyst, or enlarged caudate lobe
6. Lymphadenopathy (eg, metastases, lymphoma)
7. Pancreatic lesion (carcinoma, pseudocyst, pancreatitis)
8. [Postbulbar peptic ulcer]
9. Retroperitoneal mass
10. Superior mesenteric artery

UNCOMMON

1. Aortic aneurysm
2. Colon lesion
3. [Duodenal varices]
4. Hepatic artery dilatation
5. Idiopathic
6. Pericholecystic abscess

Reference:

Eaton SB Jr, Ferrucci JT Jr: Personal communication.

ACUTE NONOBSTRUCTIVE SMALL BOWEL DISTENSION ("PARALYTIC ILEUS")

COMMON

1. Drug induced (eg, morphine, Probanthine, hexamethonium, L-dopa, atropine)
2. Electrolyte imbalance (hypokalemia, hypochloremia, calcium and magnesium abnormalities)
3. Localized sentinel loop (eg, hepatic flexure in acute cholecystitis; terminal ileum in appendicitis; transverse colon or jejunum in acute pancreatitis; descending colon in acute diverticulitis)
4. Peritonitis
5. Pneumonia and other acute thoracic disease (eg, myocardial infarction, congestive failure)
6. Postoperative
7. Renal or ureteral calculus
8. Retroperitoneal hemorrhage
9. Shock; septicemia; hypoxia
10. Trauma (esp. spine or lower rib injury, abdominal contusion, intramural hematoma)
11. Vascular occlusion (eg, mesenteric infarction)

UNCOMMON

1. Aerophagia
2. Adrenal insufficiency
3. Diabetic acidosis; insulin shock
4. Functional (sickle cell crisis, lead colic, tabes)
5. Idiopathic intestinal pseudo-obstruction
6. Interloop abscess
7. Porphyria
8. Renal failure, acute glomerulonephritis

CHRONIC NONOBSTRUCTIVE SMALL BOWEL DISTENSION

COMMON

1. Neurogenic or muscular (eg, Parkinsonism, myotonia dystrophica)
2. Scleroderma
3. Sprue, tropical or nontropical

UNCOMMON

1. Adrenal insufficiency
2. Amyloidosis
3. Chagas' disease
4. Chronic mesenteritis
5. Hypoparathyroidism
6. Idiopathic
7. Jejunal diverticulosis
8. Mucoviscidosis
9. Myxedema
10. Renal failure
11. Spinal cord lesion

Reference:

Seaman WB: Motor dysfunction of the gastrointestinal tract. *Am J Roentgenol* 116:235–244, 1972.

GENERALIZED DILATATION OF BARIUM FILLED SMALL BOWEL
(See also Gamuts G-30 and G-31)

COMMON

1. Functional (diabetic coma, sickle cell crisis, lead colic, tabes)
2. Obstruction in distal small bowel or colon
3. "Paralytic ileus", nonobstructive distension
4. Scleroderma
5. Sprue, tropical or nontropical

UNCOMMON

1. Amyloidosis
2. Chagas' disease
3. Idiopathic
4. Myxedema

MUCOSAL DESTRUCTION OF THE SMALL INTESTINE, LOCAL OR WIDESPREAD (ALSO STRICTURED OR FIXED TUBULAR LESION)

COMMON

1. Crohn's disease; other nonspecific enteritis

UNCOMMON

1. Actinomycosis
2. Amyloidosis
3. Carcinoid
4. Carcinoma; sarcoma
5. Lymphoma
6. Mastocytosis
7. Metastatic neoplasm
8. Parasitic diseases (giardiasis, strongyloidiasis, capillariasis, hookworm disease, schistosomiasis, amebiasis)
9. Potassium enteritis
10. Radiation injury
11. Scleroderma
12. Tuberculosis
13. Typhoid fever
14. Vascular occlusion

MALABSORPTION (DEFICIENCY) PATTERN

COMMON

1. Blind loop syndrome (eg, duplication, diverticulosis of small bowel, Meckel's diverticulum, small bowel stricture with proximal dilatation, postoperative — gastroiliostomy, side-to-side anastomosis)
2. Crohn's disease
3. Idiopathic steatorrhea
4. Pancreatic disease (insufficiency, chronic pancreatitis, mucoviscidosis, pancreatic carcinoma)
5. Sprue, tropical or nontropical

UNCOMMON

1. Amyloidosis; Mediterranean fever
2. Angioneurotic edema or other gastrointestinal allergy
3. Carcinoid syndrome
4. Celiac disease
5. Diabetes mellitus
6. Disaccharidase deficiency
7. Drug induced (eg, neomycin)
8. Dysgammaglobulinemia
9. Emotional states; anorexia nervosa
10. Eosinophilic gastroenteritis
11. Fistula (esp. gastrocolic and postoperative)
12. Heavy chain disease
13. Hepatobiliary disease (biliary cirrhosis, biliary atresia)
14. Hypothyroidism; hyperthyroidism; hypoparathyroidism

(Continued)

15. Ischemia, chronic intestinal

16. Lymphangiectasia, intestinal (Gordon's enteropathy)

17. Lymphoma

18. Mastocytosis

19. Metastases, peritoneal

20. Nephrotic syndrome

21. Nutritional deficiency (kwashiorkor, pellagra)

22. Parasitic disease (hookworm disease, strongyloidiasis, giardiasis, schistosomiasis japonicum)

23. Postgastrectomy steatorrhea

24. Scleroderma; dermatomyositis

25. Small bowel resection (extensive)

26. Tuberculous peritonitis

27. Whipple's disease

28. Zollinger-Ellison syndrome

References:

1. Stacy GS, Loop JW: Unusual small bowel diseases: methods and observations. *Am J Roentgenol* 92:1072–1079, 1964.

2. Teplick JG, Haskin ME: *Roentgenologic Diagnosis*, ed 2. Philadelphia, WB Saunders Co, 1971, vol 2, p xxix.

3. Wheelock FC Jr, Bartlett MK: Case 80-1963. *N Engl J Med* 269:1374–1380, 1963.

THICKENING OF THE VALVULAE CONNIVENTES OF THE SMALL BOWEL (EDEMA, HEMORRHAGE, INFLAMMATION)

COMMON

1. Enteritis (eg, early Crohn's disease)
2. Hypoproteinemia (eg, cirrhosis, nephrotic syndrome, malnutrition)
3. Pancreatitis

UNCOMMON

1. Agammaglobulinemia
2. Amyloidosis
3. Angioneurotic edema
4. Eosinophilic gastroenteritis
5. Hematoma, intramural (trauma, anticoagulants, hemophilia, Henoch-Schönlein purpura)
6. Ischemia (thromboembolism, vasculitis, polyarteritis, hypotension)
7. Interloop abscess
8. Intussusception
9. Lymphangiectasia, intestinal (Gordon's enteropathy)
10. Malabsorption syndrome (See Gamut G-34)
11. Mastocytosis
12. Parasitic diseases (giardiasis, hookworm disease, schistosomiasis, strongyloidiasis, capillariasis)
13. Peptic ulcer; Zollinger-Ellison syndrome
14. Proximal to an obstruction
15. Radiation injury, acute
16. Retractile mesenteritis

(Continued)

17. Soft neoplasm (carcinoid, lipoma, lymphangioma, hemangioma, lymphoma)

18. Tuberculous peritonitis

19. Waldenström's primary macroglobulinemia

20. Weber-Christian disease

21. Whipple's disease

References:

1. Ellis K, McConnell DJ: Hereditary angioneurotic edema involving small intestine. *Radiology* 92:518–519, 1969.
2. Teplick JG, Haskin ME: *Roentgenologic Diagnosis*, ed 2. Philadelphia: WB Saunders Co, 1971, vol 2, p xxix.

SEPARATION OF SMALL BOWEL LOOPS

COMMON

1. Adhesions
2. Ascites or other peritoneal fluid
3. Crohn's disease
4. Peritonitis (eg, bacterial, tuberculous, typhoid)
5. Surgical resection
6. Tumor or cyst in abdomen, retroperitoneal or intraperitoneal (eg, ovarian cyst, retroperitoneal sarcoma, renal mass, intestinal neoplasm)

UNCOMMON

1. Amyloidosis
2. Hematoma (eg, abdominal wall, mesenteric, intramural)
3. Hernia
4. Interloop abscess
5. Lipomatosis of mesentery
6. Lymphoma of mesentery
7. Metastases, peritoneal
8. Radiation enteritis
9. Retractile mesenteritis
10. Vascular occlusion (mesenteric infarction)
11. Whipple's disease

SOLITARY MASS IN THE SMALL BOWEL WITH PRESERVED MUCOSA

COMMON

1. Benign tumor (angioma, carcinoid, lipoma, spindle cell tumor)
2. Foreign body, food particle, bezoar, pill
3. Polyp, adenomatous or hamartomatous (Peutz-Jeghers)

UNCOMMON

1. Gallstone
2. Intraluminal diverticulum
3. Lymphoma
4. Metastasis
5. Sarcoma

MULTIPLE INTRALUMINAL DEFECTS IN THE SMALL BOWEL
(See also Gamut G-39)

COMMON

1. Food particles, seeds
2. Parasites (ascarides, tapeworms)
3. Polyposis
   a. Adenomatous polyps
   b. Familial polyposis (colon and occasionally terminal ileum)
   c. Gardner's syndrome (colon and occasionally small bowel)
   d. Peutz-Jeghers syndrome (hamartomatous polyps)

UNCOMMON

1. Benign tumors, pedunculated
2. Foreign bodies, pills
3. Gallstones

MULTIPLE MUCOSAL OR INTRAMURAL FILLING DEFECTS IN THE SMALL BOWEL (A FINITE NUMBER, OFTEN VARYING IN SIZE AND SHAPE)

COMMON

1. Brünner's gland hyperplasia in the duodenum
2. Polyposis
   a. Adenomatous polyps
   b. Familial polyposis (colon and occasionally terminal ileum)
   c. Gardner's syndrome (colon and occasionally small bowel)
   d. Peutz-Jeghers syndrome (hamartomatous polyps)

UNCOMMON

1. Amyloidosis
2. Benign tumors (carcinoids, spindle cell tumors, hemangiomas)
3. Lymphoma
4. Mastocytosis (duodenum)
5. Metastatic neoplasm (eg, malignant melanoma, Kaposi's sarcoma)
6. Multiple myeloma
7. Submucosal hemorrhage (anticoagulants, hemophilia, purpura)
8. Typhoid fever (hyperplastic Peyer's patches in ileum)

INNUMERABLE TINY NODULES IN
THE SMALL BOWEL
(USUALLY UNIFORM AND LESS THAN 5 MM)

COMMON

1. Crohn's disease
2. [Food particles; air bubbles]
3. Normal lymph follicles; [normal folds]

UNCOMMON

1. Canada-Cronkhite syndrome
2. Intestinal lymphangiectasia
3. Lymphoid hyperplasia, usually with dysgammaglobulinemia
4. Lymphosarcoma
5. Mastocytosis
6. Mucoviscidosis
7. Waldenström's syndrome
8. Whipple's disease

TERMINAL ILEUM LESION

COMMON

1. Appendicitis
2. Carcinoid
3. Crohn's disease
4. Intussusception
5. Invasion by extrinsic inflammatory or neoplastic lesion
6. Mass, extrinsic (eg, pelvic tumor)
7. Meconium ileus

UNCOMMON

1. Benign tumor
2. Diverticulitis
3. Endometrial implant
4. Foreign body; gallstone; food particles; bezoar
5. Intramural hematoma
6. Lymphoid hyperplasia
7. Malignant neoplasm (carcinoma, sarcoma, lymphoma, metastasis)
8. Meckel's diverticulum
9. Parasitic disease
    a. Ascariasis, taeniasis (intraluminal worms)
    b. Schistosomiasis, amebiasis, strongyloidiasis (inflammatory changes)
10. Polyp
11. Radiation injury
12. Tuberculosis
13. Typhoid fever
14. Vascular occlusion, mesenteric infarction

INTESTINAL OBSTRUCTION IN A NEWBORN

COMMON

1. Congenital stenosis or atresia
2. Hirschsprung's disease
3. Imperforate anus; rectal atresia
4. Incarcerated hernia, internal or external (inguinal, femoral, umbilical, diaphragmatic)
5. Meconium ileus (mucoviscidosis)
6. Midgut volvulus with malrotation

UNCOMMON

1. Congenital band
2. Duplication
3. Intraluminal diaphragm or web
4. Intussusception
5. Meconium peritonitis with adhesions (eg, Meckel's diverticulum perforation, ruptured atretic intestine, meconium ileus)
6. Meconium plug syndrome
7. Neoplasm

POSTNEONATAL INTESTINAL OBSTRUCTION

COMMON

1. Adhesions (inflammatory, postoperative, congenital band)
2. Incarcerated hernia
3. Intussusception (ameboma, duplication, Henoch-Schönlein purpura, idiopathic, Meckel's diverticulum, lymphoma, polyp, or other tumor)

UNCOMMON

1. Congenital stenosis (eg, duodenal, rectal)
2. Duplication
3. Hirschsprung's disease
4. Midgut volvulus with malrotation
5. Mucoviscidosis
6. Neoplasm
7. Parasitic infestation (ascaris bolus)

Reference:

LoPresti JM: Personal communication.

INTESTINAL OBSTRUCTION IN AN ADULT

COMMON

1. Adhesions (postinflammatory or postoperative)
2. Crohn's disease
3. Fecal impaction
4. Hernia, internal or external
5. Malignant neoplasm (carcinoma, lymphoma, sarcoma, metastatic or invasive)
6. Volvulus

UNCOMMON

1. Benign neoplasm (mesenchymal tumor, carcinoid, cyst)
2. Bezoar
3. Diverticulitis
4. Drugs causing small bowel stricture (eg, potassium)
5. Duplication
6. Gallstone ileus
7. Infectious granulomatous disease (actinomycosis, tuberculosis, lymphogranuloma venereum)
8. Intramural hematoma
9. Intussusception
10. Malrotation
11. Parasitic disease (ascaris bolus, Chagas' disease, schistosomiasis, amebiasis)
12. Stricture
13. Vascular occlusion (see Gamut G-45)

MESENTERIC VASCULAR COMPROMISE
(INTESTINAL ISCHEMIA)

COMMON

1. Arterial embolism, thrombosis
2. Arteriosclerosis
3. Cardiac failure
4. Idiopathic
5. Intestinal obstruction or strangulation
6. Peritoneal band
7. Vascular compression by a mass involving mesenteric artery or vein
8. Venous thrombosis

UNCOMMON

1. Abdominal or pelvic inflammatory disease
2. Arteritis (eg, Takayasu's, polyarteritis nodosa)
3. Celiac axis syndrome (?)
4. Coarctation of the aorta (esp. postoperative)
5. Dissecting aneurysm
6. Fibromuscular hyperplasia of mesenteric artery
7. Iatrogenic; drug induced
8. Nonocclusive (normal blood vessels)
9. Polycythemia
10. Postoperative, surgical ligation
11. Trauma to intestine or its vessels

Reference:

Smith SL, Tutton RH, Ochsner SF: Roentgenographic aspects of intestinal ischemia. *Am J Roentgenol* 116:249–255, 1972.

GAS IN THE WALL OF THE SMALL OR LARGE BOWEL
(See also Gamut G-19)

COMMON

1. Necrosis of the intestine (eg, infarction; gangrenous, pseudomembranous, or other enterocolitis; strangulated hernia)
2. Pneumatosis cystoides intestinalis

UNCOMMON

1. Air hose injury of rectum ("goose")
2. Diabetes with infection
3. Hydrogen peroxide enema
4. Mucoviscidosis
5. Peptic ulcer with intramural perforation
6. Postoperative intramural leakage
7. Toxic megacolon (see Gamut G-51)

References:

1. Bryk D: Unusual causes of small-bowel pneumatosis: perforated duodenal ulcer and perforated jejunal diverticula. *Radiology* 106:299–302, 1973.
2. Felson B: Abdominal gas: a roentgen approach. *Ann NY Acad Sci* 150:141–161, 1968.

FISTULA INVOLVING SMALL OR LARGE BOWEL

COMMON

1. Crohn's disease
2. Diverticulitis
3. Malignant neoplasm (intrinsic, extrinsic, metastatic)
4. Postoperative

UNCOMMON

1. Actinomycosis
2. Amebiasis
3. Foreign body
4. Infection, other (eg, appendiceal perforation, pelvic in-flammatory disease)
5. Lymphogranuloma venereum
6. Pancreatitis
7. Radiation therapy
8. Tuberculosis
9. Trauma
10. Ulcerative colitis

BULL'S-EYE LESIONS (SOLITARY OR MULTIPLE NODULES IN THE GASTROINTESTINAL TRACT WITH LARGE ULCERATION)

COMMON

1. Lymphoma
2. Metastatic melanoma
3. Spindle cell tumor, benign or malignant

UNCOMMON

1. Aberrant pancreas
2. Carcinoid
3. Carcinoma
4. Eosinophilic granuloma
5. Kaposi's sarcoma
6. Metastases from kidney, breast, or other tumors

Reference:

Pomerantz H, Margolin HN: Metastases to the gastrointestinal tract from malignant melanoma. *Am J Roentgenol* 88:712–717, 1962.

CONGENITAL SYNDROMES ASSOCIATED WITH INCOMPLETE ROTATION OF THE COLON

1. Abdominal heterotaxy with or without asplenia, polysplenia, or heart disease
2. Cerebrohepatorenal S.
3. Cornelia De Lange S.
4. Down's S. (Mongolism)
5. Eagle-Barrett S.
6. Marfan's S.
7. Trisomy 13 S.
8. Trisomy 18 S.

Reference:

Smith DW: *Recognizable Patterns of Human Malformation.* Philadelphia, WB Saunders Co, 1970, p 291.

MEGACOLON IN AN INFANT OR CHILD

COMMON

1. Functional (psychogenic, idiopathic)
2. Hirschsprung's disease
3. Imperforate anus
4. Toxic megacolon

UNCOMMON

1. Anal fissure
2. Duplication
3. Neurogenic (eg, meningomyelocele, other spinal abnormality)
4. Pelvic tumor (eg, teratoma)
5. Postoperative rectal stricture

Reference:

LoPresti JM: Personal communication.

TOXIC MEGACOLON

COMMON

1. Hirschsprung's disease
2. Ulcerative colitis

UNCOMMON

1. Amebic colitis
2. Bacillary dysentery, acute
3. Cholera
4. Enterocolitis, other (staphylococcic, necrotizing, hemorrhagic, pseudomembranous)
5. Granulomatous colitis
6. Ischemic colitis
7. Typhoid fever

COLONIC DISTENSION WITHOUT OBSTRUCTION

COMMON

*1. Chronic constipation; cathartic abuse

2. Electrolyte imbalance (hypokalemia, hypochloremia, calcium and magnesium abnormalities)

*3. Hirschsprung's disease

*4. Idiopathic megacolon

5. "Paralytic ileus," acute nonobstructive distension (eg, postoperative, peritonitis)

*6. Psychogenic

7. Shock; septicemia; hypoxia

8. Toxic megacolon (see Gamut G-51)

9. Trauma (eg, spine or lower rib injury, abdominal contusion, intramural hematoma)

10. Urinary calculus

11. Vascular occlusion (eg, mesenteric infarction)

UNCOMMON

*1. Aerophagia

2. Alcoholism

*3. Amyloidosis; Mediterranean fever

*4. Chagas' disease

5. Drug induced (eg, probanthine, hexamethonium, morphine overdose, L-dopa, atropine)

*6. Endocrine disturbances (esp. adrenal insufficiency, hypothyroidism)

7. Functional (diabetic coma, lead colic, sickle cell crisis, tabes)

8. Idiopathic intestinal pseudo-obstruction

(Continued)

*9. Mucoviscidosis

*10. Neuromuscular disease (eg, amyotonia congenita, amyotrophic lateral sclerosis, multiple sclerosis, Parkinsonism, poliomyelitis, Riley-Day syndrome, senility)

*11. Pheochromocytoma; neurofibromatosis

12. Pneumonia or other acute thoracic disease (eg, myocardial infarction, congestive failure) causing reflex ileus

13. Polyarteritis nodosa

14. Porphyria

15. Renal failure, uremia

16. Retroperitoneal hemorrhage

*17. Scleroderma

*18. Spinal cord lesion

19. Sprue

*Chronic

References:

1. Bryk D, Rosenkranz W: Functional evaluation of the acute abdomen by radiological means. *CRC Crit Rev Radiol Sci* 2:1–14, 1971.
2. Bryk D, Soong KY: Colonic ileus and its differential roentgen diagnosis. *Am J Roentgenol* 101:329–337, 1967.
3. Carlson DH, Ziter FM Jr: Non-tropical sprue as a cause of megacolon: report of a case. *J Can Assoc Radiol* 21:235–237, 1970.
4. Moss AA, Goldberg HI: Intestinal pseudo-obstruction. *CRC Crit Rev Radiol Sci* 3:363, 1972.
5. Schwartz SS: The differential diagnosis of intestinal obstruction. *Semin Roentgenol* 8:323–338, 1973.

MULTIPLE FILLING DEFECTS IN THE COLON

COMMON

1. [Diverticula]
2. Familial polyposis
3. Polyps, adenomatous
4. Pseudopolyps of ulcerative colitis, granulomatous colitis, amebiasis
5. Stool; foreign bodies; air bubbles; food particles; mucus

UNCOMMON

1. Amebomas
2. Amyloidosis
3. Canada-Cronkhite syndrome
4. Carcinomas, multiple
5. Colitis cystica profunda
6. Gardner's syndrome
7. Lipomatous polyposis
8. Lymphoid hyperplasia, nodular
9. Lymphosarcoma
10. Metastases
11. Mucoviscidosis
12. Neurofibromatosis, ganglioneurofibromatosis
13. Parasites, intraluminal (ascariasis, trichuriasis)
14. Peutz-Jeghers syndrome (hamartomatous polyps)
15. Pneumatosis cystoides intestinalis
16. Polyposis, juvenile gastrointestinal (multiple juvenile polyps)

(Continued)

17. Schistosomiasis

18. Turcot syndrome

References:

1. Clemett AR: Personal communication.
2. Teplick JG, Haskin ME: *Roentgenologic Diagnosis*, ed 2. Philadelphia, WB Saunders Co, 1971, vol 2, p xxx.
3. Wolfson JJ, Goldstein G, Krivit W, et al: Lymphoid hyperplasia of the large intestine associated with dysgammaglobulinemia: report of a case. *Am J Roentgenol* 108:610–614, 1970.

SOLITARY FILLING DEFECT IN THE COLON

COMMON

1. Carcinoma
2. Fecal impaction
3. Intussusception; ileal prolapse
4. Polyp, adenomatous or hamartomatous

UNCOMMON

1. Ameboma
2. Ascaris bolus
3. Benign spindle cell tumor; angioma; lipoma
4. Carcinoid
5. Cyst, duplication or other
6. Endometrioma
7. Foreign body; gallstone; food particle
8. Lymphoma
9. Metastatic neoplasm
10. Sarcoma
11. Schistosomiasis (polypoid mass)
12. Villous adenoma

Reference:

  Teplick JG, Haskin ME: *Roentgenologic Diagnosis*, ed 2. Philadelphia, WB Saunders Co, 1971, vol 2, p xxx.

SEGMENTAL LESION OF THE COLON WITH NARROWING

COMMON

1. Carcinoma (esp. scirrhous carcinoma)
2. Crohn's disease
3. Diverticulitis
4. Extrinsic narrowing from adjacent neoplastic or inflammatory process
5. Ischemic colitis

UNCOMMON

1. Ameblasis
2. Amyloidosis
3. Carcinoid
4. Endometriosis
5. Foreign body perforation with pericolic abscess
6. Lymphogranuloma venereum
7. Lymphoma
8. Metastasis
9. Radiation fibrosis
10. Sarcoma
11. Schistosomiasis
12. Tuberculosis
13. Ulcerative colitis

COLITIS (MUCOSAL CHANGES, ULCERATION, EDEMA, SPASM, FIBROSIS)

COMMON

1. Amebiasis
2. Crohn's disease
3. Diverticulitis
4. Ischemic colitis
5. Ulcerative colitis

UNCOMMON

1. Actinomycosis
2. Amyloidosis
3. Bacillary dysentery (shigellosis)
4. [Carcinoid]
5. [Carcinoma, scirrhous]
6. [Cathartic colon]
7. Enterocolitis (drug induced, pseudomembranous, necrotizing)
8. Lymphogranuloma venereum
9. [Lymphoma, diffuse]
10. Radiation colitis
11. Salmonella colitis
12. Schistosomiasis
13. Strongyloidiasis
14. Tuberculosis

Reference:

Teplick JG, Haskin ME: *Roentgenologic Diagnosis*, ed 2. Philadelphia, WB Saunders Co, 1971, vol 2, p xxx.

"THUMBPRINTING" OF THE COLON (MULTIPLE INTRAMURAL DEFECTS)

COMMON

1. Crohn's disease
2. Diverticulitis
3. Ischemic colitis (eg, infarction, vasculitis) (see Gamut G-45)
4. Ulcerative colitis

UNCOMMON

1. Amebiasis
2. Amyloidosis
3. Endometriosis
4. Intramural hematoma
5. Lymphoma
6. Mesenteric lesion
7. Metastasis
8. Pneumatosis cystoides intestinalis

Reference:

Marshak RH, Lindner AE: Ischemia of the colon. *Semin Roentgenol* 3:81–93, 1968.

CECAL LESION

COMMON

1. Amebiasis
2. Appendiceal abscess
3. Appendiceal stump
4. Carcinoma
5. Crohn's disease
6. [Feces]
7. Ileocecal valve (normal, "lipoma")
8. Intussusception (eg, idiopathic, lymphoma, Meckel's)
9. Polyp, adenomatous
10. Ulcerative colitis

UNCOMMON

1. Actinomycosis
2. Carcinoid
3. Cathartic abuse
4. Diverticulosis; diverticulitis
5. Duplication
6. Endometriosis
7. Enterolith
8. [Foreign body]
9. [Gallstone]
10. Lymphoma
11. Mucocele; myxoglobulosis
12. Pneumatosis cystoides intestinalis
13. Schistosomiasis

(Continued)

14. Spindle cell tumor or lipoma, benign or malignant

15. Tuberculosis

16. Villous adenoma

References:

1. Felson B, Wiot JF: *Case of the Day*. Springfield, Charles C Thomas, 1967, p 3.
2. Felson B, Wiot JF: Some interesting right lower quadrant entities: myxoglobulosis of the appendix, ileal prolapse, diverticulitis, lymphoma, endometriosis. *Radiol Clin North Am* 7:83–95, 1969.

CONICAL AND/OR RAPIDLY EMPTYING CECUM (CONTRACTED CECUM)

COMMON

1. Amebiasis
2. Appendicitis, appendiceal abscess
3. Crohn's disease

UNCOMMON

1. Actinomycosis
2. Carcinoma
3. Cathartic abuse
4. Idiopathic
5. Tuberculosis
6. Typhoid fever
7. Ulcerative colitis

Reference:

Kreel L: *Outline of Radiology.* New York, Appleton-Century-Crofts, 1971, p 158.

ENLARGEMENT OF THE ILEOCECAL VALVE

COMMON

1. Crohn's disease
2. Fatty infiltration
3. Intussusception
4. Neoplasm, benign or malignant
5. Normal variant ("hypertrophy")

UNCOMMON

1. Amebiasis
2. Ileal prolapse
3. Impacted gallstone or foreign body
4. Intramural hematoma
5. Tuberculosis

RECTAL LESION

COMMON

1. Adenocarcinoma
2. Congenital anomaly (eg, Hirschsprung's disease, imperforate anus)
3. Crohn's disease
4. Endometriosis
5. Metastasis or invasion from adjacent neoplasm
6. Polyp, adenomatous or juvenile (hamartoma)
7. Ulcerative colitis
8. Villous adenoma

UNCOMMON

1. Abscess
2. Actinomycosis
3. Amebiasis
4. Amyloidosis
5. Carcinoid
6. Cloacogenic carcinoma; scirrhous carcinoma
7. Colitis cystica profunda
8. Diverticulitis
9. Ischemic colitis
10. Lymphoma
11. Lymphogranuloma venereum
12. Mesenchymal tumor
13. Pneumatosis cystoides intestinalis
14. Sarcoma
15. Schistosomiasis
16. Tuberculosis
17. Varices

INCREASED RETRORECTAL SOFT TISSUE SPACE

COMMON

1. Carcinoma of rectum or sigmoid
2. Crohn's disease
3. Diverticulitis
4. Extrinsic soft tissue mass (ovarian cyst or neoplasm, Krükenberg tumor, teratoma, uterine fibroid)
5. Lymphogranuloma venereum
6. Metastatic or invasive malignant neoplasm (esp. from prostate, cervix)
7. Pelvic abscess
8. Postresection of rectosigmoid
9. Radiation fibrosis
10. Sacral lesion (see Gamut C-21)
11. Ulcerative colitis

UNCOMMON

1. Amebiasis
2. Cushing's disease
3. Endometriosis
4. Hemorrhoid injection
5. Infarction
6. Lymphoma of rectum or retrorectal soft tissues
7. Pelvic lipomatosis
8. Retroperitoneal fibrosis
9. Retroperitoneal sarcoma
10. Schistosomiasis
11. Trauma (external, obstetrical)
12. Tuberculosis

RECTOVAGINAL FISTULA

COMMON

1. Carcinoma of rectum, cervix, or vagina; other pelvic carcinoma, invasive or metastatic
2. Crohn's disease
3. Lymphogranuloma venereum
4. Radiation therapy
5. Trauma (postoperative or postdelivery)

UNCOMMON

1. Appendiceal abscess
2. Diverticulitis
3. Endometriosis
4. Foreign body
5. Imperforate anus and other cloacal anomalies
6. Schistosomiasis
7. Ulcerative colitis

NONVISUALIZATION OF THE GALLBLADDER

COMMON

1. [Calcified gallbladder wall; milk of calcium]
2. Calculus obstructing cystic duct or infundibulum (eg, hydrops, empyema)
3. Cholecystitis
4. Failure to take contrast material
5. Gallbladder stasis
6. Liver disease with hepatocellular damage (eg, hepatitis, cirrhosis)
7. Obstruction of esophagus or pylorus
8. Obstructive jaundice (eg, carcinoma of pancreas, stone in common duct)
9. Prior cholecystectomy
10. Vomiting, diarrhea

UNCOMMON

1. [Anomalous position of gallbladder]
2. Carcinoma of gallbladder
3. Congenital absence
4. Obliterative fibrosis of gallbladder
5. Retention of contrast medium in a diverticulum or in an unobstructed stomach (eg, diabetic gastropathy)

Reference:

Shehadi WH: Radiologic examination of the biliary tract. *Radiol Clin North Am* 4:463–482, 1966.

GALLBLADDER DISEASE SECONDARY TO CYSTIC DUCT OBSTRUCTION

COMMON

1. Calcified gallbladder wall (porcelain gallbladder)
2. Hydrops; empyema; mucocele
3. Milk of calcium

UNCOMMON

1. Choledochoenteric fistula (eg, from gallstone perforation)
2. Emphysematous cholecystitis
3. Ruptured gallbladder

POLYPOID LESION OF THE GALLBLADDER

COMMON

*1. Adenomyoma, myoepithelial anomaly

*2. Calculus adherent to wall

*3. Cholesterol polyp

UNCOMMON

1. Adenoma (adenomatous polyp, papilloma, fibroadenoma, cystadenoma)

2. Angioma

3. Carcinoid

*4. Cholecystitis glandularis proliferans

5. Congenital fold or septum

6. Epithelial cyst; mucous cyst

7. Heterotopic pancreas

*8. Inflammatory polyp

9. Neurinoma

10. Polypoid malignant tumor, primary or metastatic

11. Postoperative defect

*May be multiple

Reference:

Ochsner SF: Solitary polypoid lesions of the gallbladder. *Radiol Clin North Am* 4:501–510, 1966.

FILLING DEFECT OR SEGMENTAL LESION OF BILE DUCT ON CHOLANGIOGRAPHY

COMMON

1. Air bubble
2. Calculus
3. Carcinoma of common duct, ampulla, duodenum or pancreas; metastasis
4. Edema of ampullary segment (eg, after passage of stone, pancreatitis)
5. Stricture

UNCOMMON

1. Blood clot
2. Dilated vessel
3. Ectopic cystic duct
4. Enlarged lymph node
5. Foreign body or food
6. Parasites (ascaris, clonorchis)
7. Pericholedochal adhesions
8. Polyp; adenoma
9. Postoperative defect
10. Pseudocalculus defect in distal common duct; idiopathic
11. Spasm of sphincter of Oddi; muscle hypertrophy (?)
12. [Valves of Heister]

ENLARGED PAPILLA OF VATER

COMMON

1. Calculus in distal common duct
2. Carcinoma of pancreaticoampullary region
3. Pancreatitis, pancreatic abscess

UNCOMMON

1. Edema secondary to duodenal ulcer
2. Heterotopic pancreatic tissue
3. Idiopathic; normal variant
4. Postoperative; postinstrumentation
5. Strongyloidiasis
6. Zollinger-Ellison syndrome

Reference:

Poppel MH, Jacobson HG, Smith RW: *The Roentgen Aspects of the Papilla and Ampulla of Vater.* Springfield, Charles C. Thomas, 1953.

REFLUX OF BARIUM INTO THE COMMON BILE DUCT OR PANCREATIC DUCT

COMMON

1. Carcinoma of the pancreaticoampullary region
2. Fistula from biliary tract (eg, gallstone ileus)
3. Pancreatitis
4. Physiologic (incompetent sphincter)
5. Postoperative

UNCOMMON

1. Common duct opening into a diverticulum
2. Crohn's disease of duodenum
3. Parasitic disease (strongyloidiasis, clonorchiasis, ascariasis)
4. Perforated duodenal ulcer into common duct
5. Trauma

Reference:

Eaton SB Jr, Ferruci JT Jr, Margulis AR, et al: Unfamiliar roentgeu findings in pancreatic disease. *Am J Roentgenol* 116:396–405, 1972.

GAS IN THE BILIARY TREE

COMMON

1. Carcinoma of duodenum, ampulla, bile duct, gallbladder, stomach, pancreas, or colon
2. Gallstone fistula (eg, gallstone ileus, passage of stone into bowel through gallbladder, common duct, or sphincter)
3. [Gas in portal vein]
4. Postoperative (eg, sphincterotomy, cholecystoenterostomy, choledochoduodenostomy)

UNCOMMON

1. Emphysematous cholecystitis and cholangitis
2. [Gas in gallstone]
3. Parasitic disease (strongyloidiasis, ascariasis, amebic abscess of liver)
4. Perforation of peptic ulcer into biliary tract
5. Physiologic (incompetent sphincter)

References:

1. Cummack DH: *Gastro-Intestinal X-Ray Diagnosis.* Baltimore, Williams & Wilkins, 1969.
2. Shehadi WH: Radiologic examination of the biliary tract. *Radiol Clin North Am* 4:463–482, 1966.

CYSTIC DISEASE OF THE LIVER OR HEPATIC DUCTS

DUCTS

A. Extrahepatic

1. Choledochal cyst; choledochocele
2. [Diverticulum of common duct]

B. Intrahepatic

1. Biliary cirrhosis (obstruction with dilatation of ducts)
2. Caroli's disease (communicating cavernous ectasia of the intrahepatic bile ducts)
3. Cholangiohepatitis (ascending cholangitis)
4. Clonorchiasis (liver fluke)
5. Congenital hepatic fibrosis

LIVER

1. Acquired nonparasitic cyst
2. Congenital cyst
3. Hydatid cyst
4. Polycystic disease
5. Traumatic cyst

CONGENITAL SYNDROMES WITH
HEPATOMEGALY

1. Berardinelli's S.
2. Cerebrohepatorenal S.
3. Chediak-Higashi S.
4. Cockayne's S.
5. Familial dwarfism with stiff joints
6. Homocystinuria
7. Mucopolysaccharidosis (eg, Hurler, Hunter); generalized gangliosidosis
8. Osteopetrosis
9. Rubella S.

Reference:

Smith DW: *Recognizable Patterns of Human Malformation*. Philadelphia, WB Saunders Co, 1970, p 291.

HEPATOMEGALY
(See also Gamuts G-72, G-74 to G-76)

COMMON

1. Abscess, solitary or multiple, amebic or pyogenic
2. Cardiac decompensation (congestive hepatomegaly)
3. Cirrhosis
4. Cyst (eg, congenital, traumatic, hydatid)
5. Fatty infiltration
6. Hepatitis
7. Hepatoma or other primary neoplasm, benign or malignant
8. Metastases

UNCOMMON

1. Actinomycosis
2. Anemia
3. Glycogen storage disease
4. Hematoma
5. Histiocytosis X
6. Histoplasmosis, miliary
7. Kala-azar
8. Lymphoma
9. Polycystic disease
10. Reticuloses (eg, Gaucher's disease)
11. Sarcoidosis
12. Schistosomiasis
13. Tuberculosis, miliary

HEPATIC MASS IN A CHILD

1. Abscess, amebic or bacterial
2. Adenoma
3. Cavernous hemangioma
4. Cyst (congenital, traumatic, hydatid)
5. Focal nodular hyperplasia
6. Hamartoma
7. Hemangioendothelioma
8. Hepatocarcinoma
9. Metastasis (eg, neuroblastoma, Wilms')
10. Sarcoma
11. Teratoma

AVASCULAR LESIONS OF THE LIVER, SOLITARY OR MULTIPLE

COMMON

1. Cholangiocarcinoma, hepatoma, or other primary liver tumor
2. [Extrinsic mass (eg, gallbladder, subphrenic abscess)]
*3. Fatty infiltration
*4. Hydatid cyst
*5. Liver abscess (amebic, pyogenic)
*6. Metastasis

UNCOMMON

1. Hematoma (esp. subcapsular)
*2. Hypertrophied liver nodule in cirrhosis (regenerative nodular hyperplasia)
*3. Lymphoma, including Burkitt's tumor
4. Nonparasitic cyst (congenital or acquired)
*5. Polycystic disease
6. Traumatic liver cyst

*May show multiple radiolucencies on hepatic angiogram

VASCULAR LESION OF THE LIVER

COMMON

1. Cavernous hemangioma
2. Hemangioendothelioma
3. Hepatocellular carcinoma (hepatoma, hepatoblastoma)
4. Metastasis

UNCOMMON

1. Adenoma
2. Hamartoma
3. Hemangiosarcoma (hemangioendothelial sarcoma)
4. Nodular hyperplasia, focal

HEPATIC VEIN THROMBOSIS OR OBSTRUCTION ON ANGIOGRAPHY (INCLUDES OBSTRUCTION OF UPPER INFERIOR VENA CAVA)

COMMON

1. Cirrhosis
2. Idiopathic

UNCOMMON

1. Hypercoagulation states (eg, polycythemia vera, sickle cell anemia)
2. Neoplasm (esp. hepatic, renal, pancreatic, retroperitoneal sarcoma)
3. Oral contraceptive
4. Postsplenectomy; other postoperative states
5. Pregnancy; postdelivery
6. Senecio alkaloid ingestion (bush tea disease)
7. Thrombophlebitis
8. Trauma to hepatic area

Reference:

Deutsch V, Rosenthal T, Adar R, et al: Budd-Chiari syndrome. *Am J Roentgenol* 116:430–439, 1972.

GAS IN THE PORTAL VEINS

COMMON

1. [Gas in biliary tree]
2. Mesenteric infarction
3. Necrotizing enterocolitis; gastroenterocolitis
4. Umbilical vein catheterization

UNCOMMON

1. Diabetes mellitus
2. Dilatation of gut, severe
3. Emphysematous gastritis; corrosive gastritis
4. Erythroblastosis fetalis
5. Hydrogen peroxide enema

References:

1. Fink DW, Boyden FM: Gas in the portal veins: a report of two cases due to ingestion of corrosive substances. *Radiology* 87:741–743, 1966.
2. Swaim TJ, Gerald B: Hepatic portal venous gas in infants without subsequent death. *Radiology* 94:343–345, 1970.
3. Wiot JF, Felson B: Gas in the portal venous system. *Am J Roentgenol* 86:920–929, 1961.

LIVER CALCIFICATION

COMMON

1. Granuloma (tuberculosis, histoplasmosis, brucellosis)
2. Hydatid cyst

UNCOMMON

1. Aneurysm of hepatic artery
2. Armillifer armillatus infestation
3. Chronic granulomatous disease of childhood
4. Gumma, hepar lobatum
5. Hematoma
6. [Hemochromatosis]
7. Hepatic duct calculi (intrahepatic gallstones)
8. Liver abscess, amebic or pyogenic
9. Metastasis (eg, colloid carcinoma of colon or stomach, cystadenocarcinoma of ovary)
10. Nonparasitic cyst, congenital or acquired
11. Portal vein thrombosis
12. Primary liver tumor (hemangioma, hepatoblastoma, hepatoma, cholangioma, hemangioendothelioma)
13. [Thorotrast, thallium, iron (entire liver dense)]

Reference:

Thompson WM, Chisholm DP, Tank R: Plain film roentgenographic findings in alveolar hydatid disease — *Echinococcus Multilocularis. Am J Roentgenol* 116:345–358, 1972.

SOLITARY (SOLID OR CYSTIC) LESION OF THE SPLEEN

COMMON

1. Epidermoid cyst
2. Hematoma
3. Traumatic hemorrhagic cyst

UNCOMMON

1. Abscess
2. Dermoid cyst
4. Fibroma
3. Hamartoma
5. Hemangioma; lymphangioma
6. Hydatid cyst
7. Infarct
8. Lymphoma
9. Sarcoma (esp. angiosarcoma)

SPLENOMEGALY

I. Blood dyscrasia
   COMMON
   1. Anemia (sickle cell, thalassemia, hemolytic anemia, myelofibrosis)
   2. Extramedullary hematopoiesis
   3. Leukemia

   UNCOMMON
   1. Dysgammaglobulinemia
   2. Hemochromatosis
   3. Osteopetrosis
   4. Polycythemia vera

II. Congenital
   1. Cystic lymphangioma or hemangioma
   2. Dermoid or epidermoid cyst

III. Infectious
   COMMON
   1. Parasitic (eg, malaria, schistosomiasis, hydatid cyst, kala-azar)

   UNCOMMON
   1. Bacterial (eg, miliary tuberculosis, subacute bacterial endocarditis, typhoid fever, brucellosis, typhus)
   2. Fungal (eg, histoplasmosis)
   3. Viral (eg, cytomegalic inclusion disease, infectious mononucleosis)

IV. Neoplastic
   COMMON
   1. Lymphoma

   UNCOMMON
   1. Benign neoplasm (eg, fibroma, hamartoma)
   2. Metastatic disease
   3. Sarcoma (esp. angiosarcoma)
                    (Continued)

V. Portal hypertension

COMMON

1. Nutritional or alcoholic cirrhosis

UNCOMMON

1. Splenic vein obstruction (eg, thrombosis, pancreatic neoplasm)
2. Schistosomiasis

VI. Storage diseases

1. Gaucher's disease
2. Histiocytosis X
3. Niemann-Pick disease

VII. Trauma

COMMON

1. Hematoma (subcapsular, intrasplenic, perisplenic)

UNCOMMON

1. Hemorrhagic pseudocyst

VIII. Other

COMMON

1. Amyloidosis
2. Congestive splenomegaly, cardiac failure

UNCOMMON

1. Felty's syndrome
2. Hurler's syndrome
3. Infarct
4. Juvenile rheumatoid arthritis, Still's disease
5. Lupus erythematosus

Reference:
  Teplick JG, Haskin ME: *Roentgenologic Diagnosis*, ed 2. Philadelphia, WB Saunders Co, 1971, vol 2, p xix.

ABNORMALITY ON SPLENIC ARTERIOGRAPHY

1. Accessory spleen
2. Anomalous origin of splenic or celiac artery
3. Arteriovenous fistula; angiomatous malformation
4. Avascular mass
   a. Abscess
   b. Epidermoid or dermoid cyst
   c. Hydatid cyst
   d. Infarct
   e. Lymphoma
   f. Metastasis
   g. Traumatic cyst
5. Displacement by extrinsic mass
6. Fibromuscular hyperplasia
7. Splenic artery arteriosclerosis or aneurysm, including dissecting aneurysm
8. Splenic laceration; pericapsular hematoma
9. Splenic vein abnormalities (see Gamut G-83)
10. Stenosis of splenic or celiac artery
11. Thromboembolism
12. Vascular tumor
    a. Primary sarcoma of spleen (esp. angiosarcoma)
    b. Reticulum cell sarcoma

Reference:

Kreel L: *Outline of Radiology.* New York, Appleton-Century-Crofts, 1971, pp 178–179.

ABNORMALITY ON DIRECT OR INDIRECT SPLENOPORTOGRAPHY

1. Arteriovenous fistula

2. Collateral circulation (varices)

3. Corkscrew venules (schistosomiasis)

4. Displacement or narrowing of splenic or portal vein (pancreatic, hepatic, or retroperitoneal mass)

5. Filling defect in liver (eg, abscess, cyst, neoplasm)

6. Nonfilling of portal vein (eg, flow phenomenon, thrombosis)

7. Obstruction of splenic vein (thrombosis, extrinsic compression, or infiltration)

8. Patency of portocaval shunt

9. Poor branching in liver, "pruned tree" (cirrhosis)

10. Portal vein cavernous transformation

11. Smooth narrow portal vein (eg, periphlebitis)

Reference:

Kreel L: *Outline of Radiology.* New York, Appleton-Century-Crofts, 1971, pp 171–173.

SOLITARY SPLENIC CALCIFICATION
(GREATER THAN 1 CM)

COMMON

1. Splenic artery aneurysm
2. Splenic artery atherosclerosis

UNCOMMON

1. Abscess
2. Ascites (capsular)
3. Dermoid cyst
4. Epidermoid cyst
5. Hematoma
6. Hydatid cyst
7. Infarct
8. [Sickle cell anemia]
9. [Thorotrast injection]
10. Traumatic hemorrhagic cyst
11. Tuberculosis

MULTIPLE SPLENIC CALCIFICATIONS
(LESS THAN 1 CM)

COMMON

1. Histoplasmosis
2. Phleboliths; hemangiomas
3. Tuberculosis

UNCOMMON

1. Armillifer armillatus infestation
2. Brucellosis
3. Infarcts

MASS IN REGION OF THE PANCREAS

COMMON

1. Aortic aneurysm
2. Carcinoma of duodenum, ampulla, bile duct, gallbladder
3. Gastric neoplasm (eg, carcinoma, leiomyoma, leiomyosarcoma)
4. Lymphadenopathy, inflammatory or neoplastic (eg, retroperitoneal lymphoma)
5. Pancreatic carcinoma
6. Pancreatic cyst or pseudocyst
7. Pancreatitis
8. Renal cyst or tumor
9. Splenic mass (see Gamuts G-80 and G-81)

UNCOMMON

1. Abscess of lesser sac
2. Calculus in common duct
3. Hydatid cyst
4. Pancreatic abscess
5. Retroperitoneal cyst or neoplasm (eg, sarcoma)

PANCREATIC ANGIOGRAPHIC ABNORMALITY (VIA CELIAC, SUPERIOR MESENTERIC, OR SUBSELECTIVE ARTERIOGRAPHY)

1. Arterial displacement or hypovascularity (eg, pseudocyst, pancreatitis, cystadenocarcinoma, lymphoma)

2. Gallbladder enlargement

3. Hypervascularity
   a. Carcinoma
   b. Cystadenoma and cystadenocarcinoma (florid neovascularity)
   c. Non-β islet cell tumor (Zollinger-Ellison syndrome) or insulinoma — tumor blush
   d. Pancreatitis and abscess

4. Metastases in liver

5. Narrowing of an artery
   a. Irregular (usually carcinoma)
   b. Long segment narrowing with arterial cuffing (carcinoma)
   c. Smooth (carcinoma, pancreatitis, atherosclerosis)

6. Occlusion or truncation of an artery (carcinoma or surgical ligation)

7. Small aneurysms (pancreatitis)

8. Venous narrowing, occlusion, or displacement

References:
1. Kreel L: *Outline of Radiology.* New York, Appleton-Century-Crofts, 1971, pp 145–146.
2. Eaton SB Jr, Ferrucci JT Jr: Personal communication.

PANCREATIC CALCIFICATION

COMMON

1. Chronic alcoholic pancreatitis

UNCOMMON

1. Acute pancreatitis (saponification)
2. Cavernous lymphangioma
3. Cystadenoma, cystadenocarcinoma ("sunburst" calcification)
4. Hemorrhage in pancreas
5. Hereditary pancreatitis (large clumps)
6. Hyperparathyroidism with pancreatitis
7. Idiopathic (nonspecific pancreatic ductal stenosis)
8. Islet cell tumor
9. Kwashiorkor
10. Metastatic tumor
11. Mucoviscidosis
12. Pseudocyst of pancreas

References:

1. Margulis AR, Burhenne HJ: *Alimentary Tract Roentgenology.* St. Louis, C. V. Mosby Co, 1967, p 884.
2. Ring EJ, Eaton SB Jr, Ferrucci JT Jr, et al: Differential diagnosis of pancreatic calcification. *Am J Roentgenol* 117:446–452, 1973.

ABDOMINAL CALCULI THAT LAYER IN UPRIGHT POSITION

COMMON

1. Gallstones
2. Urinary bladder calculi

UNCOMMON

1. Calculi in calyceal diverticulum or hydronephrotic kidney
2. Dermoid
3. Enteroliths
4. Meckel's diverticulum calculi
5. Milk of calcium pus (eg, Pott's abscess, granulomatous lymph node)
6. Myxoglobulosis of the appendix
7. Urachal cyst calculi

NONVISCERAL ABDOMINAL CALCIFICATION

COMMON

*1. Aneurysm, arteriovenous fistula
*2. Atherosclerotic aorta and arteries
*3. Dermoid cyst
*4. [Foreign body]
*5. [Intramuscular opaque medication]
*6. Mesenteric lymph nodes
*7. Phleboliths
*8. [Rib cartilage]

UNCOMMON

 *1. Armillifer armillatus infestation
 *2. Benign tumor (eg, lipoma)
  3. [Bone lesion]
 *4. Cysticercosis or guinea worm in abdominal wall
 *5. Epiploic appendages
 *6. Fecalith or gallstone extruded into peritoneum
  7. Hemangioma
 *8. Hydatid cyst
 *9. Lithopedion
*10. Meconium peritonitis
*11. Mesenteric cyst
*12. Mineral oil in peritoneum (lipid granuloma)
 13. Neuroblastoma
 14. Osteosarcoma or chondrosarcoma of soft tissues
(Continued)

15. Pancreatitis with saponification

16. Peritoneal metastases (colloid carcinoma, ovarian cystadenocarcinoma)

17. Pheochromocytoma

*18. Pseudomyxoma peritonei

19. Retroperitoneal hematoma

20. Retroperitoneal sarcoma

21. Tuberculous peritonitis, psoas abscess

*annular or cyst-like calcifications

ABDOMINAL CALCIFICATION IN AN INFANT OR YOUNG CHILD
(See also Gamuts G-79 and G-90)

COMMON

1. Adrenal calcification (hemorrhage, tuberculosis, histoplasmosis, tumor, Wolman's disease)
2. Appendiceal calculus
3. Duplication, atresia, or other obstruction (mural calcification)
4. [Foreign body, pills, etc.]
5. Histoplasmosis or tuberculosis in liver, spleen, or lymph nodes
6. Meconium peritonitis
7. [Minerals simulating calcium (barium, bismuth, lead, iron)]
8. Neuroblastoma and other neurogenic tumors

UNCOMMON

1. Calculi in Meckel's diverticulum, urachal cyst
2. Chronic pancreatitis
3. Cytomegalic inclusion disease (liver)
4. Dermoid cyst or teratoma
5. Enterolith
6. Gallstones (hemolytic anemias)
7. Hemangioma
8. Hematoma (spleen, retroperitoneal)
9. Liver abscess
10. Liver tumor (hepatoma, hepatoblastoma, hemangioma)
11. Mucoviscidosis

(Continued)

12. Parasites (armillifer, guinea worm, cysticercosis, hydatid cyst, schistosomiasis hematobium)

13. Renal or bladder calculus; nephrocalcinosis

14. Renal tuberculosis

15. Thrombosis of inferior vena cava or portal vein

16. Tuberculous psoas abscess

17. Wilms' tumor

Reference:

Donner MW, Weiner S: Diagnostic evaluation of abdominal calcifications in acute abdominal disorders. *Radiol Clin North Am* 2:145–159, 1964.

ABDOMINAL DISEASE ASSOCIATED WITH PLEURAL EFFUSION

COMMON

1. Cirrhosis of liver
2. Neoplasm (eg, ovarian tumor with Meig's syndrome, pleural metastasis or direct extension from pancreatic or other abdominal carcinoma)
3. Pancreatitis
4. Subphrenic abscess, perinephric abscess
5. Trauma (eg, gunshot wound, ruptured diaphragm)

UNCOMMON

1. Amebic abscess of liver
2. Aneurysm, thoracoabdominal, with rupture
3. Diaphragmatic hernia, incarcerated
4. Lymphoma of abdomen and pleura

SPONTANEOUS PNEUMOPERITONEUM WITHOUT PERITONITIS

COMMON

1. "Aspiration" per vagina; Rubin test; sudden squatting; cunnilingus
2. *Form fruste* perforation of peptic ulcer
3. Idiopathic

UNCOMMON

1. Leakage through a distended stomach (aerophagy, gastroscopy, sodium bicarbonate, misplaced oxygen tube)
2. Pneumatosis cystoides intestinalis with perforation
3. Pneumomediastinum, pulmonary emphysema

Reference:

Felson B: Abdominal gas: a roentgen approach. *Ann NY Acad Sci* 150:141–161, 1968.

ABNORMAL GAS IN THE RIGHT UPPER QUADRANT (OUTSIDE THE GUT)

COMMON

1. Biliary fistula (eg, gallstone perforation; postoperative) (see Gamut G-70)
2. [Colon interposition]
3. Pneumoperitoneum, free or loculated
4. Subphrenic or subhepatic abscess; other peritoneal abscess

UNCOMMON

1. Abdominal wall gas (postoperative, abscess)
2. Emphysematous cholecystitis
3. Liver abscess, amebic or pyogenic; gangrene of liver
4. Pancreatic abscess
5. Perinephric or flank abscess; postoperative perinephric hematoma
6. Pneumomediastinum with retroperitoneal extension
7. Portal vein gas (see Gamut G-78)
8. Renal abscess
9. Retroperitoneal rupture of duodenum (trauma, ulcer) or rectum; iatrogenic pneumoretroperitoneum
10. [Stomach (heterotaxy)]

Reference:

Love L, Baker D, Ramey R: Gas producing perinephic abscess. *Am J Roentgenol* 119:783-792, 1973.

ABNORMAL GAS IN THE LEFT UPPER QUADRANT (OUTSIDE THE GUT)

COMMON

1. Perinephric or flank abscess
2. Pneumoperitoneum, free or loculated
3. Subphrenic abscess; other peritoneal abscess

UNCOMMON

1. Abdominal wall gas (postoperative, abscess)
2. Emphysematous gastritis
3. Lesser sac abscess
4. Pancreatic abscess
5. Pneumomediastinum with retroperitoneal extension
6. Renal abscess
7. Retroperitoneal rupture of duodenum or rectum (trauma, ulcer); iatrogenic pneumoretroperitoneum
8. Splenic abscess

LARGE ABDOMINAL GAS POCKET

COMMON

1. Bladder, emphysematous cystitis
2. Cecal distension, nonobstructive "paralytic ileus" or colon obstruction
3. Gastric obstruction
4. Pneumoperitoneum, free or loculated (subphrenic, lesser sac, greater sac)
5. Volvulus of stomach, small bowel, or colon

UNCOMMON

1. Abdominal wall gas (postoperative, abscess)
2. Amnionitis, endometritis (physometria)
3. Blind loop syndrome (esp. postoperative)
4. Duplication
5. Hernia (diaphragmatic, internal, external)
6. Hydropneumometrocolpos; vaginitis emphysematosa
7. Infected fibroid
8. Liver abscess or gangrene
9. Meckel's diverticulum ("giant" size)
10. Pancreatic gas abscess
11. Pregnancy, extrauterine, perforating into colon
12. Psoas abscess
13. Small bowel obstruction, chronic (eg, Crohn's disease)
14. Subphrenic abscess
15. Tubovarian abscess

References:
1. Felson B, Wiot JF: *Case of the Day.* Springfield, Charles C Thomas, 1967, p 76.
2. Weintraub RA, Tilos F: Gas abscess within a leiomyoma of the uterus. *Am J Roentgenol* 92:400–403, 1964.

PERFORATED HOLLOW VISCUS IN A NEWBORN

COMMON

1. Gastric rupture, spontaneous
2. Iatrogenic (intubation, rectal thermometer, enema, intra-uterine transfusion, resuscitation)
3. Intestinal obstruction (eg, atresia, volvulus)
4. Meconium ileus (mucoviscidosis)

UNCOMMON

1. Hirschsprung's disease
2. Perforated peptic or stress ulcer

GASLESS ABDOMEN IN A NEWBORN

COMMON

1. Esophageal obstruction (atresia without T-E fistula, web)

UNCOMMON

1. Congenital diaphragmatic hernia
2. Continuous gastric or intestinal suction
3. Duodenal atresia
4. Gastroenteritis with vomiting
5. Midgut volvulus
6. Normal
7. Pyloric obstruction, complete

GASLESS ABDOMEN IN AN ADULT

COMMON

1. Acute pancreatitis

UNCOMMON

1. Closed loop obstruction
2. Mesenteric infarction
3. Normal
4. Obstruction of esophagus (eg, cardiospasm), stomach (eg, volvulus, pyloric obstruction), or duodenum
5. Vomiting and inanition

LARGE ABDOMINAL MASS IN AN INFANT OR CHILD

COMMON

1. Abscess (intraperitoneal, retroperitoneal, hepatic)
2. Bladder distension
3. Enlarged liver or spleen (from systemic disease)
4. Hydronephrosis, massive
5. Intestinal obstruction (fluid-filled loop)
6. Intussusception
7. Multicystic kidney
8. Neuroblastoma
9. Polycystic disease of the kidney
10. Wilms' tumor

UNCOMMON

1. Adrenal hemorrhage, cyst, or tumor
2. Anterior meningocele
3. Choledochal cyst
4. Duplication cyst
5. Hirschsprung's disease with fecal masses
6. Horseshoe kidney
7. Hydrometrocolpos
8. Liver cyst or neoplasm, primary or metastatic (see Gamut G-74)
9. Mesenteric or omental cyst
10. Multilocular cyst of the kidney
11. Ovarian cyst or tumor
12. Pancreatic pseudocyst
13. Retroperitoneal lesion (teratoma, sarcoma, hematoma)

(Continued)

14. Splenic cyst or tumor (see Gamuts G-80 and G-81)

15. Urachal cyst

Reference:

Moncada R, Wang JJ, Love L, Bush I: Neonatal ascites associated with urinary outlet obstruction (urine ascites). *Radiology* 90:1165–1170, 1968.

PERITONEAL FLUID IN AN INFANT

COMMON

1. Appendicitis with rupture
2. Cardiac disease (eg, anasarca, constrictive pericarditis)
3. Cirrhosis, portal or biliary cystic disease of the liver
4. Meconium peritonitis
5. Nephrotic syndrome, glomerulonephritis, uremia
6. Perforated Meckel's diverticulum
7. Peritonitis (eg, generalized sepsis, syphilis)
8. Portal vein obstruction, extrahepatic (tumor, lymphadenopathy, thrombosis)
9. Protein loss, malnutrition, kwashiorkor
10. Urinary outlet obstruction with hydronephrosis (urine ascites)

UNCOMMON

1. Chylous ascites (see Gamut G-102)
2. Hemolytic disease with ascites
3. Meig's syndrome
4. Preduodenal portal vein
5. Ruptured ovarian cyst
6. Ventriculoperitoneal shunt

Reference:

Moncada R, Wang JJ, Love L, Bush I: Neonatal ascites associated with urinary outlet obstruction (urine ascites). *Radiology* 90:1165–1170, 1968.

OBSTRUCTION OF ABDOMINAL LYMPHATICS, CISTERNA CHYLI, OR THORACIC DUCT ON LYMPHANGIOGRAPHY (CHYLOUS ASCITES)

COMMON

1. Benign neoplasm (esp. lymphangioma)
2. Lymphoma
3. Metastatic carcinoma in lymph nodes
4. Postoperative
5. Trauma

UNCOMMON

1. Adhesive bands
2. Cirrhosis (hepatic lymphatics visible)
3. Congenital absence of lymphatics
4. Filariasis
5. Idiopathic
6. Lymphangiomyomatosis
7. Malignant tumor compressing or invading lymphatic system (eg, carcinoma of pancreas)
8. Tuberculosis, histoplasmosis

CELIAC ARTERY ABNORMALITY

COMMON

1. Arteriosclerosis
2. Compression by median arcuate ligament of diaphragm (?)

UNCOMMON

1. Aneurysm (including dissecting)
2. Angiomatous malformation, arteriovenous fistula
3. Arteritis, Takayasu's and other
4. Congenital absence
5. Fibromuscular hyperplasia
6. Thromboembolism
7. Traumatic laceration or obstruction
8. Tumor

NOTES

NOTES

NOTES

TABLE OF CONTENTS

H. GENITOURINARY AND RETROPERITONEUM

KIDNEY

(Continued)

H

                         (Continued)

H

H

CONGENITAL SYNDROMES WITH KIDNEY MALFORMATION

1. Campomelic dwarfism
2. Cat-cry S.
3. Cerebrohepatorenal S. (Zellweger)
4. Ehlers-Danlos S.
5. Fraser's S.
6. Leprechaunism
7. Long arm 18 deletion S.
8. Long arm 21 deletion S.
9. Oculocerebral-renal S. (Lowe)
10. Pancytopenia-dysmelia S. (Fanconi)
11. Radial aplasia-thrombocytopenia S.
12. Rubinstein-Taybi S.
13. Trisomy 13 S.
14. Trisomy 18 S.
15. Turner's S.

References:

1. Felson B, Editor: Dwarfs and Other Little People. *Semin Roentgenol* **8:260,** 1973.
2. Smith DW: *Recognizable Patterns of Human Malformation.* Philadelphia, WB Saunders Co, 1970, p 291.

H

CONGENITAL SYNDROMES WITH RENAL INSUFFICIENCY

1. Cerebrohepatorenal S. (Zellweger)
2. de Toni-Fanconi S.
3. Eagle-Barrett S.
4. Fabry's S.
5. Familial hyperuricosuria
6. Laurence-Moon-Biedl S.
7. Nail-patella S. (Fong's S.)
8. Oculocerebral-renal S.
9. Oxalosis
10. Polycystic kidneys and liver
11. Potter's S.
12. von Hippel-Lindau S.
13. William's S.

Reference:

Smith DW: *Recognizable Patterns of Human Malformation.* Philadelphia, WB Saunders Co, 1970, p 291.

H

MISPLACED AND DISPLACED KIDNEYS

COMMON

1. Ectopic kidney (pelvic, thoracic, crossed)
2. Hepatomegaly or splenomegaly displacing kidney
3. Horseshoe kidney
4. Malrotation
5. Mass displacing kidney (intra- or extrarenal) (see Subgamut below)
6. Ptosis
7. Transplanted kidney

UNCOMMON

1. [Absent kidney]
2. Elevated right kidney with shrunken liver
3. Hernia

SUBGAMUT H-3A
MASS DISPLACING KIDNEY

1. Aneurysm of aorta
2. Intracapsular extrarenal mass (eg, lipoma)
3. Intrarenal neoplasm (eg, Wilms', hypernephroma)
4. Lymphoma
5. Metastases to lymph nodes (esp. from testicular tumor)
6. Other lymph node disease (eg, reticuloses, sarcoidosis, tuberculosis)
7. Retroperitoneal tumor (eg, sarcoma)
8. Suprarenal tumor (eg, neuroblastoma, adenoma, Cushing's, pheochromocytoma)

UNILATERAL ABSENCE OF RENAL OUTLINE

1. Abscess, perinephric (see Subgamut below)
2. Atrophy (eg, pyelonephritis, infarction, obstruction)
3. Congenital absence or aplasia
4. Displaced kidney (eg, by retroperitoneal tumor)
5. Ectopic kidney (eg, presacral, thoracic)
6. Hematoma, perinephric
7. Normal (eg, technical factors, insufficient perirenal fat)
8. Postnephrectomy

SUBGAMUT H-4A
PERINEPHRIC ABSCESS

1. Extraurinary infection with direct or hematogenous spread
   a. Deep infection (eg, osteomyelitis, pharyngitis, tonsillitis, perforated ulcer, diverticulitis, pancreatitis)
   b. Superficial infection (eg, furuncle, carbuncle, wound infection)
2. Instrumentation (eg, removal of ureteral calculus)
3. Obstructive uropathy
4. Trauma to kidney or ureter
5. Urinary tract infection (esp. in diabetic women)

Reference:

Love L, Baker D, Ramsey R: Gas producing perinephric abscess. *Am J Roentgenol* 119:783–792, 1973.

FOCAL OR ANNULAR CALCIFICATION IN THE KIDNEY

COMMON

*1. Aneurysm of renal artery
 2. Calculus (see Gamut H-43)
*3. Hypernephroma

UNCOMMON

 *1. Abscess, renal or perinephric
 *2. [Adrenal cyst or tumor]
 *3. Angiomatous malformation, arteriovenous fistula
 *4. Benign neoplasm (eg, dermoid, hamartoma, leiomyoma, cortical adenoma, Perlman's tumor — cystadenoma)
  5. Chronic glomerulonephritis (cortical calcification)
 *6. Cortical necrosis
 *7. Cyst (eg, simple, hydatid)
 *8. Hematoma
 *9. Hydronephrosis; pyonephrosis
 10. Infarct
*11. Multicystic kidney
 12. [Nephrocalcinosis (see Gamut H-6)]
 13. Osteosarcoma
 14. Papillary necrosis
*15. Polycystic kidney
*16. Tuberculosis
 17. Wilms' tumor

*May be annular

References:

1. Kikkawa K, Lasser EC: "Ring-like" or "rim-like" calcification in renal cell carcinoma. *Am J Roentgenol* 107:737–742, 1969.
2. Teplick JG, Haskin ME; *Roentgenologic Diagnosis*, ed 2. Philadelphia, WB Saunders Co, 1971, vol 2, p XXXII.

NEPHROCALCINOSIS

COMMON

1. Chronic pyelonephritis
2. Hyperparathyroidism
3. Idiopathic
4. Medullary sponge kidney
5. Osteoporosis (eg, immobilization, menopausal, senile)

UNCOMMON

1. Aminoaciduria
2. Cortical calcification (eg, chronic glomerulonephritis, hereditary nephritis, cortical necrosis, dialysis therapy)
3. Cushing's disease; steroid therapy
4. Cystinuria
5. Excessive calcium intake or absorption
6. Hyperthyroidism
7. Hyperuricemia (eg, gout, antimetabolic treatment of leukemia)
8. Hypervitaminosis D
9. Hypochloremic acidosis
10. Idiopathic hypercalcemia (eg, William's syndrome)
11. Idiopathic hypercalciuria
12. Metallic poisoning (eg, mercury)
13. Milk-alkali syndrome
14. Osteolytic bone metastases; multiple myeloma
15. Oxaluria
16. Paget's disease
17. Papillary necrosis (see Gamut H-8)

(Continued)

18. Renal tubular acidosis (deToni-Fanconi, cystinuria)

19. Sarcoidosis

20. Sjögren's syndrome

21. Sulfonamide intoxication

22. Tuberculosis (autonephrectomy)

References:

1. Courey WR, Pfister RC: The radiographic findings in renal tubular acidosis. *Radiology* 105:497–503, 1972.

2. Emmett JL, Witten DM: *Clinical Urography*, ed 3. Philadelphia, WB Saunders Co, 1971, vol 2, p 661–674.

3. McAlister WH, Nedelman SH: The roentgen manifestations of bilateral renal cortical necrosis. *Am J Roentgenol* 86:129–135, 1961.

4. Teplick JG, Haskin ME: *Roentgenologic Diagnosis*, ed 2. Philadelphia, WB Saunders Co, 1971, vol 2, p XXXII.

CLUBBING OR DESTRUCTION OF RENAL CALYCES

COMMON

1. Hydronephrosis
2. Localized caliectasis from obstruction of infundibulum by neoplasm, stricture, clot, or anomalous vessel
3. Papillary necrosis (see Gamut H-8)
4. Pyelonephritis
5. Tuberculosis
6. Vesicopelvic reflux

UNCOMMON

1. [Megacalyx]

PAPILLARY NECROSIS

COMMON

1. Analgesic abuse (eg, phenacetin)
2. Diabetes mellitus
3. Obstruction of urinary tract
4. Pyelonephritis
5. Sickle cell anemia

UNCOMMON

1. Cirrhosis
2. Renal vein thrombosis

References:

1. Emmett JL, Witten DM: *Clinical Urography*, ed 3. Philadelphia, WB Saunders Co, 1971, vol 3, p 1894–1907.
2. Mellins HZ: Chronic pyelonephritis and renal medullary necrosis. *Semin Roentgenol* 6:292–309, 1971.

FILLING DEFECT IN RENAL PELVIS, INFUNDIBULUM OR CALYX (SOLITARY OR MULTIPLE)

COMMON

*1. Air (from retrograde pyelogram, vesicovaginal fistula, ureterointestinal anastomosis)

*2. Blood clot (eg, trauma, neoplasm)

*3. Calculus (see Subgamut H-43A)

*4. Neoplasm (eg, hemangioma, hamartoma, papilloma, transitional cell carcinoma, hypernephroma, metastasis)

5. [Normal anatomic variation (eg, bifid pelvis, overlapping calyces, calyx seen on end)]

6. Normal renal artery and its branches

7. [Technical (incomplete filling with contrast medium; overlying intestinal gas)]

UNCOMMON

1. Aneurysm, arteriovenous fistula, collateral vessel

2. Cholesteatoma (squamous metaplasia of uroepithelium)

3. [Cyst impinging on renal pelvis (peripelvic or parenchymal)]

*4. Fungus ball (monilia)

*5. Inspissated pus, necrotic debris (eg, pyelonephritis — suppurative, xanthogranulomatous, or tuberculous)

6. Leukoplakia

7. Papilla, aberrant or sloughed (eg, papillary necrosis)

8. Pyelitis cystica

9. [Renal sinus lipomatosis]

*May fill entire renal pelvis

Reference:

Brown RC, Jones MC, Boldus R, et al: Lesions causing radiolucent defects in the renal pelvis. Am J Roentgenol 119:770–778, 1973.

PERIPELVIC EXTRAVASATION (SINUS LEAKAGE)
(See also Gamut H-34)

COMMON

1. Extrinsic abdominal compression (binder)
2. Iatrogenic (instrumentation, retrograde pyelography, accidental ureteral ligation)
3. Trauma
4. Ureteral calculus

UNCOMMON

1. Hydronephrosis from ureteral tumor or stricture
2. Increased abdominal pressure during delivery
3. Polycystic kidney
4. Tumor of renal pelvis, esp. with rupture or hemorrhage

Reference:

Bramwit, DN, Rosen LS, Cukier DS: Peripelvic extravasation in chronic ureteral obstruction by reticulum-cell sarcoma. *Radiology* 96:421–422, 1970.

AVASCULAR RENAL MASS ON ANGIOGRAPHY

COMMON

1. Abscess
2. Hematoma
3. Polycystic disease
4. Simple cyst
5. Vascular occlusion, infarct

UNCOMMON

1. Adenoma
2. Fibroma
3. Hydatid cyst
4. Lipoma
5. Lymphoma, including Burkitt's tumor
6. Malignant tumor, necrotic (eg, hypernephroma, Wilms')
7. Metastasis
8. Multilocular cyst
9. Xanthogranulomatous pyelonephritis

CYSTIC DISEASES OF THE KIDNEY

COMMON

1. Adult polycystic disease
2. Calyceal cyst or diverticulum (pyelogenic cyst)
3. [Cyst(s) secondary to tuberculosis, pyelonephritis, medullary necrosis, nephrolithiasis, trauma, or degeneration of renal cell carcinoma]
4. Medullary sponge kidney
5. Multicystic kidney
6. Parapelvic cyst
7. Simple renal cyst (solitary or multiple)

UNCOMMON

1. Cortical sponge kidney or congenital cortical cystic disease (trisomy syndromes, tuberous sclerosis)
2. Cystic dysplasia of cortex (multiple cysts associated with lower urinary tract obstruction, usually urethral valves)
3. Dermoid cyst
4. Endometrial cyst
5. Hydatid cyst
6. Infantile polycystic disease (large sponge kidneys with cystic liver)
7. Infantile polycystic disease (medullary tubular ectasia and hepatic fibrosis)
8. Medullary cystic disease (small fibrotic kidneys with uremia)
9. Multilocular cyst
10. Pericalyceal lymphangiectasis
11. Perinephric cyst (pararenal pseudocyst, urinoma)

References:

1. Elkin M, Bernstein J: Cystic diseases of the kidney — radiological and pathological considerations. *Clin Radiol* 20:65–82, 1969.
2. Gwinn JL, Landing BH: Cystic diseases of the kidneys in infants and children. *Radiol Clin North Am* 6:191–204, 1968.

RENAL PSEUDOTUMOR (NORMAL STRUCTURE)

COMMON

1. Double collecting system
2. Dromedary hump, splenic imprint
3. Enlarged column of Bertin
4. Fetal lobulation
5. Lipomatosis of renal pelvis
6. Malrotation
7. Vascular impression

UNCOMMON

1. Hypertrophy, localized (regenerated nodule from chronic pyelonephritis or infarction)
2. Renunculus

Reference:

Lopez FA: Renal pseudotumors. *Am J Roentgenol* 109:172–184, 1970.

DEPRESSION OR SCAR IN RENAL MARGIN (SOLITARY OR MULTIPLE)

COMMON

1. Arterionephrosclerosis
2. Extrinsic pressure (eg, spleen)
3. Fetal lobulation
4. Glomerulonephritis
5. Infarct
6. Pyelonephritic scarring

UNCOMMON

1. Radiation therapy
2. Tuberculosis

LOCALIZED BULGE OF RENAL OUTLINE

COMMON

1. Cyst
2. Enlarged column of Bertin
3. Localized hypertrophy (eg, in pyelonephritis)
4. Neoplasm
5. Normal (dromedary hump, fetal lobulation)

UNCOMMON

1. Abscess
2. Duplication of collecting system
3. Hematoma
4. Hypertrophy of upper pole
5. Localized hydronephrosis
6. Renunculus (supra- and infrahilar bulge)

UNILATERAL LARGE KIDNEY

COMMON

1. Compensatory hypertrophy due to disease or absence of other kidney
2. Congenital or idiopathic (opposite kidney normal)
3. Cyst, solitary
4. Double or triple collecting system
5. Multicystic kidney
6. Neoplasm (eg, hypernephroma, Wilms' tumor, metastasis, angiomyolipoma)
7. Polycystic kidneys with unilateral enlargement
8. Ureteral obstruction with hydronephrosis, any cause

UNCOMMON

1. Abscess, carbuncle
2. Crossed fused renal ectopy; horseshoe kidney
3. Renal vein thrombosis
4. Transplant rejection (acute)
5. Trauma (eg, hematoma, urinoma)

BILATERAL LARGE KIDNEYS

COMMON

1. Bilateral duplication
2. Bilateral obstructive hydronephrosis, any cause
3. Nephritis or nephrosis (eg, toxic nephrosis, acute pyelonephritis, acute or lobular glomerulonephritis, lipoid nephrosis)
4. Polycystic disease, adult or infantile

UNCOMMON

1. Acromegaly
2. Amyloidosis
3. Bartter's syndrome
4. Bilateral hamartomas (angiomyolipomas)
5. Bilateral hypernephromas
6. Bilateral metastases
7. Bilateral renal vein thrombosis
8. Bilateral simple cysts
9. Bilateral Wilms' tumors
10. Cyst in one kidney, hypernephroma in the other
11. Diabetes, lipoatrophic
12. Glycogen storage disease (von Gierke's)
13. Hereditary tyrosinosis
14. Lymphoma
15. Medullary sponge kidney; familial bilateral cystic dysplasia
16. Myelomatosis
17. Renal cortical necrosis (early)

(Continued)

18. Sarcoidosis
19. Sickle cell anemia
20. Visceromegaly, fetal
21. Work hypertrophy (eg, beer-drinker's kidneys)

UNILATERAL SMALL KIDNEY

COMMON

1. Congenital hypoplastic or dysplastic kidney
2. Obstructive renal atrophy
3. Pyelonephritis, chronic
4. Renal artery stenosis with ischemia (eg, arteriosclerosis, thromboembolism, fibromuscular hyperplasia, congenital stenosis)

UNCOMMON

1. Radiation therapy
2. Renal infarction (late)
3. Tuberculosis

References:

1. Friedland GW, Dale RL: Miniature kidneys due to obstructive atrophy. *Radiology* 99:273–277, 1971.
2. Teplick JG, Haskin ME: *Roentgenologic Diagnosis*, ed 2. Philadelphia, WB Saunders Co, 1971, vol 2, p XXXII.

BILATERAL SMALL KIDNEYS

COMMON

1. Arteriolar nephrosclerosis
2. Glomerulonephritis, chronic
3. Ischemia (eg, bilateral renal artery stenosis, fibromuscular hyperplasia)
4. Pyelonephritis, chronic

UNCOMMON

1. Back pressure atrophy from reflux or obstruction
2. Cortical necrosis (late)
3. Gouty nephritis
4. Hereditary nephritis (Alpert's disease)
5. Interstitial nephritis, chronic
6. Kimmelsteil-Wilson disease
7. Lupus erythematosus; polyarteritis nodosa; scleroderma
8. Medullary cystic disease
9. Senile atrophy

Reference:

Teplick JG, Haskin ME: *Roentgenologic Diagnosis*, ed 2. Philadelphia, WB Saunders Co, 1971, vol 2, p XXXII.

DECREASED SIZE OF PART OF A KIDNEY

COMMON

1. Ischemia, infarct
2. Pyelonephritis
3. Trauma

UNCOMMON

1. Abscess, healed
2. Radiation therapy
3. Tuberculosis

DENSE NEPHROGRAM ON IVP

COMMON

1. Contrast medium injection, rapid with large bolus
2. Extrarenal obstruction (eg, ureteral calculus, blood clot, carcinoma of cervix)
3. Glomerulonephritis, acute or chronic
4. Hypotension; shock
5. Ischemia
6. Post-traumatic reflex anuria
7. Renal failure, acute

UNCOMMON

1. Idiopathic
2. Intratubular block (eg, sulfonamide therapy, multiple myeloma, myoglobinuria, hyperuricemia, Tamm-Horsfall proteinuria)
3. Nephrosis
4. Pyelonephritis, acute
5. Renal vein thrombosis
6. Trueta phenomenon
7. Tubular necrosis, acute
8. Waldenström's macroglobulinemia

Reference:

Martin DJ, Jaffe N: Prolonged nephrogram due to hyperuricaemia. *Br J Radiol* 44:806–809, 1971.

NONVISUALIZATION OR NONFUNCTION OF ONE KIDNEY ON IVP

COMMON

1. [Ectopic kidney]
2. Fractured kidney
3. Neoplasm
4. Obstruction of ureter (eg, calculus, stricture, neoplasm)
5. Renal artery obstruction (eg, stenosis, thromboembolism, trauma)

UNCOMMON

1. Absent kidney (congenital, postnephrectomy)
2. Arteriovenous fistula of kidney
3. Multicystic kidney
4. Renal vein obstruction (eg, thrombosis, tumor)
5. Tuberculosis and other severe infection (eg, xanthogranulomatous pyelonephritis)

Reference:

Petasnick JP, Patel SK: Angiographic evaluation of the nonvisualizing kidney. *Am J Roentgenol* 119:757–766, 1973.

SUBGAMUT H-22A
NONVISUALIZATION OR NONFUNCTION OF A
SINGLE CALYX OR PART OF A KIDNEY

1. Duplication of collecting system with obstruction to one portion (eg, by stone, ectopic ureterocele)

2. Obstruction by calculus, band, vessel, neoplasm

3. Postoperative, partial nephrectomy

4. Tuberculosis or other infection

DIMINISHED CONCENTRATION OF CONTRAST MEDIUM IN PELVOCALYCEAL SYSTEM

BILATERAL

1. Arteriolar nephrosclerosis, hypertensive renal disease
2. Idiopathic
3. Inadequate dehydration or overhydration
4. Polyuria (eg, diuretic, diabetes insipidus or mellitus, renal disease)
5. Renal failure, uremia
6. Technical (eg, inadequate contrast dose)

UNILATERAL

1. Obstruction of a ureter with hydronephrosis
2. [Renal artery stenosis involving opposite kidney]
3. Renal parenchymal disease, unilateral (eg, tuberculosis, carbuncle)
4. Trauma with spasm of pelvocalyceal system

RENAL VEIN THROMBOSIS

COMMON

1. Dehydration or diarrhea (in children)
2. Extension of thrombus from inferior vena cava
3. Idiopathic
4. Obstruction or invasion by renal or extrarenal tumor

UNCOMMON

1. Amyloidosis
2. Glomerulonephritis
3. Nephrotic syndrome
4. Postpartum
5. Pyelonephritis
6. Trauma

References:

1. Coel MN, Talner LB: Obstructive nephrogram due to renal vein thrombosis. *Radiology* 101:573–574, 1971.
2. Ney C, Friedenberg RM: *Radiographic Atlas of the Genitourinary System*. Philadelphia, JB Lippincott Co, 1966.

RENAL ISCHEMIA

COMMON

1. Arteriolar nephrosclerosis
2. Atherosclerosis
3. Chronic pyelonephritis
4. Thrombosis, spasm, or stenosis of renal artery
5. Trauma (eg, fractured kidney, avulsion of renal artery)

UNCOMMON

1. Arteritis (eg, polyarteritis nodosa, Takayasu's disease)
2. Arteriovenous fistula
   a. Congenital
   b. Renal carcinoma eroding the renal vein
   c. Rupture of an aneurysm
   d. Stump fistula following nephrectomy
   e. Traumatic (eg, external trauma, operation, needle biopsy)
3. Extrinsic pressure on the renal artery (eg, neoplasm, aortic aneurysm, lymphadenopathy, bands)
4. Fibromuscular hyperplasia
   a. Intimal fibroplasia
   b. Medial fibroplasia
   c. Subadventitial fibroplasia
5. Renal artery aneurysm
6. Renal compression (eg, traumatic or spontaneous perirenal or subcapsular hematoma)

Reference:

Baum S: Renal ischemic lesions. *Radiol Clin North Am* 5:543–558, 1967.

UNILATERAL RENAL LESION THAT MAY RESULT IN HYPERTENSION

1. Lesion of renal artery or its branches
    a. Aneurysm
    b. Arteriovenous fistula
    c. Arteritis (eg, syphilis, polyarteritis nodosa, thromboangiitis obliterans, rubella, idiopathic)
    d. Atherosclerosis
    e. Congenital narrowing
    f. Fibromuscular hyperplasia
    g. Neurofibromatosis
    h. Perivascular fibrosis and subcapsular hemorrhage secondary to trauma
    i. Thrombosis or embolism

2. Renal parenchymal disease
    a. Obstructive uropathy
    b. Ptosis of the kidney
    c. Pyelonephritis
    d. Radiation nephritis
    e. Tumor (eg, carcinoma, sarcoma, Wilms' tumor)

3. Renal vein thrombosis

Reference:

Hanenson IB, Gaffney TE: Clinical recognition of renal hypertension. *Semin Roentgenol* 2:115–125, 1967.

RENAL MICROANEURYSMS ON ARTERIOGRAPHY (INCLUDING NECROTIZING ANGIITIS)

COMMON

1. Polyarteritis nodosa

UNCOMMON

1. Allergic granulomatous arteritis
2. Angiomyolipoma
3. Arteriolar necrosis of malignant hypertension
4. Collagen disease, other
5. Drug abuse angiitis
6. Homocystinuria
7. Hypernephroma
8. Hypersensitivity angiitis
9. Mycotic aneurysm
10. Neurofibromatosis
11. Rheumatic arteritis

Reference:

  Halpern M, Citron BP: Necrotizing angiitis associated with drug abuse. *Am J Roentgenol* 111:663–671, 1971.

RAPID RENAL CIRCULATION (LESS THAN 5 SEC) WITH EARLY RENAL VEIN OPACIFICATION

COMMON

1. Renal arteriovenous fistula, congenital or acquired (traumatic, postbiopsy, postoperative)
2. Renal neoplasm

UNCOMMON

1. Acute renal artery obstruction (eg, by catheter in wedge position)
2. Inflammatory disease, severe diffuse (absence or marked decrease of cortical tissue and perfusion — Trueta phenomenon)
3. Localized inflammatory lesion (renal carbuncle, perirenal abscess)

Reference:

Becker JA, Kanter IE, Perl S: Rapid intrarenal circulation. *Am J Roentgenol* 109:167–171, 1970.

SOLITARY URETERAL DEFECT

COMMON

1. Air bubble from retrograde study
2. Blood clot
3. Calculus

UNCOMMON

1. Benign mesenchymal tumor (eg, fibroma, lipoma, hamartoma, hemangioma)
2. Benign stricture
3. Carcinoma, primary or metastatic
4. Compression or invasion from adjacent malignancy or nodes
5. Endometrioma
6. Granuloma
7. Papillary tumor (papilloma)
8. Polyp
9. Seeding from transitional cell carcinoma of kidney
10. Varicosity

Reference:

Emmett JL, Witten DM: *Clinical Urography*, ed 3.   Philadelphia, WB Saunders Co, 1971, vol 2, pp 1145–1185.

MULTIPLE URETERAL DEFECTS

COMMON

1. Air bubbles from retrograde study
2. Blood clots
3. Extrinsic indentations from blood vessels (see Gamut H-44)

UNCOMMON

1. Endometriosis
2. Granulomas (eg, schistosomiasis)
3. Malakoplakia
4. Multiple calculi
5. Papillomatosis; multiple polyps
6. Seeding from transitional cell carcinoma of kidney
7. Tuberculous ureteritis
8. [Ureteral peristalsis]
9. Ureteritis cystica

Reference:

Chait A, Matasar KW, Fabian CE, Mellins HZ: Vascular impressions on the ureters. *Am J Roentgenol* 111:729–749, 1971.

OBSTRUCTION OF THE URETER

COMMON

1. Blood clot or inspissated pus
2. Calculus
3. Congenital ureteropelvic junction obstruction (eg, band, valve, vessel)
4. Cystitis or carcinoma of bladder with compression or obstruction of intramural ureter
5. Inflammation, edema (eg, pelvic inflammatory disease)
6. Invasion or compression by extrinsic malignancy (eg, retroperitoneal lymphoma or sarcoma; carcinoma of pancreas, cervix, or other pelvic organ)
7. Postoperative (eg, ligature, edema)
8. Pregnancy
9. Stricture (eg, congenital, traumatic, postoperative, radiation therapy, inflammatory — tuberculosis, schistosomiasis)
10. Ureterocele
11. Vascular compression by normal or abnormal vessel or aneurysm

UNCOMMON

1. Benign ureteral tumor (eg, polyp, papilloma, mesenchymal tumor)
2. Bladder diverticulum
3. Carcinoma of ureter, primary or metastatic
4. Endometriosis
5. Megacolon
6. Papillary necrosis with sloughed papilla
7. Pelvic lipomatosis
8. Retroperitoneal fibrosis (Ormond's disease)

URETERECTASIS, SEGMENTAL OR DIFFUSE

COMMON

1. Congenital or idiopathic (eg, fusiform terminal ureterectasis)
2. Infection
3. Neurogenic bladder
4. Obstruction of ureter, intrinsic or extrinsic (see Gamut H-31)
5. Obstruction of urethra (eg, valve, stricture, diverticulum) or bladder outlet
6. Reflux

UNCOMMON

1. Absent abdominal musculature or "prune belly" (Eagle-Barrett syndrome)
2. Aganglionosis, Chagas' disease

Reference:

Emmett JL, Witten DM: *Clinical Urography,* ed 3. Philadelphia, WB Saunders Co, 1971, vol 1, pp 432–451.

VESICOURETERAL REFLUX

COMMON

1. Infection
2. Neurogenic bladder

UNCOMMON

1. Absent abdominal musculature or "prune belly" (Eagle-Barrett syndrome)
2. Aganglionosis of colon (Hirschsprung)
3. Anomaly of kidney or ureterovesical junction
4. Constipation
5. Ectopic anus
6. Exstrophy of bladder
7. Iatrogenic; irritative contrast agent
8. Pelvic mass
9. Urethral valve or stenosis

Reference:

Shopfner CE: Vesicoureteral reflux. *Radiology* 95:637–648, 1970.

URETERAL EXTRAVASATION OR FISTULA
(See also Gamut H-10)

COMMON

1. Instrumentation (eg, retrograde pyelography)
2. Postoperative

UNCOMMON

1. Amebiasis of colon
2. Calculus in ureter
3. Carcinoma of ureter
4. Crohn's disease
5. Diverticulitis
6. Endometriosis
7. Trauma
8. Tuberculosis

FILLING DEFECT IN THE BLADDER
(WALL OR LUMEN)

COMMON

1. Blood clot
2. Calculus
3. Instrument (eg, Foley catheter, cystoscope)
4. Neoplasm, intrinsic or invasive
5. Polyp
6. Prostatic enlargement
7. Ureterocele, simple or ectopic

UNCOMMON

1. Endometriosis
2. Foreign body
3. Fungus ball (eg, monilia)
4. Hematoma, intramural
5. Hydatid cyst
6. Infection, fistula, abscess (eg, Crohn's disease, diverticulitis)
7. Postoperative
8. Schistosomiasis hematobium (granuloma or papilloma)

EXTRINSIC PRESSURE DEFORMITY OF THE BLADDER

COMMON

1. Colon distension
2. Pelvic abscess (eg, pelvic inflammatory disease, tubovarian abscess)
3. Pelvic hematoma
4. Pelvic tumor (eg, uterine, ovarian)
5. Pregnancy
6. Prostatic enlargement
7. Uterine enlargement

UNCOMMON

1. Carcinoma in a bladder diverticulum
2. Ectopic ureterocele
3. Extrauterine pregnancy
4. Lymphadenopathy, any cause
5. Normal levator ani muscle or sacrospinous ligament
6. Pelvic lipomatosis
7. Retroperitoneal sarcoma, teratoma, or lymphoma

Reference:

Levene G, Kaufman SA: The diagnostic significance of roentgenologic soft tissue shadows in the pelvis. *Am J Roentgenol* 79:697–704, 1958.

NEUROGENIC BLADDER

COMMON

1. Cerebral palsy
2. Neoplasm of spine, spinal cord, or brain
3. Spina bifida vera with meningomyelocele
4. Spinal cord injury or hematoma

UNCOMMON

1. Arteriovenous malformation of spinal cord
2. Block vertebrae
3. Diastematomyelia
4. Neurofibromatosis
5. Neurosyphilis
6. Sacral anomaly, caudal regression syndrome (eg, sacral agenesis, hypoplasia, scoliosis, hemisacrum)
7. Syringomyelia
8. Transverse myelitis
9. Tuberculosis (Pott's disease)

Reference:

Grossman H, Winchester PH, Colston WC: Neurogenic bladder in childhood. *Radiol Clin North Am* 6:155–163, 1968.

CONTRACTED BLADDER

COMMON

1. Carcinoma, infiltrating
2. Cystitis, severe
3. [Ileal conduit]
4. Neurogenic bladder (see Gamut H-37)
5. Pelvic hematoma
6. Pelvic inflammatory disease
7. Postoperative; postradiation therapy

UNCOMMON

1. Cystitis glandularis
2. Eosinophilic cystitis
3. Interstitial cystitis
4. Pelvic lipomatosis
5. Schistosomiasis
6. Tuberculosis

BLADDER CALCIFICATION (WALL OR LUMEN)

COMMON

1. Calculus

UNCOMMON

1. Benign tumor
2. [Calculus in urachal cyst]
3. Carcinoma (encrusted)
4. Cystitis (encrusted)
5. Foreign body, blood clot (encrusted)
6. Hemangioma
7. Hematoma
8. Metastatic or invasive ovarian cystadenocarcinoma or rectal colloid carcinoma
9. Neuroblastoma
10. Postradiation therapy
11. Schistosomiasis hematobium (commonest cause in Africa)
12. Tuberculosis

Reference:

Ferris EJ, O'Connor SJ: Calcification in urinary bladder tumors. *Am J Roentgenol* 95:447–449, 1965.

GAS IN THE BLADDER (WALL OR LUMEN)

COMMON

1. Cystitis caused by gas-forming organism (emphysematous cystitis)
2. Iatrogenic (eg, air cystogram, cystoscopy)
3. Trauma or surgical complication

UNCOMMON

1. Bladder fistula (see Gamut H-41)
2. Fungus ball in bladder

BLADDER FISTULA

COMMON

1. Congenital anal atresia
2. Crohn's disease
3. Diverticulitis
4. Malignant neoplasm of colon, bladder, or reproductive system
5. Postoperative, postpartum
6. Radiation therapy
7. Trauma

UNCOMMON

1. Appendicitis
2. Embedded bladder stone eroding through bladder wall
3. Foreign body
4. Lymphogranuloma venereum
5. Pelvic inflammatory disease; endometritis
6. Schistosomiasis hematobium
7. Tuberculous enterocolitis
8. Ulcerative colitis

URINARY TRACT OBSTRUCTION BELOW THE BLADDER IN A CHILD

COMMON

1. Ectopic ureterocele
2. Foreign body
3. Meatal stenosis
4. [Neurogenic]
5. Posterior urethral valve
6. Trauma
7. Urethral stricture

UNCOMMON

1. Anterior urethral valve
2. Congenital bladder neck obstruction (?)
3. Congenital urethral duplication
4. Fibroelastosis of the prostate
5. Hydrometrocolpos
6. Hypertrophy of the verumontanum
7. Tumor
8. Urethral calculus
9. Urethral diverticulum

SUBGAMUT H-42A
THE OBSTRUCTIVE UROPATHIES IN CHILDREN

1. All of the above
2. Congenital ureteropelvic obstruction (stricture, band, anomalous vessel)
3. Congenital ureterovesical obstruction

URINARY TRACT CALCULI
(See also Gamut H-6)

COMMON

1. Chronic urinary infection
2. Hyperparathyroidism
3. Osteoporosis (eg, immobilization, menopausal, senile)
4. Stasis of urine (eg, urinary tract obstruction, neurogenic bladder)

UNCOMMON

1. Cushing's disease; steroid therapy
2. Dehydration
3. Excessive calcium intake or absorption
4. Hypervitaminosis D
5. Idiopathic hypercalcemia (eg, William's syndrome)
6. Idiopathic hypercalciuria
7. Medullary sponge kidney
8. Milk-alkali syndrome
9. Osteolytic bone metastases; multiple myeloma
10. Osteomalacia
11. Paget's disease
12. Papillary necrosis
13. Renal tubular acidosis
14. Sarcoidosis
15. Schistosomiasis

Reference:

Kreel L: *Outline of Radiology.*   New York, Appleton-Century-Crofts, 1971, p 187.

SUBGAMUT H-43A
RADIOLUCENT URINARY TRACT CALCULI

1. Cystine stones
2. Matrix stones composed of mucoproteinaceous material
3. Urates of ammonium, sodium, magnesium, or potassium
4. Uric acid stones
5. Xanthine stones

VASCULAR IMPRESSIONS ON THE URINARY TRACT

COMMON

1. Collateral arterial circulation (eg, secondary to renal artery stenosis, aortic or iliac artery occlusion)
2. Collateral venous circulation (eg, secondary to obstruction of inferior or superior vena cava, renal, gonadal, azygos, splenic, or portal vein)
3. Normal accessory renal artery
4. Normal iliac artery

UNCOMMON

1. Aortic or hypogastric artery aneurysm
2. Arteriovenous fistula of renal or juxtarenal vessels
3. Cirsoid aneurysm of renal artery
4. Normal gonadal vein
5. Right ovarian vein syndrome (?)
6. Ureteral varices
7. Varicocele of gonad and varices of the broad ligament

Reference:

Chait A, Matasar KW, Fabian CE, Mellins HZ: Vascular impressions on the ureters. *Am J Roentgenol* 111:729–749, 1971.

SUPRARENAL CALCIFICATION

COMMON

1. Hemorrhage (neonatal, sepsis)
2. Idiopathic
3. Neuroblastoma
4. Tuberculosis

UNCOMMON

1. Addison's disease
2. Histoplasmosis
3. Other adrenal tumors (eg, adenoma, carcinoma, dermoid)
4. Pheochromocytoma
5. Waterhouse-Friderichsen syndrome
6. Wolman's disease (xanthomatosis)

Reference:

Queloz JM, Capitanio MA, Kirkpatrick JA: Wolman's disease. *Radiology* 104:357-359, 1972.

PELVIC OR LOWER QUADRANT CALCIFICATION

COMMON

1. Appendiceal calculus (fecalith)
2. Dermoid cyst, teratoma
3. [Foreign material: foreign body, intrauterine device, vaginal pessary, medicinal injections (bismuth) in buttocks, residual barium in bowel especially in appendix or diverticula, pills in intestines, pantopaque in lower spinal canal, ethiodol in lymph nodes, radon seeds, metallic clips, wire sutures, catheter, gauze sponge, etc.]
4. Leiomyoma of uterus
5. Lymph node, often presacral
6. Pregnancy, lithopedion
7. Prostatic calculi
8. Urinary tract calculus (ureter, bladder, bladder diverticulum, urethra, pelvic kidney)
9. Vas deferens, seminal vesicle, fallopian tube (eg, tuberculosis, diabetes)
10. Vascular (eg, arteries, phleboliths)

UNCOMMON

1. Bladder or ureteral wall calcification (Schistosomiasis hematobium, tuberculosis) — see Gamut H-39
2. Bladder tumor (encrustation)
3. Bone tumor
4. Calcified epiploic appendage (attached or detached)
5. Calculus in Meckel's diverticulum
6. Colloid carcinoma of colon
7. Cystadenoma or cystadenocarcinoma of ovary with psammomatous calcifications

(Continued)

8. Enterolith
9. Gallstone in ileum
10. Hemangioma
11. Myxoglobulosis, mucocele of appendix
12. Parasites (cysticercus, armillifer, guinea worm)

CALCIFICATION IN THE VAS DEFERENS OR SEMINAL VESICLE

COMMON

1. Aging (?)
2. Diabetes
3. Idiopathic

UNCOMMON

1. Chronic nonspecific urinary tract infection
2. Paraplegia
3. Schistosomiasis
4. Syphilis
5. Tuberculosis

Reference:

King JC Jr, Rosenbaum HD: Calcification of the vasa deferentia in non-diabetics. *Radiology* 100:603–606, 1971.

CALCIFICATION IN THE SCROTUM

COMMON

1. Diabetes
2. Trauma (hemorrhage)
3. Varicocele (phleboliths)

UNCOMMON

1. Meconium peritonitis
2. Sebaceous cyst (steatoma)
3. Testicular atrophy
4. Tuberculosis
5. Tumor

LARGE SOFT TISSUE MASS IN THE PELVIS

COMMON

1. Abscess
2. Distended bladder
3. Distended fluid-filled loop of bowel
4. [Feces in rectosigmoid colon]
5. Hematoma
6. Ovarian cyst or neoplasm
7. Pregnancy
8. Uterine fibroids, hydatid mole, other uterine neoplasm

UNCOMMON

1. Anterior sacral meningocele
2. Bone tumor
3. Extraperitoneal neoplasm (lymphoma, teratoma, chondro-sarcoma, fibrosarcoma, liposarcoma)
4. Hydatid cyst
5. Pelvic kidney
6. Pelvic lipomatosis

ABNORMAL GAS SHADOWS IN THE PELVIS

COMMON

1. Abscess
2. Perforated diverticulum, appendix, or colon
3. Pneumatosis cystoides of pelvic colon
4. Rectal laceration

UNCOMMON

1. Bowel necrosis
2. Clostridium infection of abdominal wall
3. Emphysematous cystitis (see Gamut H-40)
4. Emphysematous vaginitis
5. Gas in dead fetus
6. Giant colon diverticulum
7. Hydrogen peroxide enema
8. Infected uterine fibroid
9. Intestinal fistula into bladder or elsewhere
10. Ovarian gas abscess
11. Perforation of extrauterine pregnancy into colon
12. Uterine emphysema due to Clostridium infection

Reference:

Seaman WB, Fleming RJ: Pneumatosis of pelvic viscera. *Semin Roentgenol* 4:202–211, 1969.

GAS IN THE EXTRAPERITONEAL SPACE

COMMON

1. Abscess (appendiceal, perinephric, subphrenic, pancreatic, splenic, abdominal wall; gas gangrene)
2. Gastrointestinal tract perforation (peptic ulcer, diverticulum, carcinoma, inflammatory disease — eg, Crohn's disease)
3. Iatrogenic (eg, postoperative, postrectal biopsy, retroperitoneal gas insufflation, diagnostic retropneumoperitoneum)
4. Trauma (eg, gunshot wound, duodenal or colonic rupture)

UNCOMMON

1. Gallbladder rupture secondary to emphysematous cholecystitis
2. Pneumatosis intestinalis with rupture
3. Pneumomediastinum with downward dissection (eg, spontaneous, traumatic, post-tracheotomy)

Reference:

Calenoff L, Poticha SM: Combined occurrence of retropneumoperitoneum and pneumoperitoneum. *Am J Roentgenol* 117:366–372, 1973.

RETROPERITONEAL FIBROSIS

COMMON

1. Drug (eg, Sansert)
2. Idiopathic

UNCOMMON

1. Crohn's disease
2. Radiation therapy
3. Retroperitoneal scirrhous carcinoma
4. Sclerosing agents for hemorrhoids
5. Sclerosing lymphoma
6. Tuberculosis

CONGENITAL SYNDROMES WITH HYPOSPADIAS OR OTHER AMBIGUOUS EXTERNAL GENITALIA

COMMON

1. Fraser's S.
2. Long arm 21 deletion S.
3. Short arm 4 deletion S.
4. Smith-Lemli-Opitz S.
5. William's S.

UNCOMMON

1. Cerebrohepatorenal S.
2. Ellis-van Creveld S.
3. Fanconi's S.
4. Laurence-Moon-Biedl S.
5. Popliteal web S.
6. Russell-Silver S.
7. Trisomy 13 S.
8. Trisomy 18 S.
9. XXXXY S.

Reference:

Smith DW: *Recognizable Patterns of Human Malformation.* Philadelphia, WB Saunders Co, p 291, 1970.

LARGE FETAL ABDOMEN DURING LAST TRIMESTER

COMMON

1. Generalized edema (eg, hemolytic disease or maternal diabetes)
2. Massive hydronephrosis
3. Polycystic kidneys

UNCOMMON

1. Absent abdominal musculature or "prune belly" (Eagle-Barrett syndrome)
2. Ascites
3. Enterogenous tumor or cyst
4. Hepatic tumor or cyst (eg, polycystic disease)
5. Hydrometrocolpos
6. Neuroblastoma
7. Ovarian tumor or cyst
8. Teratoma
9. Wilms' tumor

Reference:

Moncado R, Wang JJ, Love L, Bush I: Neonatal ascites associated with urinary outlet obstruction (urine ascites). *Radiology* 90:1165–1170, 1968.

FAILURE OF FETAL HEAD TO ENGAGE DURING LABOR

COMMON

1. Cephalopelvic disproportion
2. Extrauterine pregnancy
3. Fetal hydrops, hydrocephalus, or other fetal deformity
4. Multiple pregnancy
5. Pelvic tumor or cyst

UNCOMMON

1. Distended bladder or rectum
2. Low lying placenta
3. Maternal spondylolisthesis or other pelvic girdle deformity
4. Prominent ischial spines
5. Short or twisted umbilical cord
6. Uterine malformation, persistent uterine contraction ring

Reference:

Bishop PA: *Radiologic Studies of the Gravid Uterus.* New York, Harper & Row, 1965, p 39–84, 268–269.

STRAIGHT FETAL SPINE IN UTERO

COMMON

1. Abdominal pregnancy
2. Abnormal size or position of placenta
3. Breech presentation
4. Hydramnios; anencephalic fetus
5. Hydrops fetalis
6. Multiple fetuses

UNCOMMON

1. Intraabdominal fetal tumor (eg, Wilms' tumor, polycystic kidneys, hydronephrosis, hepatic tumor)
2. Maternal pelvic tumor (eg, uterine fibroids)
3. Meconium or urinary peritonitis

Reference:

1. Barnett E, Nairn A: A study of foetal attitude. *Br J Radiol* 38:338–349, 1965.
2. Daw E: Generalized deflexion of the foetal spine. *Br J Radiol* 43:240–241, 1970.

NOTES

NOTES

NOTES

NOTES

NOTES

NOTES

NOTES